Pocket Companion for

Medical-Surgical Nursing

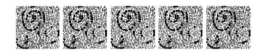

Pocket Companion for

Medical-Surgical Nursing

Foundations for Clinical Practice

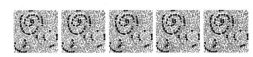

2nd Edition

Frances Donovan Monahan, PhD, RN

Professor and Director
Department of Nursing
Rockland Community College
State University of New York
Suffern, New York

Marianne Neighbors, EdD, RN

Professor
Eleanor Mann School of Nursing
College of Education
University of Arkansas
Fayetteville, Arkansas

W.B. SAUNDERS COMPANY
A Division of Harcourt Brace & Company
Philadelphia   London   Toronto   Montreal   Sydney   Tokyo

W.B. SAUNDERS COMPANY

A Division of Harcourt Brace & Company

The Curtis Center
Independence Square West
Philadelphia, Pennsylvania 19106

Pocket Companion for
MEDICAL-SURGICAL NURSING: FOUNDATIONS
FOR CLINICAL PRACTICE   ISBN: 0-7216-7334-1

Printed in the United States of America.

Last digit is the print number: 9   8   7   6   5   4   3   2

Dedicated to:

William Thomas Monahan, my husband
Michael McCain Monahan, my son
Kerryane Torpey Monahan, my daughter
with all my love

FDM

This book is dedicated to my sons, nieces, and nephews — Joey Butler, Jeremy Neighbors, Melissa and Laura Schwickrath, Tony, Jessica, and Michael Zadra, Sheryl Campbell, Teresa, Steven, and Cameron Jones — may you always be healthy; you are loved.

Marianne Neighbors

Preface

◆◆ ◆◆ ◆◆ ◆◆

This book was written in recognition of every nursing student who has carried a large heavy text to clinical only to find there is no easily accessible, safe place to leave it. It is also written in recognition of all those nursing students who are juggling family responsibilities, work, and school, and as a result must study at little league games, in the dentist's office, even at traffic lights, as well as in the more traditional environments.

This book is designed as an easily carried quick reference and study aid. As such it contains information on the nursing care of patients with commonly occurring medical-surgical disorders and the nursing care of patients undergoing common diagnostic and therapeutic interventions. It also contains information presented in medication card format, on more than 75 of the most commonly prescribed medications. To make accessing needed information easy, the book is divided into three sections: Disorders, Diagnostic and Therapeutic Interventions, and Drugs, each of which is alphabetized. Reference data found in the appendices include normal laboratory values, Fahrenheit to Centigrade temperature conversions, standard precautions, electrolyte values, and respiratory and metabolic acid-base information.

It is the authors' hope that this pocket companion will serve as a convenient reference guide for student nurses and practicing nurses in the clinical setting. Please inform us if the handbook has achieved this objective.

Contributors

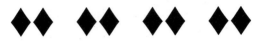

Cheryl Brady, RN, MSN
Assistant Professor
Department of Nursing
Kent State University
East Liverpool Campus
East Liverpool, Ohio

Sue-Ann Eitches, MA, RN
Associate Professor
Department of Nursing
Rockland Community College
State University of New York
Suffern, New York

John Hutchcroft, MNSC, CCM, CRRN
Adjunct Faculty
Eleanor Mann School of Nursing
College of Education and Health Professions
University of Arkansas
Fayetteville, Arkansas

Margaret Rateau, RN, MSN
Assistant Professor
Department of Nursing
Kent State University
East Liverpool Campus
East Liverpool, Ohio

Contents

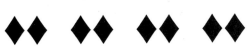

Section I—Common Disorders

Acute Renal Failure 3

Adult Respiratory Distress Syndrome 5

Alzheimer's Disease 7

Anaphylaxis 10

Anemias (Hemorrhagic, Hypoproliferative,
          Hemolytic) 11

Aneurysm 13

Angina 17

Appendicitis 19

Asthma 22

Atherosclerosis 25

Benign Prostatic Hyperplasia 30

Bone Tumors 31

Brain Tumors 35

Breast Cancer 36

Cancer 40

Cardiac Dysrhythmias 42

Cerebrovascular Accident 44

Cervical Cancer 47

Cholecystitis 50

Chronic Arterial Occlusive Disease
          (Arteriosclerosis Obliterans) 51

Chronic Bronchitis 52

Chronic Renal Failure 56

Cirrhosis 59

Colorectal Cancer 62

Coronary Artery Disease 62

Crohn's Disease 63

Diabetes Mellitus 66

Disseminated Intravascular Coagulation (DIC) 71

Diverticular Disease 72

Emphysema 74

Encephalitis 75

Endocarditis, Myocarditis, and Pericarditis ... 76

Endometrial Cancer 80

Fractures 80

Gastric Cancer 85

Glomerulonephritis 85

Heart Failure 88

Herniated Disk Disease 94

Hodgkin's Disease 97

Hydronephrosis 101

Hyperglycemic Hyperosmolar Non-Ketotic

      Syndrome 101

Hypertension 103

Hyperthyroidism 109

Hypothyroidism 112

Increased Intracranial Pressure 115

Intestinal Obstruction 117

Ischemic Cardiac Disease 119

Laryngeal Cancer 119

Leukemia 119

Liver Cancer 124

Lung Cancer 125

Mechanical Obstruction 125

Meningitis 127

Mitral Valve Prolapse 130

Mitral Valve Stenosis 130

Multiple Myeloma 132

Myocardial Infarction 134

Nephrotic Syndrome 138

Osteoarthritis 139

Osteomalacia 139

Osteomyelitis 141

Osteoporosis 144

Pancreatic Cancer 147

Pancreatitis 147

Parkinson's Disease 150

Peptic Ulcer Disease 155

Peripheral Vascular Disease 159

Peritonitis 159

Pheocromocytoma 161

Pneumonia 163

Pneumothorax, Hemothorax, and Hydrothorax 166

Prostate Cancer 168

Pulmonary Embolism 169

Rheumatoid Arthritis 170

Shock 174

Spinal Cord Injury 176

Testicular Cancer 179

Thromboangiitis Obliterans (Buerger's
        Disease) 182

Thrombocytopenic Purpura 184

Thrombophlebitis (Venous Thrombosis) 186

Thyroid Cancer 189

Tuberculosis 190

Ulcerative Colitis 194

Urinary Tract Infections 195

Varicose Veins 198

Vasospastic Disorder (Raynaud's Disease) 199

Venous Stasis Ulcers 199

Viral Hepatitis 202

Section II— Diagnostic and Therapeutic Procedures

Amputation 209

Arterial Blood Gases 214

Arterial Lines 216

Arteriography (Angiography) 217

Arthroscopy 218

Biopsy 218

Blood Transfusion 220

Bronchoscopy 223

Cardiac Catheterization 224

Casts 227

Chemotherapy 232

Chest Drainage 243

Cholecystectomy 245

Colonoscopy 249

Colostomy 250

Computed Tomography 257

Craniotomy 259

Cystoscopy 262

Dilation and Curettage 263

Electrocardiography (ECG, EKG) 264

Endoscopy 265

Enteral Nutrition (Tube Feedings) 265

Esophagogastroduodenoscopy 268

Fixation Devices 269

Gastrectomy 274

Hysterectomy 277

Ileostomy 280

Intestinal Resection 281

Joint Replacement 284

Laparoscopy 289

Lobectomy 290

Lumbar Puncture 292

Magnetic Resonance Imaging 293

Mechanical Ventilation 293

Modified Radical Mastectomy 298

Nasogastric Intubation 302

Pneumonectomy 305

Preoperative Nursing Care 310

Postoperative Nursing Care 312

Prostatectomy 315

Pulmonary Function Studies 321

Pulse Oximetry 321

Radiation Therapy 322

Thoracentesis 325

Thyroidectomy 325

Total Parenteral Nutrition
    (Hyperalimentation) 327

Tracheostomy 330

Traction 333

Treadmill 336

Ultrasonography 338

Wounds/Grafts 339

Section III—Pharmacologic Agents

Acetaminophen/Codeine 343

Albuterol 344

Alprazolam 345

Aminophylline 346

Amoxicillin Trihydrate 348

Ampicillin 350

Atenolol 351

Atropine Sulfate 353

Azithromycin 354

Buspirone 355

Captopril 357

Cefaclor 359

Cefadroxil Monohydrate 360

Cefuroxime Sodium 361

Cephalexin 363

Cimetidine Hydrochloride 364

Ciprofloxacin 365

Clarithromycin 367

Co-Trimoxazole, Sulfamethoxazole-
    Trimethoprim 369

Diazepam 370

Diclofenac Sodium 372

Digoxin 373

Diltiazem Hydrochloride 375

Doxepin Hydrochloride 377

Doxycycline Hyclate 378

Enalopril Maleate 380

Erythromycin 382

Etodolac (Ultradol) 383

Famotidine 385

Ferrous Sulfate 386

Fluoxetine Hydrochloride 387

Furosemide 388

Gemfibrozil 390

Glipizide 392

Glyburide 393

Heparin 395

Human Insulin 397

Hydrochlorathiazide 399

Hydrocodone Bitartrate 401

Hydrocortisone 402

Ibuprofen 404

Imipramine 406

Indapamide 407

Levothyroxine Sodium 409

Lisinopril 410

Lorazepam 412

Lovastatin 413

Meclizine Hydrochloride 414

Meperidine Hydrochloride 415

Metoprolol 417

Nabumetone 419

Naproxen 420

Nifedipine 421

Nortriptyline Hydrochloride 423

Ofloxacin 424

Oxaprozin 425

Paroxetine Hydrochloride 427

Penicillin V Potassium 428

Pentoxifylline 429

Phenobarbital 430

Piroxicam 432

Potassium Chloride 433

Prednisone 434

Propoxyphene Hydrochloride 436

Propoxyphene Napsylate 437

Ranitidine 438

Sertraline Hydrochloride 440

Tetracycline Hydrochloride 441

Timolol Maleate 443

Triamcinolone 445

Triamterene 447

Verapamil Hydrochloride 448

Warfarin Sodium 450

References 451

Appendices

Standard Precautions 454

Temperature Conversion Table 458

Reference Values for Laboratory Tests 460

Acid-Base 488

Electrolytes: Normal Values and Imbalances . 490

Index 493

Section I

Common Disorders

◆◆ ◆◆ ◆◆ ◆◆

◆ Acute Renal Failure (ARF)

ARF is the sudden, usually reversible, partial or total loss of kidney function, which occurs only when there is functional loss of at least 75% of the nephrons, the functioning unit of the kidney. The causes of ARF have three distinct sources: prerenal — interference with blood flow such as hemorrhage or obstruction; renal—conditions that cause direct kidney damage such as nephrotoxic substances; and postrenal—relating to obstruction of the urinary tract from the renal tubules to the urinary meatus. Management of acute renal failure includes preventing hyperkalemia, fluid overload, acidosis, and pulmonary edema, and restricting dietary intake of protein, potassium, sodium, and fluids. Pharmacologic agents are also prescribed to correct or prevent the complications of the disorder.

ASSESSMENT

- Assess subjective data: patient's voiding patterns, weight gain in recent weeks, nausea, family history of renal disease, recent history of flu-like symptoms, and any medications taken recently.
- Check objective data: amount of urine excreted in 24 hours, blood pressure (including postural changes), daily weight, fluid status, peripheral edema, breath sounds, skin turgor, changes in mental status, changes in pulse rate and rhythm, and laboratory studies (especially electrolytes).
- Determine the patient's knowledge level regarding renal failure and the prescribed treatment.
- Assess the patient's and family's coping mechanisms and identify any support systems.

NURSING DIAGNOSES, PLANNING, AND NURSING INTERVENTIONS

NDx: Fluid volume excess related to malfunctioning kidneys

Planning: Patient outcomes

1. Patient exhibits decreased peripheral, facial, and sacral edema.

2. Systemic signs of fluid overload are absent.
3. Patient states causative factors and treatments to alleviate overload.
4. Patient has a balanced intake and output.
5. Patient's electrolytes are within safe limits.

Nursing Interventions

Report signs and symptoms of fluid volume excess, which include significant weight gain, increased BP and pulse, change in mental status, dyspnea, orthopnea, crackles in the lungs, edema, distended neck veins, and elevated CVP.

Monitor chest x-ray results.

Measure fluid intake and output.

Maintain fluid restrictions and restrict sodium intake as ordered.

Monitor and document the therapeutic effect and side effects of prescribed medications.

Weigh the patient at the same time each day.

Alert the physician if signs and symptoms persist or worsen.

Prepare the patient and family for dialysis if needed.

NDx: Altered nutrition: less than body requirement related to renal failure and dietary restrictions

Planning: Patient outcomes

1. Patient's weight is within accepted range.
2. Patient verbalizes need for dietary changes.
3. Patient follows prescribed diet.
4. Patient eats 75% of meals.

Nursing Interventions

Document the patient's food intake.

Weigh the patient daily.

Monitor fluid intake and output.

Assess the patient for any problems that could be associated with poor intake, such as anorexia, nausea, vomiting, fatigue, and mouth discomfort.

Administer antiemetics as ordered.

Provide oral hygiene frequently.

Provide small, frequent meals and ensure the environment is clean, relaxed, and pleasant.

Provide a rest period before meals to minimize fatigue.

Provide basic nutritional information and refer to a dietitian as needed for further counseling.

Encourage the family to bring in favorite foods that meet dietary requirements.

◆ Adult Respiratory Distress Syndrome (ARDS)

Adult respiratory distress syndrome (ARDS) is a life threatening condition manifested by severe hypoxemia and decreased lung compliance. It is frequently referred to as noncardiogenic pulmonary edema; pulmonary edema not due to heart failure. ARDS develops in response to a direct or indirect injury to the lung causing increased pulmonary capillary permeability. Potential causes include trauma, oxygen toxicity, drug overdose, disseminated intravascular coagulation (DIC), complications of coronary artery bypass grafting (CABG), inhalation of noxious gases, sepsis, multiple blood transfusions, shock, hemolytic disorders, cerebrovascular accident (CVA), brain tumors, and sudden increase in intracranial pressure. Management is directed at supporting the patient's vital functions while identifying and treating the precipitating problem. Treatment includes the administration of supplemental oxygen and possible intubation and mechanical ventilation with positive end-expiratory pressure (PEEP) or pressure controlled inverse ratio ventilation (PC-IRV). Intravenous fluids, crystalloids, and colloids are also administered.

ASSESSMENT

- Identify patients at risk.
- Assess for the following clinical manifestations:
  - Initial or latent stage—there may be no evidence of respiratory distress (unless the underlying or precipitating disorder responsible for triggering the ARDS response is pulmonary).

- Second or interstitial edema stage—breathlessness, tachypnea, feeling of impending doom, restlessness, apprehension.
- Third or acute intra-alveolar edema stage—severe dyspnea, use of accessory muscles of respiration, intercostal retraction, agitation, depressed mental status, diffuse fine crackles and diminished breath sounds on auscultation.
- Fourth stage or the chronic or fibrotic stage—continued hypoxemia despite treatment.

NURSING DIAGNOSES, PLANNING, AND NURSING INTERVENTIONS

NDx: Impaired gas exchange related to oxygenation and ventilation failure and increased oxygen consumption

Planning: Patient outcomes

1. Arterial oxygen level remains equal to or greater than 60 to 70 mm Hg.
2. Arterial oxygen saturation remains equal to or greater than 90%.
3. Arterial carbon dioxide remains equal to or less than 45 to 50 mm Hg.

Nursing Interventions

Position the patient to promote oxygenation and ventilation.
Pace and limit activities and care measures to decrease risk for oxygen depletion.
Monitor ABGs.

NDx: Inability to sustain spontaneous ventilation related to increased intrapulmonary shunt and decreased V/Q ratio

Planning: Patient outcomes

1. Patient maintains spontaneous ventilation.
2. Intrapulmonary shunt is improved.
3. V/Q ratio is improved.

Nursing Interventions

Administer supplemental oxygen as ordered.
Maintain mechanical ventilation.
Monitor breathing pattern, respiratory rate, and cardiac function.
Monitor airway pressures for decreasing lung compliance.

Additional Interventions

Suction the airway as needed to decrease secretions and maintain a patent airway.
Maintain a clean environment.
Monitor temperature.
Administer analgesics as ordered.
Provide paper and pencil, alphabet, picture, or electronic communication board.
Assist family members with communication methods.

Alzheimer's Disease

Alzheimer's disease is a chronic, progressive, neurodegenerative condition characterized by marked cognitive dysfunction. The exact cause is unknown, but possible etiologic factors include genetic tendency, autoimmune reaction, slow virus, and dysfunction of the neurotransmitters. Management is symptomatic and supportive. Vasodilators or psychostimulants may be used in an attempt to improve mental status.

ASSESSMENT

- Assess for signs of progressive mental and physical deterioration such as forgetfulness, memory loss, contusion, difficulty comprehending, wandering behavior, antisocial behavior, emotional outbursts, paranoia, lack of awareness of the environment, depression, and gait disturbance.
- Explore the impact of the disease on family functioning.

NURSING DIAGNOSES, PLANNING, AND NURSING INTERVENTIONS

NDx: Altered thought processes related to cognitive decline

Planning: Patient outcomes

1.   Displays of behavioral dysfunction are minimal.

Nursing Interventions

Provide a consistent, structured environment.
Allow the patient to have familiar objects around.
Establish daily routines; avoid variations in day to day activities.
Anticipate the patient's needs.
Minimize stress, noise, and disruption of physical surroundings.

NDx: Chronic confusion related to effects of progressive cerebral degeneration

Planning: Patient outcomes

1.   Patient participates in activities of daily living.
2.   Patient frustrations appear decreased when environmental stressors are reduced.

Nursing Interventions

Promote communication by talking in simple sentences, presenting one idea at a time, asking questions the patient can answer, and using eye contact.
Identify fears and frustrations associated with combative episodes.
Keep the environment simple and uncluttered.
Maintain a consistent routine.
Monitor for increasing fatigue and anxiety.

NDx: Self-care deficit: feeding, hygiene, grooming related to cognitive decline

Planning: Patient outcomes

1. Patient performs self care within limits of ability.
2. Patient wears neat, clean clothes during daytime.
3. Patient maintains acceptable personal hygiene.
4. Family or significant others identify personal and community resources that can provide support and assistance.

Nursing Interventions

Monitor the patient's ability to perform ADL.
Ensure that the patient attends to daily personal hygiene, wears clean clothing, and eats adequate diet.
Allow the patient to maintain self-care activities as long as possible.
Encourage the patient to complete self care.
Supervise the patient and provide direct care when necessary.
Consult with nutritionist as necessary.

NDx: Risk for injury related to cognitive decline

Planning: Patient outcomes

1. Patient remains free from injury.

Nursing Interventions

Monitor the patient's cognitive functioning.
Identify changes that increase risk of injury.
Provide a consistent, familiar and safe environment.
Supervise the patient as necessary.
Ensure that the patient carries identification.

Additional Interventions

Support family members in developing effective coping mechanisms.
Encourage expression of feelings such as anxiety, fear, and hopelessness.
Teach the family strategies that are effective in managing the patient's behavior.

Refer to support groups, day care centers, and respite centers.

◆ Anaphylaxis

Anaphylaxis is a sudden, life threatening overreaction to an antigen mediated by IgE antibody, which is produced following first exposure to the antigen. On subsequent exposure, the antigen binds with the cell-bound IgE causing release of chemical mediators, which produce bronchoconstriction, vasodilation, and increased capillary permeability. Management must begin immediately if respiratory arrest and shock are to be prevented. It consists of drug therapy to reverse effects of chemical mediators (epinephrine to stop bronchospasm, Benadryl to block histamine, steroids to reduce capillary permeability and maintain blood volume, and dopamine or isoproterenol to maintain blood pressure), fluid replacement, and airway maintenance.

NURSING CARE

Be alert to symptoms of anaphylaxis: feelings of anxiety and uneasiness, flushing, diaphoresis, itching, hypotension, edema of face, hands, and feet, and bronchospasm.

Limit exposure to antigen if identified (e.g., if an IV medication, stop the infusion)

Obtain emergency help and equipment for intubation and emergency tracheostomy immediately.

Do not leave the patient alone if at all possible.

Suction airway PRN and give O_2.

Lay patient flat and elevate legs if hypotensive.

Establish an IV line if not already in place.

Following the incident, explain the following to the patient:

What the precipitating factor was.

What related substances may cause a similar reaction.

Ways to avoid the antigen and related substances in the future.

Importance of informing all health care providers of the problem and wearing a Medic Alert identification.

◆ Anemias (Hemorrhagic, Hypoproliferative, Hemolytic)

The hematologic conditions of low red blood cell (RBC) count and a low hemoglobin (Hgb) or hematocrit (Hct) level are categorized as anemias. Anemias may be classified according to their etiology or their morbidity. Etiologic classification is as follows: (1) hemorrhagic or blood loss anemia, which results from trauma, rupture of an aneurysm, tearing of an artery, or from a progressive internal bleed; (2) hypoproliferative or decreased RBC production anemia, which results when the marrow is unable to produce an adequate number of cells caused by drugs, chemicals, or the lack of iron, vitamin B12, or folic acid; and (3) hemolytic or RBC destruction anemia, which results from inherited conditions such as thalassemia, sickle cell disease, or G6PD deficiency. Medical therapy depends on the cause and may include oxygen administration, blood transfusions, nutritional and pharmaceutical supplements, and administration of erythropoietin.

ASSESSMENT

- Check for fatigue, shortness of breath, and weakness and the patient's ability to complete activities of daily living.
- Note vital signs before and after exertion.
- Check for signs of bleeding such as ecchymoses or petechiae.
- Assess for bloody urine or stools.
- Observe for pallor, cyanosis, and hydration.
- Review the patient's nutritional status, checking for signs of deficiencies.
- Assess the patient's level of understanding about the disorder.

NURSING DIAGNOSES, PLANNING, AND NURSING INTERVENTIONS

NDx: Activity intolerance related to decreased oxygen-carrying capacity of the blood

Planning: Patient outcomes

1. Patient follows a regimen of planned activities and rest periods each day.
2. Patient reports feeling less fatigued and demonstrates increased activity.
3. Patient is able to complete activities of daily living.
4. Patient denies shortness of breath with mild exercise.
5. Patient's vital signs are within normal ranges for the patient.

Nursing Interventions

Instruct patient to develop a regimen of daily activity with frequent rest periods.

Teach energy-saving techniques to use during daily self-care activities.

Encourage good nutritional habits to increase the patient's energy level.

Teach the patient how to gradually increase the amount of exercise tolerated without dyspnea.

Have the patient practice deep breathing exercises to increase oxygen and blood to the brain.

Provide warm clothes and blankets to prevent chilling secondary to peripheral vasoconstriction.

NDx: Knowledge deficit: Nature of the disease, nutritional needs, treatment, and prevention of fatigue

Planning: Patient outcomes

1. Patient describes the cause, effects, and clinical course of anemia.
2. Patient relates the nutritional therapy for the disorder.
3. Patient states the self care needed to prevent fatigue and other complications.

Nursing Interventions

Explain the disorder, effects, and clinical course in understandable terms.

Allow the patient to ask questions and verbalize concerns.

Teach the patient how to conserve oxygen needs and to prevent fatigue.

Alert the patient to signs of bleeding and oxygen deficiency.

Encourage good nutritional patterns with frequent small meals, to prevent gastric distention, and high-protein, high-vitamin foods.

Explain the dosage, route, time, side effects, and therapeutic effects of any medication prescribed.

◆ Aneurysm

An aneurysm is a dilation or out-pouching of an artery that is usually caused by atherosclerosis, but may also be caused by other pathologic processes that cause arterial changes, resulting in weakened vessel walls, or they may be of unknown etiology. Aneurysms are most frequently found in the aorta and are classified by location, cause, and shape. *True* aneurysms, fusiform, saccular, and dissecting types, consist of an out-pouching or sac composed of at least one unbroken layer of the vessel wall. *False* aneurysms, usually the result of trauma, do not have an intact wall. Blood therefore forms a channel within the walls of the aneurysm, which is likely to rupture and leak into surrounding tissue. Surgical resection with a graft is the treatment of choice for most aneurysms, especially abdominal aortic aneurysms.

GRAFTS

A patch graft removes the diseased part of the vessel and replaces it with a *patch* from the patient's vein, usually the saphenous vein. A bypass graft leaves the diseased area intact but bypasses it with a graft, using either the patient's saphenous vein or a synthetic material. Bypass grafting is preferred over excision and replacement grafting because collateral circulation is maintained. The successful reestablishment of blood flow is evidenced by return of pulses, warming of the extremity, and decreased ischemic pain.

PREOPERATIVE NURSING CARE

Assessment

- Assess and document vital signs and vascular and neurovascular status.
- Check for a signed informed consent.
- Determine the patient's level of understanding about the surgery.
- Determine risk factors presented by nutritional deficits, lifestyle, and involvement of cardiac, respiratory, or endocrine systems that could complicate surgery and postoperative course.

Nursing Diagnoses, Planning and Nursing Interventions

NDx: Knowledge deficit: Surgical procedure and postoperative course

Planning: Patient outcomes

1. Patient states accurate information about the surgical procedure and expected results.
2. Patient describes the typical postoperative course.

Nursing Interventions

Assess the patient's understanding about the surgical procedure, its risks, the usual postoperative course, and self-care responsibilities after discharge.

Explain all facets of the procedure, the recovery period, and the postoperative care required.

Teach the patient about medications, activity progression, and routine postoperative deep breathing exercises.

Provide time for the patient and family to ask questions or verbalize concerns.

POSTOPERATIVE NURSING CARE

Assessment

- Assess the patient's vital signs, level of consciousness, respiratory pattern, skin temperature and color, and check the dressing for bleeding.
- Check the integrity of the intravenous site.
- Monitor blood coagulation; study results for abnormal bleeding times.
- Evaluate the patient's pain, noting location, intensity, and duration.
- Complete a critical assessment of pulses and other parameters of neurovascular compromise that indicate complications.

Nursing Diagnoses, Planning, and Nursing Interventions

NDx: Altered tissue perfusion, peripheral, related to thrombus formation or reocclusion induced by the previous existing vascular dysfunction or excessive bleeding

Planning: Patient outcomes

1. Patient exhibits palpable pulses, adequate temperature, sensation and color in extremities.
2. Patient develops no excessive bleeding or ischemic pain.
3. Patient's laboratory coagulation studies are within safe range.

Nursing Interventions

Monitor neurocirculatory status for signs of reocclusion.

Ask the patient to report changes in color or sensation.

Assess pulses, mark location of distal pulses, Doppler ultrasound nonpalpable pulses.

Check color, sensation, temperature, and motor ability in the affected extremities and document the changes.

Notify the physician of abnormalities since sudden changes indicate acute occlusion requiring emergency medical intervention.

Observe for edema, which may be caused from hemorrhage into the tissues from a leaking graft.

Position the patient off of the graft site or drains to prevent damage to the graft and promote optimal circulation.

Monitor vital signs for evidence of shock.

Maintain blood pressure at the prescribed level to prevent stress on the graft, which may cause rupture and hemorrhage.

NDx: Risk for infection related to surgical incision, location, length, and presurgical tissue integrity

Planning: Patient outcomes

1. Patient demonstrates a dry nondraining wound with no evidence of erythema or swelling.
2. Patient is free of signs of infection (afebrile, normal WBC).

Nursing Interventions

Use strict aseptic techniques when changing dressings or handling IV equipment.

Monitor temperature and WBC reports.

Inspect the incision for warmth, erythema, swelling, unusual drainage, and wound approximation.

Observe for and prevent skin breakdown by position changes and early mobilization of the patient.

Have the patient cough and deep breathe every 2 hours to prevent respiratory infection.

NDx: Pain related to incision and surgical manipulation

Planning: Patient outcomes

1. Patient states pain is relieved.
2. Patient is able to mobilize freely without extreme discomfort.
3. Patient is able to participate in self-care.

Nursing Interventions

Manage operative pain with prescribed analgesics and note patient responses.

Explain that revascularization pain is sometimes experienced as a throbbing sensation, but the return of ischemic pain indicates reocclusion, and the nurse should be notified immediately.

Reposition the patient in bed as needed for comfort, handling operative area carefully.

NDx: Risk for altered health maintenance related to lack of knowledge of self-care after discharge

Planning: Patient outcomes

1. Patient relates accurate information on wound care, medications, potential complications, and the need to seek medical attention if these occur.
2. Patient palpates pulses and inspects incision and skin daily for changes in color, temperature, and integrity.
3. Patient is able to increase activity as prescribed.
4. Patient states the importance of follow-up care.

Nursing Interventions

Teach the patient about the care of the surgical incision and how to complete an aseptic dressing change.

Explain the signs and symptoms of complications and when to seek medical intervention.

Inform the patient of activity restriction such as avoiding heavy lifting.

Reinforce teaching of the prescribed progression of ambulation.

Teach how to perform pulse checks and assessment of extremities.

Obtain referrals for home health or other transitional home care needs as determined by a self-care needs assessment.

◆ Angina

Angina is chest pain associated with temporarily decreased oxygen supply to the myocardium, resulting in ischemic muscle tissue. Angina may be caused by multiple factors, such as previous heart disease or atherosclerosis, but typically it is triggered by something that increases the workload of the heart and, thus, the oxygen demand. Pain is usually relieved by rest and/or vasodilation by pharmacologic agents. Patients usually describe the pain as a heaviness or tightness of the chest. Unstable angina is characterized by increasing frequency, severity, or duration of symptoms, and indicates severe coronary artery disease.

ASSESSMENT

- Ask the patient to describe the location, intensity, duration, severity, and radiation of the chest pain.
- Check the vital signs.
- Determine the precipitating factors and relief methods.
- Assess the skin for paleness, cyanosis, and diaphoresis.
- Monitor the electrocardiogram for abnormal patterns in rate or rhythm.

NURSING DIAGNOSES, PLANNING, AND NURSING INTERVENTIONS

NDx: Pain related to inadequate oxygenation of cardiac tissue

Planning: Patient outcomes

1. Patient experiences pain relief (absent or diminished) within 15 minutes of onset.
2. Patient describes and demonstrates methods of pain relief.

Nursing Interventions

Place the patient at rest immediately upon the onset of chest pain.

Loosen any restrictive/constrictive clothing.

Administer oxygen and nitroglycerin, or other prescribed medications.

If the pain is unrelieved, notify the physician.

Obtain a 12-lead electrocardiogram.

Ask the patient to describe the pain and document the
description.

Observe the patient for non-verbal signs of pain.

Instruct the patient about pain relief measures and the use
of the prescribed medications.

NDx: Anxiety related to pain, the threat of death, and/
or the threat to health status or self-concept

Planning: Patient outcomes

1. Patient uses effective coping mechanisms to man-
    age anxiety.
2. Patient verbalizes knowledge of the risks, complica-
    tions, and incidence of the chest pain.
3. Patient reports reduced anxiety and fear of chest
    pain episodes.
4. Patient exhibits behaviors associated with reducing
    the risks and complications of the disorder.

Nursing Interventions

Teach the patient relaxation exercises.

Refer the patient and significant others for cardiac education regarding the pathophysiology of chest pain
and cardiac risk factor identification and reduction.

Provide immediate and continuous means to summon
assistance when anginal episodes occur.

Instruct the patient about medications (at the bedside) to
take with the onset of pain.

Allow the patient to ask questions and voice concerns.

◆ Appendicitis

Appendicitis is an acute inflammation of the appendix,
believed to result from invasion of its wall by local bacteria. Obstruction of the appendix appears to be the precipitating factor in appendicitis. Possible causes of obstruction include calculi in the appendix, parasites, viral

infections, adhesions, and a malfunction of the valve at the opening of the appendix. Management consists of IV antibiotics and appendectomy. Prior to confirmation of the diagnosis, the patient is NPO. No analgesics are given as they can mask symptoms. No cathartics or enemas are given to avoid stimulation and irritation which could cause perforation. Intravenous antibiotics are begun and an appendectomy is performed as soon as possible.

PREOPERATIVE CARE

Assess for clinical manifestations of appendicitis: abdominal pain, classically beginning in the perium-bilical or epigastric area but localizing as intense colicky pain in the right lower quadrant (RLQ); anorexia; nausea with or without vomiting; low-grade fever; tenderness over McBurney's point; rebound tenderness; rigidity of the right rectus muscle; exacerbation of pain on coughing; RLQ pain triggered by palpation of the left lower quadrant, leukocytosis with elevated neutrophil count.

Position for comfort: bending the right knee on the abdomen is helpful.

Keep all instructions brief and to the point since the patient is usually too uncomfortable for long explanations.

Provide other care as described in the Preoperative entry.

POSTOPERATIVE CARE

Assessment

- Make usual postoperative assessments related to physiologic stabilization.
- Measure vital signs, measure intake and output, and check dressing for intactness and drainage.
- Assess for pain and good respiratory excursion and airway clearance.
- Check bowel sounds and assess tolerance of oral intake when resumed.

Nursing Diagnoses, Planning, and Nursing Interventions

NDx:　　Risk for altered health maintenance related to insufficient knowledge of postoperative activities and discharge instructions

Planning: Patient outcomes

1.　Patient coughs, deep breathes, splints the incision, and ambulates as directed.
2.　Patient describes self care at home as presented below.

Nursing Interventions

Guide the patient in splinting the incision, coughing, and deep breathing every 2 hours.

Instruct the patient in self care as follows.

- Gently wash the incision with soap and water daily, and pat dry.
- Be aware that if Steri-Strips are in place they will eventually fall off by themselves, and this is expected.
- Inspect the incision daily, and report any incisional redness, swelling, or drainage.
- Avoid clothing that places pressure on the incision line, such as bikini underwear and pantyhose.
- Avoid heavy lifting and strenuous exercises. Resume normal activities gradually over 2 to 3 weeks.
- Eat small, frequent, high-calorie meals and gradually increase as tolerated.
- Report any chills, fever, or increased pain.
- Return for follow-up visit on (specify date and place).

Additional Interventions

Place the patient in Fowler's position after recovery from anesthesia.

Medicate patient every 3 to 4 hours as needed and prescribed.

Give oral fluids as desired when alert and progress to a regular diet as tolerated.

Assist patient out of bed and begin to ambulate when alert and condition is stable.

◆ Asthma

Asthma is an immunologic allergic disease characterized by chronic inflammation of the lower airways with episodes of hyperresponsiveness to respiratory irritants, the end result of which can be permanent structural damage in the lungs. Asthma is believed to be basically an allergic response in which airways sensitized by allergens become more reactive to a variety of stimuli that can trigger an attack. Identified triggers include cold or dry air; air pollutants such as cigarette smoke, perfumes, feathers, animal danders, molds, and pollens; foods such as eggs and those containing sulfates; stress; exercise; and upper respiratory viral infections. Medical management aimed at prevention includes identification of allergens followed by avoidance of allergens and/or desensitization. Pharmacologic treatment of asthma follows the step-care approach based on the severity classification of the disease and includes non-steroidal anti-inflammatory medications such as cromolyn sodium, bronchodilators such as Ventolin, and inhaled corticosteroids such as Vanceril. Persons with severe asthma may require theophylline or oral corticosteroids. Sedatives, tranquilizers, and antibiotics may also be prescribed. Management of severe asthmatic attacks includes oxygen, IV aminophylline or theophylline, IV steroids, and hydration. Breathing exercises, postural drainage, and aerosol therapy assist in removing retained secretions.

ASSESSMENT

- Determine time of onset of the attack, any identifiable precipitating factors, and the name, dose, and time of any drug taken prior to admission.
- Assess respiratory status including breath sounds and presence of tachypnea, dyspnea, tightness in the chest, paroxysmal attacks of cough, thick tenacious mucus, prolonged expiration, and use of accessory muscles of respiration.

- Observe for symptoms of hypoxia (restlessness, tachycardia, confusion, hypotension, and cyanosis).
- Review results of laboratory tests such as ABGs.
- Question the patient about history of allergy; previous asthmatic episodes, including precipitating factors and treatment; understanding of the disease and prescribed medications; and effect of disease on lifestyle.

NURSING DIAGNOSES, PLANNING, AND NURSING INTERVENTIONS

NDx: Ineffective breathing pattern related to bronchial spasm and hypersecretion of mucus

Planning: Patient outcomes

1. Respiratory rate returns to baseline.
2. Complaints of dyspnea are absent.
3. Audible expiratory wheeze is absent.
4. Cyanosis is absent.
5. Pulse oximeter values are within normal range.

Nursing Interventions

Administer medications as ordered to relieve respiratory distress.

Monitor for side effects (cardiac dysrhythmias, tremor, nervousness, nausea, and headaches) of prescribed medications.

Position the patient to ease respiratory effort; e.g., sitting position with upper body bent slightly forward using the over-bed table for support.

Maintain a quiet environment.

Protect from drafts and chills.

Assist with bronchial toilet: breathing exercises, postural drainage, and suctioning.

Note and document color, odor, quantity, and consistency of expectorated sputum.

Encourage 2 to 3 L of fluid per day to liquefy secretions.

Monitor I & O.

NDx: Risk for altered health maintenance related to insufficient knowledge of disease process; ways to avoid

23

allergen; contributing factors such as smoking, lack of sleep, and stress; medication regimen; and other self-care measures.

Planning: Patient outcomes

1. Patient identifies trigger factors.
2. Patient lists ways to eliminate or reduce exposure to trigger factors.
3. Patient states name, dose, route, time of administration, and use of prescribed medication.
4. Patient demonstrates correct use of metered dose inhaler medications.
5. Patient demonstrates use of peak flow meter.
6. Patient wears a Medic Alert tag or similar device.

Nursing Interventions

Explain what triggers the symptoms and what happens in the lungs to cause the symptoms.

Assist the patient to identify ways to avoid the causative antigen and to incorporate them into daily living.

Recommend a stress management program if emotional stress is a frequent cause of the attacks.

Recommend a smoking cessation program if the patient smokes.

Teach self-administration of prescribed drugs including the use of a metered dose inhaler, spacer, and peak flow meter; have the patient perform a return demonstration.

Instruct patient in the following precautions:

- Do not discontinue, increase, or take newly prescribed or OTC drugs without consulting the physician treating the asthma.
- Do not exceed 4 to 6 inhalation treatments per day.
- Follow physician's orders for changes in medication regimen based on peak flow values precisely.
- Inform all health care providers about the asthma and name and dose of medications being taken.
- Wear a Medic Alert or similar identification.

Additional Interventions

Assure the patient that he or she will not be left unattended and carefully explain each aspect of care during an acute episode.

Provide high-nutrient supplemental feedings if shortness of breath precludes adequate nutritional intake.

Encourage participation in exercise, sports, and other activities, stressing that no activities need to be restricted except those that precipitate an attack.

Stress the importance of avoiding fatigue.

Refer the patient to appropriate agencies and support groups.

Atherosclerosis

Atherosclerosis is a vascular condition in which the walls of arteries become calcified from fatty plaques, causing obstruction of the vessels. Calcification, necrosis, and rupture of the vessel may occur. Any vessel may be involved, but the aorta, iliac carotid, and the coronary arteries are most commonly affected. Atherosclerosis is the most common occlusive disorder of the arteries and is the major cause of death in individuals over 65 years of age. Risk factors associated with atherosclerosis include increased cholesterol, cigarette smoking, hypertension, diabetes, and a family history of heart disease. Management of atherosclerosis depends on the location and severity of the disorder. It may consist of palliative treatment, supportive care, and pharmacologic or surgical intervention. The patient is educated about lifestyle changes needed such as diet modifications, cessation of smoking, and the initiation of a mild exercise regimen. Antiplatelet therapy may be prescribed for carotid artery occlusion. Sympathectomy, angioplasty, and grafts are the most common surgeries performed for atherosclerotic disorders.

ASSESSMENT

- Assess for pain, noting the onset, intensity, duration, radiation, and location.

- Determine if the pain is present only during exercise or at rest.
- Look for signs of pain such as grimacing, clenching of hands, moaning, or guarding when the patient is moving in bed or ambulating, or after ambulation when the patient is at rest.
- Ask the patient about numbness, tingling, or paresthesia of the extremities.
- Check the temperature and color of the extremities when elevated and when in a dependent position.
- Observe the condition of the skin and feet.
- Palpate for pulses and compare bilaterally.
- Auscultate for bruits over occluded arteries.
- Monitor serum cholesterol levels and other laboratory data.
- Check the patient's physical mobility.
- Ask about assistance needed to perform activities of daily living.
- Determine the patient's flexibility, range of motion, and strength in the extremities.
- Assess the patient's level of knowledge about the disorder and treatment.
- Ask about the patient's lifestyle and associated risk factors.
- Assess the level of adaptation to the disorder and ability to manage the disease process and its manifestations.

NURSING DIAGNOSES, PLANNING, AND NURSING INTERVENTIONS

NDx: Pain related to ischemic tissues secondary to decreased circulation from disease process

Planning: Patient outcomes

1. Patient reports an absence or reduction in pain with ambulation or at rest.
2. Nonverbal signs of pain such as grimacing, clenching hands, or guarding are absent.
3. Patient describes methods of relaxation to reduce pain and coping strategies to deal with the pain.

Nursing Interventions

Instruct the patient to cease smoking since it causes an increased demand for blood and oxygen to tissues, as well as vasoconstriction.

Use diversional activities to decrease the patient's awareness of pain.

Determine coping strategies that help the patient deal with the pain, especially when it is severe.

Be sure the patient avoids constricting clothing that interferes with circulation in the extremities.

Administer pain medication as prescribed.

Teach the patient about the effects of the medication, frequency of use and potential side effects.

Help the patient decrease stress and tension through the use of relaxation methods to relieve the pain caused by increased vasoconstriction.

Allow for periods of rest during episodes of intermittent claudication.

NDx: Impaired physical mobility related to pain and decreased strength and sensation secondary to disease state

Planning: Patient outcomes

1. Patient reports increased mobility, strength, and endurance.
2. Patient is able to perform activities of daily living.

Nursing Interventions

Assist the patient when getting out of bed and ambulating.

Use durable medical equipment accessories, when appropriate, to assist the patient in maintaining mobility.

Teach the patient to perform range of motion exercises to increase circulation and to maintain or improve strength and endurance.

Prepare a daily exercise schedule for the patient, increasing the level as tolerated.

Tell the patient to walk slowly and avoid stairs or inclines at first, if necessary, and to stop for a few minutes when pain occurs.

Encourage the patient to persist in the exercise regimen, even if it must be moderated at times of pain or lack of endurance.

Praise the patient on achievements made.

NDx: Altered health maintenance related to knowledge deficit about the disease, nutritional needs, treatments, and measures to reduce risk

Planning: Patient outcomes

1. Patient describes cause, effects, and risk factors associated with atherosclerosis.
2. Patient lists symptoms and treatments for the complications of the disorder.
3. Patient relates the nutritional therapy for lowering cholesterol levels.
4. Patient states the self care needed to prevent risk or complications of atherosclerosis.

Nursing Interventions

Explain the cause, effects, and clinical course of atherosclerosis to the patient.

Allow time for questions from the patient or significant others.

Provide appropriate literature about atherosclerosis for the patient and family to review.

Allow patient to verbalize concerns and fears.

Evaluate discharge needs of the patient and family and obtain referrals as indicated.

Alert the patient to signs and symptoms of atherosclerosis and the complications such as impaired mobility, skin breakdown, and infection or gangrene of the extremities.

Teach the patient to use safety measures or ask for assistance when out of bed or when ambulating.

Instruct the patient about dietary modifications needed to promote good health, decrease dietary fats and cholesterol, and reduce risk or prevent complications of the disorder.

Initiate counseling with a dietitian to assist with meal planning if needed.

Teach the patient how to achieve comfort by frequent repositioning and padding bony prominences.

Show family members how to massage the patient with lotion to promote circulation and prevent skin breakdown.

Tell the patient to avoid using heating pads since thermoreceptors in the tissue may be dulled from oxygen deprivation.

Explain the use of a bed cradle to prevent pressure on joints and sensitive areas.

Teach the patient the dosage, route, time, frequency, side effects, and toxic effects of any medication prescribed.

Explain the diagnostic studies completed and the need for any follow-up studies after discharge.

Include the family in any of the teaching sessions when applicable.

NDx: Self-esteem disturbance related to chronic illness, changes in lifestyle to manage disease and reduce risk factors, and/or inability to perform activities of daily living

Planning: Patient outcomes

1. Patient identifies methods to cope with illness.
2. Patient denies feelings of inadequacy, helplessness, or dependency.
3. Patient appears positive, friendly, cheerful, and actively participates in plans for discharge and patient education sessions.
4. Patient takes responsibility for self care.

Nursing Interventions

Teach the patient self-care measures, encouraging participation and decision-making by the patient to increase independence and self-esteem.

Explain how changes in lifestyle can benefit the patient and significant others.

Allow time for expression of concerns, questions, and clarification of misunderstandings.

Praise the patient for knowledge gained about the disorder, for attempts at lifestyle change, and for participation in self care.

Seek assistance from clergy, family members, or other professionals when appropriate.

Make referrals for the patient upon discharge, as needed.

Benign Prostatic Hyperplasia

Benign prostatic hyperplasia (BPH) is an overgrowth of cells in the prostate gland that occurs only in aging males with normal testicular function. Classic manifestations of symptomatic BPH, all of which are secondary to compression of the urethra, are frequency of urination, nocturia, difficulty starting and stopping the stream of urine, weak stream, and dribbling. The increased resistance to outflow of urine from the bladder results in hypertrophy of the detrusor muscles and to trabeculation and bladder diverticula. This predisposes to urinary retention and places the patient at risk for bladder infection and calculi.

In evaluating the patient, the American Urological Association (AUA) Symptom Index is used to help quantify symptom severity. In accord with the Agency for Health Policy and Research (AHCPR) policy, the initial evaluation of the patient should also include a detailed medical history, a physical examination including a digital rectal exam, a focused neurological examination, a urinalysis, and a protein-specific antigen (PSA) level.

When few symptoms of obstruction are present (AUA score of 7 or less) management consists of watchful waiting with regular prostatic massage and sexual intercourse to help decrease prostatic congestion; limiting amount of fluids taken at any one time to avoid distending the bladder; urinating at the first urge; and avoiding drugs that can precipitate acute urinary retention. When major symptoms of obstruction exist, management options include alpha blocker therapy, which relaxes the smooth muscle of the prostate, thereby facilitating bladder emptying; finasteride therapy, which shrinks the prostate due to its anti-androgen action; balloon dilatation of the prostatic urethra; and prostatectomy. The latter is recommended by AHCPR guidelines for patients with intractable urinary retention, recurrent urinary infection, or gross hematuria, bladder stones, or renal insufficiency.

See Prostatectomy in Section II for specific nursing care related to this method of management.

◆ Bone Tumors

A bone tumor or neoplasm is any abnormal bone cell growth that serves no useful purpose and derives its nutrition from, and often destroys, healthy surrounding tissues. Bone tumors may be either osteoblastic, bone-forming, or osteolytic, bone-destroying. The exact cause of the formation and growth of bone tumors is not known. They are classified by the type of tissue they arise from. Most benign bone tumors occur in children and young adults, grow slowly, and do not metastasize. Malignant bone tumors grow rapidly, metastasize to other parts of the body via the blood and lymph systems, and destroy surrounding tissue. Malignant tumors are further classified as primary tumors that arise directly from musculoskeletal tissue, such as Ewing's sarcomas, chondrosarcomas, fibrosarcomas, and histiocytomas, or secondary tumors, which spread to the bone from a malignancy in another part of the body. Chemotherapy, radiation therapy, and surgical excision are the treatments of choice for most malignant bone tumors, but amputation may be necessary in some cases.

ASSESSMENT

- Review the patient's history, diagnostic studies, and presenting problems.
- Assess the affected area, noting any swelling, deformity, or pain.
- Ask the patient about ability to perform activities of daily living, including range of motion and any mobility problems.
- Determine when the pain is most significant.
- Note problems with weight bearing and mobility.
- Determine the patient's and family's understanding about the diagnosis and possible treatment alternatives.

31

- Assess the patient's coping strategies, support systems that are available to the patient, and their effectiveness.

NURSING DIAGNOSES, PLANNING, AND NURSING INTERVENTIONS

NDx: Self-esteem disturbance related to deformity, effects of chemotherapy, or amputation

Planning: Patient outcomes

1. Patient relates feelings of self-worth.
2. Patient maintains social activity.
3. Patient is able to look at self with understanding and acceptance.

Nursing Interventions

Allow the patient to vent feelings about the diagnosis.
Provide information about cancer support groups.
Seek assistance from clergy or professional counseling.
Provide diversional activities for the patient when bedfast due to exacerbations from the disease or the treatment regimen.
Involve support from the family and other friends.
Seek effective coping strategies for the patient.
Assist the patient in finding the positive aspects of life to focus on during periods of depression.
Help the patient cope with the altered appearance by suggesting methods of concealment, such as the use of appropriate clothing, makeup, or natural-looking prosthetic devices.

NDx: Fear related to forthcoming treatments, prognosis, and uncertain future

Planning: Patient outcomes

1. Patient appears relaxed and is able to rest and sleep at intervals.
2. Patient denies extreme fear about the diagnosis, prognosis, and the future.

3. Patient freely expresses concerns about the diagnosis and prognosis.
4. Patient states acceptable coping mechanisms to reduce the fear.

Nursing Interventions

Help the patient cope with the diagnosis and uncertain future.

Provide referral to professional counseling services.

Assist the patient in the identification of support systems.

Talk with clergy and/or significant others about support for the patient.

Explain and reinforce all information regarding the diagnosis and treatment modalities provided by the physician.

Allow time for questions and concerns from the patient and family.

Provide opportunity for the patient and family to talk with others who have coped with similar circumstances successfully.

Inform the patient about organizations such as the American Cancer Society, which provide psychological support, educational services, and other assistance for patients and families.

NDx: Pain related to effects of the tumor, swelling, and deformity

Planning: Patient outcomes

1. Patient reports an absence or tolerable level of pain.
2. Patient identifies methods to decrease pain, such as reduction of swelling, relaxation strategies, and appropriate use of analgesics.

Nursing Interventions

Give prescribed analgesics and explain the dosage, frequency, side effects, and expected therapeutic effects of the medications.

Caution the patient not to perform tasks that require mental alertness while under the effects of the pain medication.

Tell the patient to elevate the part to reduce swelling and, thus, reduce pain.

Caution the patient about weight-bearing, if contraindicated, since that might increase the pain significantly.

NDx: Knowledge deficit: Nature of disorder, prognosis, management, and prevention of injury of weakened part

Planning: Patient outcomes

1. Patient states accurate information about the cause of the tumor, prognosis, treatment, and methods to prevent injury.
2. Patient reports an understanding of the disorder and the information presented by the physician for management of the condition.

Nursing Interventions

Tell the patient about the tumor type, the prognosis, methods of prevention of injury, and appropriate treatment.

Explain that increased swelling, discoloration, or decreased sensation in the affected part may be signs of complications or increased tumor growth, and that the physician should be notified.

Reinforce the physician's instruction about weight-bearing since the bone structure may be weakened or necrosis may have developed.

Demonstrate prescribed exercises to the patient and encourage participation in the exercise regimen to prevent loss of strength and joint motion.

NDx: Anxiety related to diagnosis, potential permanent loss of limb, and pain

Planning: Patient outcomes

1. Patient demonstrates manageable levels of anxiety, fear, or nervousness about the diagnosis, therapy, and potential outcome of therapy.

2. Patient appears relaxed and is able to rest at intervals and to sleep well.
3. Patient does not display signs of increased anxiety such as twitching, increased respirations and pulse, or withdrawal from self-care activities.

Nursing Interventions

Explain the purpose of all treatments to the patient.

Allow the patient time to ask questions and relay concerns.

Reinforce information from the physician to the patient.

Give support without offering unrealistic reassurances.

Teach the patient relaxation methods and coping strategies.

Assess vital signs and watch for changes indicating increased anxiety.

Brain Tumors

Intracranial tumors can be either primary or secondary (metastatic). Primary brain tumors arise from brain tissue and the etiology is unknown; secondary (metastatic) brain tumors arise from tissue elsewhere in the body and spread to the brain. The origin (primary malignancy) of metastatic brain tumors is most often the lung, breast, skin, gastrointestinal tract, and kidneys. All tumors compress and invade surrounding brain tissue resulting in pathophysiologic changes in the brain and increased intracranial pressure. Headache, vomiting, and papilledema are general symptoms associated with intracranial tumors. Management of brain tumors involves surgery, radiotherapy, or chemotherapy alone or in combination.

For specific guides to nursing care see entries under Increased Intracranial Pressure, Cancer, Craniotomy, Chemotherapy, and Radiation Therapy.

◆ Breast Cancer

Most breast cancers arise in the epithelial tissues of the ductal system in the UOQ and the tail of the breast. Metastasis is via the lymphatic system and blood stream to sites such as the lungs, liver, and bones. Management consists of surgery, chemotherapy, hormonal therapy, and irradiation alone or in combination, depending on the stage of the disease and characteristics of the tumor. The most common surgery is modified radical mastectomy, with lumpectomy and chemotherapy becoming increasingly common. Antiestrogen therapy is used for tumors that are estrogen receptor positive.

See entries under Modified Radical Mastectomy, Chemotherapy, and Radiation Therapy in Section II for information on related nursing care.

◆ Burns

A burn is an injury to the skin, tissues, and/or mucous membranes due to thermal, chemical, or electrical insult. Approach to the care of burns requires a concerted team effort. Burns are categorized by the depth of the burn: partial thickness (superficial or deep) and full thickness; and by the percentage of total body surface injured, areas involved, and presence of complications (major, minor, or moderate). Burn management involves immediate care, emergency care, long-term care, and rehabilitation. Burns are treated in a variety of ways depending upon the type of burn and its severity. The treatments include open and closed treatment, application of topical agents, skin flaps, and skin grafts (homografts, heterografts, and autografts).

ASSESSMENT

- Assess for life-threatening injuries.
- Check vital signs.
- Obtain a history of the burn injury.
- Determine the severity of the injury: size, body part affected, depth.
- Determine the type of agent that caused the burn.

- Assess for associated injuries.
- Determine the immediate care necessary and initiate the emergency process.

NURSING DIAGNOSES, PLANNING, AND NURSING INTERVENTIONS

NDx: Risk for ineffective airway clearance related to possible upper airway edema secondary to inhalation of superheated air

Planning: Patient outcomes

1. Patient maintains patent airway with regular, unlabored respirations within normal rate.

Nursing Interventions

Examine nasal and oral airways for signs of burns.
Auscultate breath sounds and assess respiratory status and voice quality.
Administer humidified oxygen as needed.
Elevate the head of the bed.
Administer pain medication if needed.
Encourage the patient to cough and take deep slow breaths to clear airways.
Monitor pulmonary blood gases.
Suction patient as necessary.
Plan for emergency interventions if respiratory distress occurs.

NDx: Risk for fluid volume deficit related to inadequate replacement of fluids lost through evaporation from the burn wound and fluid shifts into interstitial spaces

Planning: Patient outcomes

1. Patient maintains adequate hydration as evidenced by:
   mental alertness
   urine output >30 ml/hr.
   blood pressure 90/60 mm Hg

heart rate between 60 and 100 bpm
CVP 4 to 15 mm H_2O pressure
moist mucous membranes
good skin turgor

Nursing Interventions

Weigh the patient daily.
Monitor vital signs, level of consciousness, CVP, urine
output, and skin appearance.
Maintain intravenous infusion as prescribed.
Auscultate and evaluate breath sounds.

NDx: Pain related to burn injury

Planning: Patient outcomes

1. Patient states pain is relieved or within tolerable
    limits.
2. Patient appears relaxed and is able to rest well.

Nursing Interventions

Administer intravenous pain medication as ordered, es-
pecially prior to necessary procedures or manipula-
tions of the patient.
Monitor respirations and level of consciousness.
Assist the patient to move to a position of comfort.
Teach the patient relaxation methods.
Provide diversional activities.
Provide emotional support.

NDx: Risk for infection related to open burn wounds
and suppressed immune response

Planning: Patient outcomes

1. Patient remains free of infection as evidenced by
    absence of fever, daily increase in wound granula-
    tion and healing, and lack of signs of infection in the
    wound.
2. Patient demonstrates correct wound care prior to
    discharge.

Nursing Interventions

Maintain strict cleanliness and asepsis when handling
patient or performing wound care.

Cleanse wound as ordered, and assess and record untoward findings.

Teach the patient appropriate wound care and observe the
technique prior to discharge.

NDx: Anxiety related to appearance of wounds, excessive treatments necessary, pain, and unknown outcome of
treatments

Planning: Patient outcomes

1. Patient and family verbalize an understanding of
    the treatment needed and the uncertainty of the
    outcome.
2. Family is prepared for the appearance of the patient.
3. Patient and family verbalize concerns and ask ques-
    tions freely.

Nursing Interventions

Discuss the patient's appearance before the family members are allowed into the patient's room.

Explain the equipment, treatments, and other necessary
medical interventions to the patient and family.

Encourage the patient and family to verbalize their concerns and thoughts, and to ask questions.

Offer spiritual support and consult clergy, if appropriate.

Answer questions in an honest manner without express-
ing false hopes.

Reinforce the physician's explanation.

NDx: Risk for fluid volume excess related to mobilization of fluids from the interstitial spaces into the intravascular circulation

Planning: Patient outcomes

1. Patient maintains fluid balance as evidenced by:
    urine output of 30 to 100 ml/hr.

blood pressure between 90/60 and 140/90 mm Hg
heart rate 60 to 100 bpm
CVP 4 to 15 mm H_2O pressure
lungs clear to auscultation
body weight within 5% of preinjury weight

Nursing Interventions

Auscultate for respiratory status frequently, and ask the
    patient to report any respiratory distress.
Check vital signs frequently.
Weigh daily and compare with previous weights.
Monitor electrolyte levels.

◆ Cancer

Cancer is a malignant neoplasm that is composed of
undifferentiated cells that have little resemblance to the
tissue of origin. Cancers tend to grow rapidly, expanding
at the periphery and invading and destroying surrounding tissues; tend to recur when removed; metastasize by
way of blood and lymph to distant areas of the body; and
cause systemic manifestations such as altered taste,
anorexia, weight loss, weakness, and ultimately death if
not controlled.

Cancers of epithelial tissue are called carcinomas. Cancers of connective tissue, muscle, or bone are sarcomas,
and cancers of the blood and lymphatics are leukemias,
myelomas, and lymphomas.

Cancers are graded histologically based on the similar-
ity of tumor cells to normal cells of that tissue as follows:

Grade 1 - Well-differentiated (looks like normal cells)
Grade 2 - Moderately well-differentiated
Grade 3 - Poorly differentiated
Grade 4 - Anaplastic

Higher grade tumors, i.e., those with more immature
cells are considered more malignant and more likely to
grow and spread.

Cancer is also staged to identify the extent of disease. An
internationally accepted staging system is the TNM. With
this system each anatomic site of cancer is classified based
on three components: tumor size (T), characteristics of

regional lymph nodes and the presence or absence of malignant cells in the nodes (N), and the presence or absence of metastatic disease (M).

The warning signs of cancer that all patients should be taught are:

C   Change in bowel or bladder habits
A   A sore that does not heal
U   Unusual bleeding or discharge
T   Thickening or lump in breast or elsewhere
I   Indigestion or difficulty swallowing
O   Obvious change in a wart or mole
N   Nagging cough or horseness

Guidelines for patient screening tests for cancer are:

Monthly breast self-examination after age 20.

Annual professional breast examination after age 40, every third year between ages 20 and 40.

Baseline mammography between ages 35 and 40, every 1 to 2 years between ages 40 and 49, annually after age 50.

Monthly teslicular examination.

Annual digital rectal examination for prostate cancer after age 40. Prostate-specific antigen level and rectal examination after age 50, earlier if in a high risk group.

Annual test for occult blood in the stool after age 50.

Skin inspection

Papanicolaou smear after two negative smears 1 year apart, every third year between ages 20 (or when sexually active, whichever comes first) and 65.

Pelvic exam every third year between ages 20 and 40, annually after age 40.

Management of oncologic disorders is complex and involves the treatment modalities of surgery, radiotherapy, chemotherapy, and immunotherapy, alone or in combination, for prevention, control, elimination, or palliation.

See following entries for information on specific cancers:

Brain Tumor
Laryngeal Cancer
Breast Cancer
Lung Cancer
Cervical Cancer
Pancreatic Cancer
Colorectal Cancer
Prostate Cancer

Endometrial Cancer
Testicular Cancer
Gastric Cancer

See entries under Chemotherapy and Radiation for specific information on these treatment modalities as well as nursing care related to them.

Cardiac Dysrhythmias

Cardiac dysrhythmias are disturbances in the conduction of electrical activity in the heart. These disturbances may be caused by electrolyte and acid-base imbalances, cardiac edema, surgical incision of conduction pathways, cardiac ischemia or infarct, metabolic alterations, and medications. Basic dysrhythmias are classified as bradycardia or tachycardia. Dysrhythmias may arise from the sinoatrial node, the atrioventicular node, or the ventricular conductive tissue. Although all dysrhythmias can be potentially life-threatening, ventricular tachycardia is a true emergency that may rapidly result in death and therefore must be treated without delay. Dysrhythmias are detected through pulse monitoring and are diagnosed by electrocardiac monitoring. Drug therapy is usually the treatment of choice, although a pacemaker may be inserted. Patients in ventricular fibrillation may be defibrillated by electric shock.

ASSESSMENT

- Review medical history and diagnostic data for the type of dysrhythmia being exhibited.
- Assess for unexplained fatigue and weakness.
- Perform a thorough cardiopulmonary physical assessment.
- Evaluate the mental status and behaviors of the patient.
- Check vital signs and electrocardiograph monitoring.
- Check mental status, circulation, urine output, and observe for signs of respiratory distress.

NURSING DIAGNOSES, PLANNING, AND NURSING INTERVENTIONS

NDx: Decreased cardiac output related to altered electrical conduction

Planning: Patient outcomes

1. Patient achieves adequate cardiac output as evidenced by electrical conduction.
2. Patient demonstrates reduced frequency of dysrhythmias.

Nursing Interventions

Monitor vital signs at rest and during activity.
Evaluate sleep and rest patterns.
Encourage activity alternated with periods of rest.
Monitor the electrocardiograph readings.
Observe for signs of decreased cardiac output such as shortness of breath, poor skin color, diminishing pulses, mental confusion, and decreased urine output.
Monitor laboratory values and the patient's fluid intake and urine output.

NDx: Anxiety related to potentially life-threatening dysrhythmias, treatment regimen, and fear of death

Planning: Patient outcomes

1. Patient reports reduced anxiety and fear.
2. Patient rests well and does not present signs of anxiety such as restlessness, withdrawal, or changes in vital signs.

Nursing Interventions

Assist the patient to learn effective coping techniques.
Teach the patient relaxation methods.
Explain the dysrhythmia and the treatment plan.
Allow the patient to verbalize concerns and ask questions.
Refer to appropriate support resources as needed.

◆ Cerebrovascular Accident

The term *cerebrovascular accident* (CVA), or *stroke*, describes a condition in which there is an interruption of blood flow to the brain resulting in temporary or permanent dysfunction of motor, sensory, perceptual, emotional, or cognitive abilities. CVAs result from occlusive disease of the cerebral arteries and vessels caused by thrombosis or embolism, or from hemorrhage that occurs in the space surrounding the brain (subarachnoid) or within the brain (intracerebral). Risk factors include hypertension, heart disease, atherosclerosis, smoking, hypercholesterolemia, hypercoagulopathies, diabetes mellitus, cerebral aneurysm, arteriovenous malformation, and hemorrhagic disorders. Major classes of stroke include transient ischemic attack (TIA), reversible ischemic neurologic deficit (RIND), progressive stroke (PS), and complete stroke (CS). Management involves treatment of predisposing conditions, control of hypertension with antihypertensive agents, anticoagulant therapy with heparin followed by Coumadin and antiaggregation therapy with aspirin and dipyridamole (Persantine) in nonhemorrhagic events, and possibly surgical intervention.

ASSESSMENT

- Assess for headache, nausea, vomiting, seizures, changes in vital signs, and level of consciousness.
- Assess for hemiplegia, facial paralysis, numbness, paresthesia, hemianopia, monocular blindness, dysphasia, aphasia, agnosia, alexia, dysphagia, and spatial perceptual dysfunctions.
- Assess for cognitive decline, mental changes with memory impairment, impaired judgment, behavioral changes, and emotional instability.
- Observe for bowel and bladder incontinence and one-sided neglect.
- Check respiratory rate and rhythm, ability to clear secretions, breath sounds, and gag reflex. Assess the patient's ability to perform ADL, to be free from injury, to communicate, and to maintain appropriate social interaction.

NURSING DIAGNOSES, PLANNING, AND NURSING INTERVENTIONS

NDx: Risk for ineffective breathing pattern related to muscle weakness and immobility

Planning: Patient outcomes

1. Cyanosis is absent.
2. ABG values are within normal range for patient.
3. Bilateral breath sounds are clear.

Nursing Interventions

Monitor respiratory pattern and auscultate lung fields.
Monitor vital signs.
Position the patient at a 30° head elevation.
Suction the airway and perform chest physiotherapy as necessary.
Encourage and teach the patient to perform coughing and deep-breathing exercises every 2 hours and to use the incentive spirometer.
Review ABG values.
Administer O_2 as ordered.
Have emergency intubation and mechanical ventilation readily available.

NDx: Risk for aspiration related to dysphagia

Planning: Patient outcomes

1. Patient avoids aspiration.

Nursing Interventions

Monitor the patient's ability to clear secretions from airway and for intactness of gag reflex.
Maintain working suction equipment at bedside and suction as needed.
Position the patient with head elevated to 30°.
Monitor the patient during feeding.
Encourage the patient to eat semi-solids and soft foods.

NDx: Impaired physical mobility related to plegia

Planning: Patient outcomes

1. Patient participates in ADL.
2. Patient ambulates, transfers, or moves self with or without assistance.
3. Complications of immobility: deep venous thrombosis, pulmonary embolism, decubitus formation, and subluxation of joints are absent.

Nursing Interventions

During the acute phase, position the patient semi-prone with the head of the bed elevated 30°.

Maintain proper body alignment with use of splints, trochanter rolls, footboard, and pillows.

Turn and position every 2 hours; avoid positioning the patient on the affected side.

Position the patient flat and prone for 30 minutes each day.

Perform active or passive range of motion exercises at least every 6 hours.

Provide good skin care and air mattress.

Encourage the patient to wear an arm sling if ordered.

Prepare the patient for ambulation by teaching standing balance, standing pivot, to look at extremities and assess position, to lean and move toward the unaffected side, and to bear weight on the unaffected side.

Consult with the physical and occupational therapists to obtain supportive and assistive devices.

Apply thigh-length antiembolic stockings as ordered.

Monitor for edema and redness of calves and Homans' sign.

Additional Interventions

Encourage the patient to participate actively in self care.

Monitor I & O.

Weigh weekly.

Place food tray on the unaffected side and encourage patient to chew on the unaffected side.

Consult with the nutritionist regarding the patient's dietary needs and ability to ingest required calories.

Draw attention to, and reorient the patient to, the neglected side.

Establish a bowel regimen based on the patient's usual pattern of elimination.

Identify alternate strategies that can be used to foster the patient's understanding and/or expression of needs.

Anticipate the patient's needs, reduce environmental distractions, and allow time to give one direction at a time, and allow time to process messages and respond.

Consult with social services to assist with discharge planning and identifying available resources.

Cervical Cancer

Almost all cervical cancers are squamous cell carcinomas that have a gradual onset originating with a dysplastic precursor lesion. Precursor lesions are referred to as cervical intraepithelial neoplasia (CIN) and graded on a scale of I to III depending on the amount of dysplasia present. The main routes of spread are into the vaginal mucosa, into the myometrium of the uterus, into the lymph nodes around the cervix and by direct extension into other structures of the pelvis such as the bladder, rectum, and pelvic wall. Distant metastases can occur although a predilection to spread within the pelvis seems to exist. Management depends on the stage of the disease, the patient's age, desire for child bearing and general health status. It may consist of surgery (conization, hysterectomy, radical hysterectomy with pelvic lymph node dissection), internal and/or external radiation, and chemotherapy alone or in combination. Nursing care of patients receiving internal radiation is discussed below.

See entries in Part 2 under chemotherapy, hysterectomy, and radiation therapy for additional information on nursing care applicable to individual patients.

Internal or intracavity radiation is used to irradiate malignant cells in the cervix and endometrial cavity. Preparation for the procedure includes a low-residue diet and cleansing enema, a cleansing douche, insertion of a Foley catheter, as well as general measures applying to any preoperative patient. The applicator is inserted in the OR; placement is confirmed with x-ray; and the radiation source is inserted when the patient returns to her room. It is left in place for 48–72 hours, during which time nursing care is as follows.

ASSESSMENT

- Check VS. Expect temperature elevation over 100°F on first evening.
- Observe for vaginal bleeding and erythema of the buttocks and perineum, which can be the precursor to radiation-induced desquamation, and signs of skin breakdown over pressure points.
- Assess for vaginal cramping, discomfort due to limited mobility and effectiveness of medications in providing relief.
- Monitor for signs of cystitis, proctitis, phlebitis, dehydration, and radiation sickness, all of which are potential complications of intracavity radiation therapy.

NURSING DIAGNOSES, PLANNING, AND NURSING INTERVENTIONS

NDx: Risk for injury related to accidental movement of radiation source.

Planning: Patient outcomes

1. Patient stays in flat dorsal position.
2. Bladder distention is absent.

Nursing Interventions

Maintain patient on absolute bedrest in the dorsal position.

Elevate head of bed to a maximum of 10–15° for comfort.

Avoid turning patient but, if absolutely necessary, place pillow between her knees and roll her like a log.

Maintain free flowing urinary drainage.

Give fracture pan if patient needs to have BM despite bowel prep.

NDx: Pain related to uterine contractions and limited movement

Planning: Patient outcomes

1. Patient appears comfortable: does not grimace, moan, clench fist or hold abdomen.
2. Patient states she has less cramping.

Nursing Interventions

Give narcotics as ordered.
Encourage use of relaxation exercises.
Provide distraction (e.g., radio, TV) in accordance with patient's wishes.

NDx: Risk for fluid volume deficit related to normal fluid loss secondary to tissue destruction at the site of radiation

Planning: Patient outcomes

1. Patient has at least 3000 ml fluid intake per day.
2. Mucous membranes are moist.
3. Skin turgor is firm.

Nursing Interventions

Encourage patient to drink at least 3000 ml per day.
Keep fluids of the patient's choice within her reach.
Record I & O.

NDx: Risk for altered health maintenance related to insufficient knowledge of discharge instructions

Planning: Patient outcomes

1. Patient describes/demonstrates douche procedure.
2. Patient states when sexual intercourse can be resumed.
3. Patient lists symptoms to be reported.

Nursing Interventions

Provide the patient with the following information:
- Some vaginal bleeding may occur for 1 to 3 months after irradiation.

- Foul-smelling vaginal discharge will occur for some time.
- Douches are to be taken in accordance with physician's orders while discharge persists. (Specify the solution and the frequency with which douching should be done. Demonstrate proper technique for performing the procedure and for cleansing the equipment).
- Emollient cream may be used to ease pruritus.
- Sexual intercourse may be resumed in 7 to 10 days; intercourse may be difficult because radiation can cause vaginal atrophy.

Instruct the patient to:
- Report continued sexual difficulties as dilation of the vagina may be required.
- Report persistent rectal irritation.

Additional Interventions

Place patient in private room, preferably at end of corridor. If this is not an option, place patient with a postmenopausal woman.

Do not allow any pregnant woman or anyone under age 18 in the room.

Work as far from the radiation source as possible, always keeping the lead shield between it and you.

Be well organized and provide quality care in the least possible time.

Orient patient on admission to call system, exercises, etc., to decrease need for time spent at bedside after the radiation is in place.

Bathe patient's upper body for comfort. Do not bathe below waist unless soiled.

Use air mattress or egg crate for comfort.

Encourage ROM exercises for upper extremities.

Provide a foot board and encourage foot exercises while awake.

◆ Cholecystitis

Cholecystitis is an inflammation of the gallbladder that is almost always associated with cholelithiasis (the presence of stones in the gallbladder, cystic duct, or common bile duct). The exact cause of stone formation is unknown, however; bile stasis, imbalances in cholesterol metabolism, and infection seem to be precipitating factors. Stones, once formed, may remain in the gallbladder or migrate to the cystic or common bile duct, causing inflammation and obstruction. Cholecystitis may be acute or chronic. Management of the acute form includes supportive measures such as the use of analgesics, anticholinergics, and antibiotics, and maintaining the patient NPO with a NG tube to gastric suction progressing to a low-fat, soft diet. Supportive measures for chronic cholecystitis include a low-fat diet and, in some cases, the use of oral gallstone dissolving drugs. The most common surgical intervention is the cholecystectomy, which may be a conventional open cholecystectomy or a laparoscopic cholecystectomy (see entry under Cholecystectomy). Stones in the common bile duct may also be removed endoscopically, a procedure called mechanical litholysis.

 # Chronic Arterial Occlusive Disease (Arteriosclerosis Obliterans)

Arteriosclerosis obliterans is the occlusion of arterial vessels such as the distal aorta and iliac, femoral, and popliteal arteries. It is usually caused by atherosclerosis, resulting in gradual blockage of the large vessels, which results in ischemia distal to the occlusion. The superficial femoral artery is most commonly affected. This produces intermittent claudication in the calf muscles, thighs, buttocks, lower back, and feet. The pain increases with exercise. The goal of treatment is to restore blood flow through the narrowed vessels and to relieve the patient's symptoms. Reduction of risk factors is recommended. Vasodilators and anticoagulants are prescribed, but surgical intervention may be required to bypass the occluded artery. Amputation may be necessary if the artery is completely occluded or if gangrene is present.

NURSING CARE

The nursing care for the patient with chronic arterial occlusive disease is similar to that for a patient with *atherosclerosis*. If the treatment requires surgery, refer to the preoperative and postoperative entries in this handbook and Chapter 9 in the textbook for a discussion of endarterectomy, sympathectomy, and amputation.

◆ Chronic Bronchitis

Chronic bronchitis is classified as a chronic obstructive pulmonary disease (COPD). It is characterized by expiratory airflow obstruction resulting from inflammation of the bronchi with enlargement and hypersecretion of the mucous glands. Chronic bronchitis is clinically defined as excess production of mucus, accompanied by a chronic cough that lasts 3 months of the year for 2 consecutive years. It is caused by prolonged exposure to bronchial irritants such as smoking, secondhand smoke, air pollution, toxic fumes, and dust. Management is aimed at reversing airway narrowing, reducing mucus production, controlling symptoms, and maintaining general health. Pharmacologic management includes bronchodilators to treat bronchospasm and increase airway size and in some cases oral or inhaled corticosteroids and/or antibiotics. Measures to promote pulmonary hygiene include deep breathing, coughing, chest percussion and vibration, postural drainage, hydration, and suctioning as necessary. Low-flow oxygen is administered to maintain a PaO_2 between 50 and 60 mm Hg, and a program of exercise is prescribed unless contraindicated.

ASSESSMENT

- Assess for heavy, productive cough, particularly upon awakening, which is worse in the cold, damp weather, after intake of alcohol, or after talking for an extended time.
- Observe for dyspnea on exertion and at rest, cyanosis (secondary to hypoxemia and hypercapnea),

peripheral pedal edema, digital clubbing, distended neck veins on expiration, use of accessory muscles of respiration, abdominal breathing, pursed lip breathing, and prolonged expiration.

- Auscultate the chest for musical wheezes.
- Assess for signs of hypoxia and hypercapnea: increased shortness of breath, restlessness, lethargy, headache, confusion.
- Review results of all diagnostic tests such as ABGs, pulmonary function tests, and x-ray films.
- Assess general physical status, emotional response to the illness, and available support systems.

NURSING DIAGNOSES, PLANNING, AND NURSING INTERVENTIONS

NDx: Ineffective airway clearance related to excessive viscous secretions

Planning: Patient outcomes

1. Patient uses nebulizer and medication as ordered.
2. Patient uses breathing exercise techniques during treatments.
3. Patient coughs productively following treatments.
4. Patient uses positioning techniques to help drain lungs after treatments.

Nursing Interventions

Administer oral, subcutaneous, intravenous, rectal, or nebulized bronchodilator drugs as ordered.

Teach the patient to self-administer drugs, i.e., inhalation therapy and how to obtain needed equipment for home use.

Instruct the patient to follow inhalation of bronchodilator aerosols with postural drainage and coughing and oral hygiene.

Instruct the patient to use the nebulizer before meals to improve lung ventilation and to reduce fatigue associated with eating.

Monitor for therapeutic effect of bronchodilator drugs and for side effects such as tachycardia, cardiac dysrhythmias, and CNS excitation.

Force fluids to 2 to 3 L/day unless contraindicated.

NDx: Impaired gas exchange related to prolonged expiration and carbon dioxide retention

Planning: Patient outcomes

1. Carbon dioxide levels range between 40 and 55 mm Hg. (35–45 mm Hg is normal).
2. Arterial oxygen saturation remains greater than 92%.
3. Arterial oxygen level remains greater than 55 mm Hg (normal 80–100 mm Hg).
4. Patient uses oxygen therapy equipment correctly and safely.
5. Patient lists signs of hypoxia and hypercapnia to be reported.

Nursing Interventions

Administer O_2 as ordered and teach appropriate safety measures.

Explain the hypoxic drive and the need for ABG value monitoring to the patient requiring home oxygen therapy; caution not to increase the flow unless ordered.

Review the signs and symptoms of hypoxia and hypercapnia with patient and significant others (see assessments); stress the need to report them immediately.

NDx: Activity intolerance related to muscular fatigue

Planning: Patient outcomes

1. Patient participates in a program of aerobic exercises.
2. Patient describes four basic techniques of energy conservation.
3. Patient practices energy conservation techniques in daily living.

Nursing Interventions

Encourage the patient to perform aerobic exercises as prescribed.

Review the purpose of the exercise program and emphasize the benefits.

Explore methods of energy conservation with the patient.

Review stress management and relaxation techniques.

Assist the patient to identify work simplification strategies and measures to promote restful sleep.

Encourage the patient to adopt a slower pace of living and
to plan for regular rest periods.

NDx: Risk for altered health maintenance related to
insufficient knowledge of prevention, identification, and
treatment of respiratory complications of COPD

Planning: Patient outcomes

1. Patient lists ways to avoid irritation of the respira-
    tory tract.
2. Patient identifies methods of avoiding respiratory
    tract infection.
3. Patient lists symptoms to be reported.
4. Patient acknowledges need for smoking cessation.

Nursing Interventions

Instruct the patient in the prevention and treatment of
respiratory irritation and infection as follows:

Avoid exposure to cigarette, pipe, and cigar smoke as well
as to dusts and powders.

Avoid use of aerosol sprays.

Stay indoors when the pollen count is high.

Use air conditioning to help decrease pollutants and control temperature.

Avoid exposure to persons known to have colds or other
respiratory tract infections.

Avoid enclosed, crowded areas during cold and flu season.

Obtain immunization against influenza and pneumococcal pneumonia.

Report any changes in sputum color or character, increased tightness of the chest, increased dyspnea, or
fatigue.

Call the physician if ordered antibiotics do not relieve
symptoms within 24 hours.

Provide the patient with information on available smoking cessation programs.

Teach the patient to identify symptoms of right-sided heart failure, to weigh himself or herself daily, and to report a gain of 5.5 lbs. or more.

Additional Interventions

Instruct the patient in the use of the I:E ratio breathing technique, diaphragmatic breathing, and pursed lip breathing.

Provide an opportunity for the patient to verbalize his or her feelings, answer questions honestly, and provide clear concise information about the condition.

Suggest the following strategies to help the patient meet nutritional needs:

- Use a microwave oven to conserve energy.
- Use convenience foods if appropriate.
- Sit at a table with elbows supported.
- Plan rest periods for 30 minutes before eating.
- Avoid large meals and gas-forming foods.

◆ Chronic Renal Failure (CRF)

CRF is an irreversible condition of partial or total loss of kidney function characterized by progressive reduction of nephrons until the remaining nephrons can no longer maintain the body's internal environment. Causes of chronic renal failure include glomerulonephritis, acute renal failure, polycystic kidney disease, obstruction, systemic disorders, pyelonephritis, and nephrotoxins. Treatment for chronic renal failure focuses on regulating fluids, electrolytes, and metabolic wastes through dietary and volume controls along with medication, control of concurrent disorders, and patient comfort.

ASSESSMENT

- Assess the patient's voiding patterns, weight gain in recent weeks, nausea, family history of renal disease, history of flu-like symptoms, and any medications taken recently.
- Check the amount of urine excreted in 24 hours, blood pressure (including postural changes), daily weight, fluid status, peripheral edema, breath

sounds, skin turgor, changes in mental status and changes in pulse rate and rhythm.

- Assess for nausea, often one of the first signs exhibited with retention of metabolic wastes.
- Check for discomforts such as muscle cramps, itching or skin irritations, and paresthesia.
- Observe for edema and decreased or wet breath sounds, which are signs of fluid retention.
- Observe for changes in mentation, which are symptoms of uremia and electrolyte imbalances.
- Check for changes in cardiac rate and rhythm, which may be indicative of hyperkalemia or hypokalemia.
- Note the laboratory studies, especially electrolytes.
- Determine the patient's knowledge level regarding renal failure and the prescribed treatment.
- Assess the patient and family's emotional status, coping mechanisms, and any support systems.

NURSING DIAGNOSES, PLANNING, AND NURSING INTERVENTIONS

NDx: Fluid volume excess related to retention of sodium and water secondary to decreased number of functioning nephrons and decreased glomerular filtration

Planning: Patient outcomes

1. Patient exhibits decreased peripheral, facial, and sacral edema.
2. Patient is free of systemic signs of fluid overload.
3. Patient relates causative factors and treatments to alleviate overload.
4. Patient has a balanced fluid intake and output.
5. Patient's electrolytes are within safe limits.

Nursing Interventions

Report signs and symptoms of fluid volume excess, which include significant weight gain, increased BP and pulse, change in mental status, dyspnea, orthopnea, crackles in the lungs, edema, distended neck veins, and elevated CVP.

Monitor chest x-ray results.

Measure fluid intake and output.

Maintain fluid restrictions and restrict sodium intake as ordered.

Monitor and document the therapeutic effect and side
effects of prescribed medications.

Weigh the patient at the same time each day.

Alert the physician if signs and symptoms persist or
worsen.

Prepare the patient and family for dialysis if needed.

NDx: Pain related to muscle cramps, burning, tingling,
itching, and restless leg syndrome secondary to peripheral neuropathies associated with electrolyte imbalances
and nitrogenous waste accumulation and atrophy of sweat
glands with accumulation of crystals on the skin

Planning: Patient outcomes

1. Patient denies muscle cramps, burning, itching, and
restless leg syndrome.
2. Patient completes activities of daily living without
complaints of discomfort.
3. Patient refrains from scratching skin and presents
no evidence of skin irritation.

Nursing Interventions

Explain the cause of the discomfort to the patient.

Provide a footboard and instruct the patient to push feet
against the board.

Tell the patient to move the legs frequently while in bed.

Apply cool packs, as needed, for comfort.

Give prescribed analgesics.

Apply lotions to dry skin frequently.

Instruct the patient about the effects of continued scratching of the skin.

Use mild soap and tepid water for bathing to prevent
further skin irritation.

Provide diversional activities.

Teach relaxation techniques and encourage their use.

NDx: Altered thought processes related to accumulation of toxic wastes

Planning: Patient outcomes

1. Patient is oriented to time, place and person.

2. Patient remains alert and responds to questions appropriately.
3. Patient is in a safe environment and is protected when mental processes are not functioning appropriately.

Nursing Interventions

Orient the patient to person, place and time frequently.

Place familiar objects near the patient to prevent further confusion.

Encourage the family to visit frequently and explain the need for continually orienting the patient to time, place, and person.

Check laboratory data, noting electrolyte and other imbalances, relate this to the patient's mentation status, and document the information.

Provide a safe environment for the patient.

Assist the patient to perform activities of daily living and to ambulate.

Refer patient to home health services upon discharge.

◆ Cirrhosis

Cirrhosis is a chronic degenerative process affecting the liver that is characterized by nodule formation and generalized liver fibrosis. Major types of cirrhosis include (1) Laennec's cirrhosis, which results from excessive chronic alcohol ingestion, (2) primary biliary cirrhosis, which may be caused by genetic factors or may be related to estrogen and progesterone levels, and (3) postnecrotic cirrhosis of unknown cause. Regardless of the type or etiology, the end result is massive destruction of hepatocytes, which are replaced by dense fibrous scar tissue and nodules. This progresses through a cascade of anatomic and physiologic changes including splenomegaly and disrupted coagulation. Management of cirrhosis depends on the stage of the disease and presenting symptoms, but is aimed at reducing any physiologic liver stressors and early detection and treatment of complications.

ASSESSMENT

- Observe for jaundice, weakness, gastrointestinal disturbances, varices, ascites, and peripheral edema.
- Assess mental status to determine presence of hepatic encephalopathy.
- Question the patient regarding alcohol use.
- Observe for signs of bleeding such as petechiae and ecchymoses.
- Determine the patient's level of understanding about the disorder, its complications, and medical management.
- Assess the patient's nutritional status.

NURSING DIAGNOSES, PLANNING, AND NURSING INTERVENTIONS

NDx: Altered tissue perfusion — cerebral, cardiopulmonary, and/or peripheral — related to risk of hemorrhage secondary to portal hypertension, varices, and impaired coagulation

Planning: Patient outcomes

1. Patient exhibits improved blood supply to ischemic areas.
2. Patient identifies signs of bleeding for early detection.
3. Patient presents stable vital signs, palpable pulses, warm, dry skin, and appropriate level of consciousness.

Nursing Interventions

Help the patient conserve oxygen needs by encouraging rest and limiting activities.

Utilize range-of-motion exercises to stimulate circulation.

Observe for petechiae, ecchymoses, varices, and bleeding gums.

Check the patient's orientation to person, place, and time.

Monitor vital signs and laboratory data.

Check secretions and excretion for frank and occult blood.

Describe the early signs of bleeding to the patient.

NDx: Altered thought processes related to encephalopathy

Planning: Patient outcomes

1. Patient responds appropriately and is oriented to person, place, and time.
2. Patient's laboratory studies remain stable or improve.
3. Patient remains free of injury.

Nursing Interventions

Monitor neurologic status and orient the patient to person, place, and time.

Monitor laboratory studies, observing for signs of improvement or reduced liver function.

Maintain a hazard-free environment.

Assist the patient to perform self care and to ambulate, if needed, to prevent injury.

NDx: Knowledge deficit: Nature of the disease, the treatment, and prognosis

Planning: Patient outcomes

1. Patient verbalizes knowledge of causative factors, treatments, and prognosis.
2. Patient states behaviors that decrease complications and disease progression.

Nursing Interventions

Explore the patient's lifestyle related to alcohol intake and dietary or pharmacologic liver stressors, and explain the relationship of lifestyle to liver function problems.

Provide alternative measures to improve liver function and explain the lifestyle changes needed.

Refer the patient to health education and support programs to assist with the necessary treatments and lifestyle changes.

♦ Colorectal Cancer

Colorectal cancers are primarily adenomas that develop from the colonic epithelium. These tumors may project into the lumen of the bowel or encircle the bowel, causing stenosis, ulceration, or perforation. Spread occurs by invasion through the colon wall into adjacent organs such as the small intestine and uterus and by metastasis via the portal vein and lymphatic system to the liver and sometimes the lungs, kidneys, and bone. Management depends on the location of the tumor and the stage of the disease. It may involve surgery, e.g., intestinal resection with reanastomosis, a colostomy proximal to the tumor for palliation in advanced disease, chemotherapy, and/or radiation or, late in the disease, simply comfort measures and nutritional support. These latter may include continuous analgesic infusion via implantable pump and tube feedings or TPN given in the home, hospital, or hospice.

Risk factors for colorectal cancer include familial history, familial polyposis, rectal polyps, active inflammatory bowel disease of more than 10 years' duration, and a low-fiber, high-fat diet.

See entries under Chemotherapy, Colostomy, Intestinal Resection, and Radiation Therapy in Section II for information on related nursing care.

♦ Coronary Artery Disease (CAD)

Coronary artery disease is the most common form of heart disease. CAD usually results from atherosclerosis but may also be caused by collagen-vascular disease, coronary spasm, or embolic events. The process develops slowly over many years but eventually impairs the blood flow through the coronary arteries to the heart. This may result in angina, myocardial infarction, dysrhythmias, congestive heart failure, or even death. The management of CAD is based on reducing risk factors and managing the effects of the disease process.

NURSING CARE

The nursing care for a patient with CAD is similar to that for a patient with *atherosclerosis*. Also refer to the following entries in this text: Angina, Myocardial Infarction, Cardiac Dysrhythmias, and Congestive Heart Failure for additional nursing diagnoses, planning, and nursing interventions.

Crohn's Disease

Crohn's disease is a form of inflammatory bowel disease (IBD) most often involving the terminal ileum and the adjacent right colon. It is chronic and characterized by exacerbations and remissions. Its cause is unknown but immunologic dysfunction, food allergy, and infection are considered possible etiologic factors. Management is palliative and varies with the severity of disease. To support nutrition, TPN or enteral feedings with a low-residue defined formula are given in the acute stage of disease; a low-fat, low-fiber diet is given during mild stages of disease. Pharmacologic therapy includes corticosteroids to suppress inflammation and parenteral antiinfectives given for acute disease and oral antiinfectives for mild disease. Other drugs used include immunosuppressant and antidiarrheal agents. Surgery is rarely done as the disease almost always recurs in the remaining bowel.

ASSESSMENT

- Assess for abdominal pain (type, location, severity, duration and relationship to eating, stress or other identifiable factor), diarrhea (number of stools per day, color, consistency, and odor), blood in the stool, nutritional status (weight loss, appetite, usual diet), signs of fluid and electrolyte imbalance, and elevated temperature.
- Assess for weakness, fatigue, anorexia, anemia, and other symptoms of malabsorption.
- Inspect the perineal area for irritation, skin breakdown, and fistula formation.

- Observe for extraintestinal signs of Crohn's disease: dull red, raised nodules on the legs, joint stiffness and pain, and inflamed conjunctiva.
- Explore sources of stress, relationship of stress to disease exacerbation, methods of coping with stress, and support systems.
- Question about a family history of Crohn's disease and about any known allergies, particularly to milk.

NURSING DIAGNOSES, PLANNING, AND NURSING INTERVENTIONS

NDx: Pain related to the inflammation of the intestinal wall

Planning: Patient outcomes

1. Patient reports pain has decreased.
2. Nonverbal signs of abdominal pain are absent.

Nursing Interventions

Encourage patient to report abdominal pain.
Administer analgesics and antispasmodics as prescribed.
Position the patient with knees flexed.
Apply heat to the abdomen if ordered.
Encourage deep breathing and other relaxation exercises.

NDx: Diarrhea related to impaired absorption of sodium and water secondary to mucosal inflammation

Planning: Patient outcomes

1. Patient passes no more than three stools per day.
2. Stools are formed.

Nursing Interventions

Maintain bedrest during severe exacerbations to decrease peristalsis.
Keep bedpan readily accessible since episodes of diarrhea are sudden.
Place a deodorizer in the room to control odor.
Keep patient NPO or give small frequent low-residue meals as prescribed.

Administer prescribed antidiarrheal agents.

NDx: Risk for impaired skin integrity related to perianal irritation secondary to diarrhea

Planning: Patient outcomes

1. Patient denies perirectal soreness.
2. Perirectal skin is free of redness.
3. Perirectal skin is intact.

Nursing Interventions

Monitor for perianal skin irritation and fissures.
Wash rectal area well after each bowel movement using
    tap water for irritated areas and mild, soapy water
    for surrounding areas.
Rinse and pat dry thoroughly.
Apply an emollient or topical anesthetic for comfort.

NDx: Risk for altered nutrition: less than body requirements related to limited intake of nutrients secondary to anorexia, fear of exacerbating symptoms, and malabsorption

Planning: Patient outcomes

1. Patient is in positive nitrogen balance.
2. Patient maintains or regains normal weight.
3. Patient explains nutritional guidelines for self care
    as presented below.

Nursing Interventions

Administer IV solutions, TPN, or nutritional supplements
    as prescribed.
Administer prescribed anticholinergics one-half hour be-
    fore meals to decrease bowel motility.
Encourage patient to avoid smoking since it increases
    peristalsis.
Record I & O and weight daily.
Instruct the patient in the following nutritional guide-
    lines:
*   Eat foods that are high in protein (eggs, meat, cheese)
    and calories to promote healing.

- Limit fat intake, especially if steatorrhea (fatty stools) is present, by avoiding all fried foods and most dairy products except skim milk.
- Eat a low- or minimum-residue diet to reduce fecal output. Avoid raw vegetables and fruits, dried fruits and beans, whole-grain breads and cereals, bran, seeds, and nuts.
- Avoid foods that stimulate intestinal peristalsis such as prune juice, coffee, and carbonated beverages.
- Take note of which foods cause discomfort or diarrhea because individual food intolerances are common. Eliminate these foods from diet.
- Ensure adequate intake of vitamins and minerals, especially vitamin C (found in citrus fruits and juices), folic acid (found in green, leafy vegetables), and zinc (found in red meat). If foods high in these substances are not tolerated in the diet, take supplements as directed.
- Promote a restful environment while eating.
- Eat slowly, and chew foods well.

◆ Diabetes Mellitus

Diabetes mellitus is a chronic disorder of altered carbohydrate, fat, and protein metabolism caused by either a relative or absolute lack of insulin or the inability of the tissues to respond to insulin. It is characterized by persistent hyperglycemia, leukocyte activity, and long-term vascular and neurologic degeneration.

Type 1 diabetes, or insulin-dependent diabetes mellitus, occurs most often in persons under age 40. The blood glucose is elevated due to lack of insulin, so daily insulin injections are required.

Type 2 diabetes, non-insulin-dependent diabetes mellitus , is characterized by insulin resistance at the cellular level. It is the most common form of diabetes. It occurs in adults over 40 years of age. Insulin supplements may be required only at specific times, such as during illness or high-stress periods, but are generally not necessary.

Diabetes may also be classified as "other types" such as temporary carbohydrate and glucose intolerance, as occurs in gestational diabetes, some endocrine disorders, and as a response to some medications. Diagnosis of diabetes is made by the presence of hyperglycemia and the classic signs of the disorder (polydipsia, polyuria, polyphagia, and weight loss). A fasting blood sugar of >140 mg/dL, random blood glucose of >200 mg/dL, and an oral glucose tolerance test may confirm the disease. Medical management includes diet, exercise, insulin, or oral hypoglycemic agents.

ASSESSMENT

- Obtain a history and perform a physical exam of the patient, noting any complications of the disorder.
- Check the patient's diet history, exercise habits, and any present medications.
- Assess the patient's level of knowledge about the disease, complications, and management regimen.
- Determine the patient's level of compliance (if already a diabetic), and readiness and ability to learn the self-care regimen (if a newly diagnosed diabetic).
- Identify support systems and their willingness to become involved in the patient's self-care regimen.

NURSING DIAGNOSES, PLANNING, AND NURSING INTERVENTIONS

NDx: Anticipatory and/or dysfunctional grieving related to loss of freedom and required changes in lifestyle

Planning: Patient outcomes

1. Patient appropriately verbalizes feelings about diabetes.
2. Patient asks questions and states concerns freely.
3. Patient states desire to participate in self-care.
4. Patient states plans to incorporate changes into lifestyle.

Nursing Interventions

Determine the patient's perception of the disease and its impact on lifestyle and the future.
Allow the patient to have time to deal with the grief while promoting trust and providing support by showing care and concern.

Use therapeutic communication techniques to assist the patient through this period of time.

Allow the patient to voice concerns and ask questions.

Seek assistance from clergy or other professional counselors.

Review expectations from both the patient and family.

NDx: Altered tissue perfusion related to degenerative vascular changes of diabetes

Planning: Patient outcomes

1. Patient maintains adequate systemic perfusion as evidenced by:
   a. blood pressure and pulse within normal ranges for the patient.
   b. palpable peripheral pulses.
   c. warm skin of normal color.
   d. capillary refill time of less than three seconds.
   e. verbalization of increased sensation and decreased numbness and tingling in the extremities.
   f. decreased edema in extremities.
   g. verbalization of increased comfort.
   h. appropriate skin integrity.

Nursing Interventions

Monitor tissue perfusion status by:
   checking vital signs and peripheral pulses.
   observing the warmth and color of the skin.
   checking capillary refill.
   palpating for edema in the extremities.
   asking the patient about decreased sensation in the periphery.

Turn the patient frequently and assist the patient to get out of bed as tolerated to maintain skin integrity.

Ask the patient to perform active foot and leg exercises for 10 minutes every 2 hours.

Alternate activity with rest periods.

Provide a warm, comfortable environment.

Instruct the patient to avoid any activities that could restrict blood flow in the extremities, such as gatching the knee of the bed, crossing the legs, sitting with the legs in a dependent position, or wearing constricting clothing.

Tell the patient to wear antiembolic hose to promote
    venous return.
Instruct the patient in the signs and symptoms of poor tissue
    perfusion and to report the presence of any symptoms.

NDx: Fluid volume deficit related to loss of fluids
associated with diarrhea, vomiting, and osmotic diuresis
from hyperglycemia

Planning: Patient outcomes

1. Patient maintains adequate intake of fluids and
    electrolytes as evidenced by:
    a. normal skin turgor.
    b. moist mucous membranes.
    c. blood pressure and pulse within normal limits
        for the patient.
    d. balanced intake and output.
    e. urine specific gravity between 1.010 and 1.030.
    f. normal electrolyte values.
    g. absence of nausea, vomiting, and diarrhea.

Nursing Interventions

Monitor the patient for signs of dehydration, such as dry skin
    and mucous membranes, changes in vital signs and
    laboratory data, and continued vomiting and diar-
    rhea.
Monitor the blood glucose levels, administer insulin as
    prescribed, and maintain appropriate fluid intake.
Encourage slow, deep breathing.
Provide frequent oral hygiene and encourage the patient
    to increase fluid intake.

NDx: Risk for trauma related to muscle weakness and
atrophy, sensory and motor loss due to peripheral neuropathy, and symptoms of hypoglycemic insulin reactions

Planning: Patient outcomes

1. Patient identifies factors that increase potential for
    trauma and verbalizes the desire to prevent injury.
2. Patient maintains blood glucose levels within target
    range to prevent or delay the onset of degenerative
    changes.

3. Patient utilizes measures to maintain adequate blood glucose levels.

Nursing Interventions

Instruct the patient in daily foot care routine.
Teach the patient measures to prevent hypoglycemic reactions and how to test the glucose level.
Explain the symptoms of an insulin reaction.
Have the patient verbalize the instructions and provide demonstrations of the self-care techniques.

NDx: Risk for altered health maintenance related to lack of knowledge or understanding of self care needed

Planning: Patient outcomes

1. Patient verbalizes basic understanding of the pathophysiology of diabetes mellitus.
2. Patient verbalizes an understanding of the prescribed regimen.
3. Patient demonstrates ability to prepare and administer insulin correctly.
4. Patient verbalizes knowledge of diet and use of the exchange list.
5. Patient demonstrates the proper technique for testing for glucose levels.
6. Patient states the treatment, signs, and symptoms of a hyperglycemic and hypoglycemic reaction.
7. Patient demonstrates proper foot care.
8. Patient describes how the treatment plan can fit into the patient's lifestyle.
9. Patient identifies and utilizes support systems.

Nursing Interventions

Explain the pathophysiology of diabetes to the patient in understandable terms and allow time for questions.
Instruct the patient in the use of insulin therapy, or other medications prescribed, and have the patient demonstrate the technique.
Have the dietitian work with the patient and family for appropriate meal planning.
Instruct the patient in the proper glucose testing method that will be used in the home.

Teach the patient the signs and symptoms of a hyperglycemic and hypoglycemic reaction and what to do if
one occurs.

Explain the foot care procedure.

Have the patient explain how he or she will incorporate
the treatment plan into lifestyle, and plans for compliance with the regimen.

Encourage the patient to utilize support systems.

Provide referral for continued follow-up and support
after discharge.

◆ Disseminated Intravascular Coagulation (DIC)

DIC is a bleeding disorder characterized by widespread
coagulation in the arterioles and capillaries throughout
the body. This results in disseminated fibrin deposits and
microthrombi formation with subsequent depletion of clotting factors causing prolonged bleeding. Although the
exact cause of DIC is unknown, it is usually associated with
serious illnesses and may follow massive tissue trauma,
surgery, septic shock, abruptio placentae, septicemia, transfusion reactions, leukemia, or cancers. Management involves diagnosing and correcting the underlying condition, controlling the bleeding, and slowing the widespread
coagulation. Severe hemorrhage may be treated by transfusions of platelet concentrate, fresh frozen plasma, cryoprecipitate, and red blood cell concentrates.

NURSING CARE

- Assess the patient at risk for bleeding tendencies,
  internal bleeding, pain caused by pressure from
  hematomas, oliguria, and altered level of consciousness.
- Look for changes in vital signs, which indicates
  shock from hemorrhage.
- Check laboratory data for coagulation studies.
- Prepare to manage an acute hemorrhage episode.

◆ Diverticular Disease

Diverticula are outpouchings of mucosa through the muscular wall of the intestine. They are found most often in the sigmoid colon. When these diverticula are not inflamed the condition is called diverticulosis and is largely asymptomatic. When there is inflammation present the condition is referred to as diverticulitis. Basic management of diverticulosis is aimed at increasing stool bulk and preventing constipation and increased intraluminal pressure in the bowel. It includes a high fiber diet, bulk-forming laxatives, stool softeners, and spasmolytic anticholinergics. Management of diverticulitis includes clear fluids to rest the bowel and parenteral antibiotics, or in more severe cases, NPO status, IV fluids, and NG suction. Bowel resection and sometimes temporary colostomy may be required if hemorrhage, obstruction, abscess formation, or perforation occurs.

ASSESSMENT

- Check for abdominal pain (onset, type, location, intensity), abdominal distention, and fever.
- Assess elimination pattern: appearance, size, and consistency of stool, frequency, time, and ease of defecation, occurrence of bleeding, and use of laxatives or enemas.
- Review dietary patterns including type, amount, and time of foods eaten.
- Monitor for abdominal rigidity and tenderness, tachycardia, and hypotension, which can indicate perforation.
- Review white blood cell count and sedimentation rate values for indication of infection.

NURSING DIAGNOSES, PLANNING, AND NURSING INTERVENTIONS

NDx: Pain related to increased pressure within an area of the intestine

Planning: Patient outcomes

1. Patient reports decrease in pain.
2. Signs of abdominal discomfort, such as pressing on abdomen or flexing legs on abdomen, are absent.

Nursing Interventions

Administer nonopiate analgesics (opiates increase pressure in the bowel lumen) and spasmolytics as prescribed.

Encourage rhythmic deep breathing and progressive relaxation exercises to promote relief.

Give clear fluids or a low-residue diet as ordered to rest the bowel in patients with diverticulitis.

If an NG tube is in place, keep the patient NPO and monitor the suction apparatus for proper function.

NDx: Risk for altered health maintenance related to insufficient knowledge of prevention of recurrence

Planning: Patient outcomes

1. Patient describes self-care measures to prevent recurrence of symptoms.
2. Patient states time of follow-up visit.

Nursing Interventions

Instruct the patient in self care as follows:

Eat high-fiber foods to add bulk to stool and speed its passage through the bowel. Examples of foods to include are fresh fruits with skins such as apples, pears, and plums; bananas; dried fruits; whole-wheat bread and crackers; and raw vegetables such as lettuce, carrots, and cauliflower.

Add bran to food on a daily basis. Begin with one teaspoon per day and gradually progress to two teaspoons per day.

Avoid high-roughage foods such as nuts, popcorn, and raw celery.

Drink 8 to 10 glasses of water per day (unless otherwise contraindicated) because fiber retains water and decreases its absorption.

Avoid large meals and the consumption of alcohol.

Maintain weight within the accepted range for age and sex.

Avoid activities such as lifting, bending, stooping, coughing, vomiting, and straining at stool that increase intraabdominal pressure.

Avoid strong enemas or purgative products: Use hydrophilic colloid laxatives (Metamucil) and stool softeners such as dioctyl sodium sulfosuccinate if needed to prevent constipation and straining at stool.

Encourage frequent turning and foot and leg exercises in order to prevent venous stasis if the patient is on bedrest.

 # Emphysema

Emphysema, a chronic obstructive pulmonary disease (COPD), is a progressive disease with enlarged air spaces distal to the terminal nonrespiratory bronchioles and destruction of the alveolar walls and supporting structures. It is the direct affect of cigarette smoking and may have a genetic component related to its development. A deficiency of alpha-antitrypsin, an enzyme inhibitor, has been shown to produce emphysema in very young people. Emphysema is usually complicated by a coexisting disease such as chronic bronchitis. The management of emphysema is the same as that for the patient with chronic bronchitis. When all medical therapies have been exhausted, lung volume reduction surgery (LVRS) may be an option for those who meet the criteria.

ASSESSMENT

- Assess for dyspnea that worsens over time and is initially present with exertion and eventually at rest.
- Observe for increased anteroposterior diameter of the chest (barrel chest), use of accessory muscles of respiration (sternocleidomastoid, scalene, and trapezius), and pursed lip breathing with prolonged expiration.
- Check for hyperresonance of the chest to percussion.
- Auscultate for breath sounds and heart sounds that are distant, absent, or dull.
- Assess for anorexia, muscle mass wasting, weight loss.
- Observe for signs of carbon dioxide narcosis: occipital headache, decreased ability to concentrate, drowsiness, bounding pulse, $PaCO_2$ levels greater than 75 mm Hg, asterixis, confusion, and coma.

- Assess for chronic cough, wheezing, inspirational coarse crackles, and frequent respiratory infections.

NURSING DIAGNOSES, PLANNING, AND NURSING INTERVENTIONS

Same as that for patient with chronic bronchitis. See entry under that heading.

◆ Encephalitis

Encephalitis is an inflammation of the brain most often caused by a virus, although cases caused by bacteria, fungi, and parasites occur. Herpes simplex encephalitis is a common, nonepidemic form of the disease caused by herpes simplex virus 1 or 2. Management involves supportive care and includes the use of steroids, anticonvulsants, antipyretics, and analgesics. Herpes simplex encephalitis may be treated with antiviral agents such as acyclovir (Zovirax).

ASSESSMENT

- Assess for fever, malaise, headache, listlessness, joint pain, nausea, vomiting, altered mentation, and decreasing level of consciousness.
- Observe for hemiparesis, ataxia, tremors, seizures, bizarre behavioral manifestations, aphasia, stiff neck, photophobia, and cranial nerve dysfunction.

NURSING DIAGNOSES, PLANNING, AND NURSING INTERVENTIONS

See information under Meningitis as well as that which follows.

NDx: Risk for impaired skin integrity related to immobility, dehydration and diaphoresis

Planning: Patient outcomes

1. Skin remains intact.
2. Irritation and redness are absent.

Nursing Interventions

Change linen frequently to avoid wetness against the skin.
Minimize covers and blankets to avoid excess moisture.
Turn and position the patient every 2 hours PRN.
Inspect bony prominences for signs of redness or pressure.
Protect the heels and elbows.

NDx: Altered family processes related to critical nature of situation and uncertain prognosis

Planning: Patient outcomes

1. Family members acknowledge difficulty in accepting the illness.
2. Family members identify coping patterns.

Nursing Interventions

Encourage family members to express their feelings of fear, anger, and concern.
Offer explanations regarding the disease process.
Help family members to identify their strengths as well as behaviors that interfere with their ability to be supportive.
Refer family members to a social worker and spiritual counselor as needed.

◆ Endocarditis, Myocarditis, Pericarditis

Endocarditis is an inflammatory or infective process involving the endocardial surface of the heart, which includes the valves. Inflammatory endocarditis may be the result of collagen vascular disease and rheumatic fever. Infective endocarditis can be an acute or subacute process from direct bacterial, fungal, or rickettsial invasion, and is classified according to the causative organism.

Myocarditis is an inflammation of the heart muscle itself that can be caused by a variety of agents such as bacteria, viruses, fungi, or parasites. It may be acute or chronic. This leads to degeneration of the cardiac muscle fibers, which results in dilation, hypertrophy, and eventually heart failure.

Broad-spectrum antibiotics such as high-dose intravenous penicillin or a semisynthetic penicillin, plus streptomycin, vancomycin, or gentamicin are used to treat cardiac infections/inflammations such as endocarditis and myocarditis. Anti-inflammatory agents such as salicylates and corticosteroids are given concurrently to reduce the edema, pain, and general inflammation of the joints. If bacterial destruction of the valve is widespread, valvular replacement may be needed within 1 year of the acute illness.

Pericarditis is the inflammation of the pericardium, the sac surrounding the heart. Many conditions may cause pericarditis, including open heart surgery, viral, bacterial, fungal, or parasitic infections, MI, and trauma. Inflammatory causes of pericarditis include rheumatic and collagen-vascular diseases. Metabolic causes include uremia, myxedema, and amyloidosis. Autoimmune pericarditis is a response to nonspecific pericardial trauma such as myocardial infarction. The most common type of pericarditis is *acute idiopathic pericarditis*, which has no apparent predisposing or causative factors.

Immediate removal of this excess pericardial fluid (pericardiocentesis) is done by needle aspiration of the fluid through needle puncture of the chest wall into the pericardium. Antipyretics are used to treat fever associated with pericarditis as well as the inflammatory process. Antibiotics specific for the causative agent of pericarditis are prescribed.

ASSESSMENT

- Review the patient's history, present symptoms, and diagnostic test results.
- Assess the patient's vital signs.
- Obtain a thorough history of strep throat, rheumatic fever, congenital heart disease, and cardiac surgery.
- Assess for fatigue, weakness, dyspnea, palpitations, and fainting spells.
- Auscultate the heart sounds to determine whether any abnormal sounds are present such as S3 or S4 rubs or murmurs.
- Examine the patient for evidence of painful or swollen joints to determine whether there are systemic symptoms as well as cardiac symptoms.

NURSING DIAGNOSES, PLANNING, AND NURSING INTERVENTIONS

NDx: Pain related to inflammation of the myocardium, pericardium, and local or systemic infection

Planning: Patient outcomes

1. Patient verbalizes relief or controlled pain levels.
2. Patient demonstrates use of relaxation skills and diversional activities that decrease the sense of pain.
3. Patient's vital signs are within normal ranges for the patient.

Nursing Interventions

Investigate all complaints of chest and joint pain.

Document onset of pain as well as factors that aggravate and relieve the pain.

Provide a quiet environment for the patient with comfort measures, which may include medications, positioning, back rubs, and emotional support.

Teach relaxation exercises to assist in the relief of pain.

Give prescribed medications for pain as necessary.

NDx: Activity intolerance related to inflammation and degeneration of myocardial muscle cells, reduced cardiac output, and painful, inflamed joints

Planning: Patient outcomes

1. Patient demonstrates a decrease in physiologic signs of activity intolerance.
2. Patient demonstrates an increase in physiologic signs of activity tolerance, such as stable blood pressure, normal pulse rate, and absence of dyspnea with increased activity levels.

Nursing Interventions

Assess the patient's response to activity and the types of activity that may not be possible.

Note accompanying symptoms of dyspnea, weakness, and fatigue.

Maintain bedrest during febrile periods and until painful, edematous joints can tolerate increased movement.

Note the response of blood pressure, heart rate, and respiratory rate to increased activity as the patient becomes more mobile.

Allow uninterrupted sleep periods to reduce the fatigue.

Limit interruptions and restrict visitors as needed, so patient can have lengthy periods of rest.

Have the patient perform range-of-motion exercises frequently during the day to maintain and increase strength and endurance.

Assist patient with activities as necessary.

Provide six small meals during the day to conserve strength and energy.

NDx: Altered health maintenance related to a knowledge deficit about inflammatory cardiac diseases and the need for long-term therapy and follow-up, and ways to prevent recurrence or complications

Planning: Patient outcomes

1. Patient verbalizes understanding of inflammatory process, treatment program, possible complications, and prevention plan.
2. Patient displays behavior changes in lifestyle that will prevent recurrence and complications of inflammatory cardiac processes.

Nursing Interventions

Explain the effects of inflammation upon the heart and other affected tissues.

Educate the patient about signs and symptoms of recurrence, symptoms to report, and actions to take that will reduce the possibility of future recurrence.

Discuss the use of prophylactic antibiotics, the time period of their use, and procedures that require prophylaxis throughout the lifetime, i.e., dental procedures.

♦ Endometrial Cancer

Cancer of the uterus, the most common cancer of the female reproductive tract, is most commonly an adenocarcinoma that appears to develop in areas of hyperplastic endometrium. This is a slow growing tumor that metastasizes to the pelvic lymph nodes. Basic management consists of total abdominal hysterectomy and bilateral salpingo-oophorectomy (TAH & BSO), often in conjunction with radiation and/or chemotherapy.

See entries under Hysterectomy, Chemotherapy, and Radiation Therapy in Section II for information on related nursing care. See entry under Cervical Cancer for information on the care of patients receiving internal radiation.

♦ Fractures

A fracture is a crack or break in the continuity of a bone. It may be caused by a direct blow or trauma to the bone, a sudden strong muscle contraction that bends the bone to the breaking point, continuous extreme stress on the bone, demineralization secondary to pathologic conditions, prolonged bedrest, decreased weight bearing, and the aging process. Fractures are described by the type of break, the part of the bone involved, and the direction of the fracture line. A closed fracture is one in which the bone is broken but there is no external injury, and is not usually considered life-threatening. An open or compound fracture is one in which the bone fragments have broken through or penetrated the skin. This type is associated with severe tissue damage and blood loss, as well as high risk of infection, and may be life-threatening. Management of the fracture is dependent upon the type, amount of blood loss, the severity of associated soft tissue injuries, and the patient's general condition. Reduction, restoration of displaced bone to the normal position, may be achieved by traction or surgery. Immobilization and proper alignment of the part are maintained through the healing process.

Immediate Nursing Care

Control bleeding by direct pressure.

Protect known or suspected fractures from further injury until medical intervention is possible.

Cover open wounds with sterile or clean, white, or light-colored lint-free material to prevent further contamination.

Splint extremities by the application of bandages or well padded improvised or commercial splints.

If the injured part is in a deformed position, splint nin the shape of the deformity because movement of the bone fragments may cause further damage to soft tissues, nerves, and blood vessels.

Assess distal neurovascular function before and after splinting.

Stabilize the patient with known or suspected spine or pelvic injuries with sandbags on a firm board before movement or transport.

After injured parts are adequately splinted, position the patient for comfort and transport to an appropriate health care facility.

ASSESSMENT

- After the immediate care to stabilize the patient has been provided, continue to assess the patient's affected part for pain, swelling, discoloration or malalignment.
- Look for signs of continued bleeding.
- Check the neurovascular status proximal and distal to the injury by palpating for pulses, feeling for warmth of the part and assessing for decreased sensation.
- Assess vital signs noting changes reflective of ensuing shock such as decreasing blood pressure and rapid weak pulse with increased respiratory effort.
- Ask the patient about numbness or tingling in the extremity.
- After the patient's fracture has been treated medically, continue to assess neurovascular status of the affected part.
- Look for signs of decreased tissue perfusion due to constriction from the immobilization device or edema.
- In the case of forearm fractures and lower leg fractures, assess for symptoms of compartment syndrome, a limb-threatening complication.

- Determine the patient's understanding of the injury and treatment necessary.
- Assess the patient's ability to perform self care and to be mobile if a lower extremity is affected.

NURSING DIAGNOSES, PLANNING, AND NURSING INTERVENTIONS

NDx: Altered tissue perfusion; peripheral, related to the interruption of blood flow secondary to the trauma, edema, thrombus formation, or pressure from the attached device (wrap, cast, traction, or immobilizer)

Planning: Patient outcomes

1. Affected part has good color, sensation and pulses are present, and part is free of signs of compromised circulation.
2. Patient denies numbness, tingling, or decreased sensation in the affected part.

Nursing Interventions

Help the patient conserve oxygen needs by encouraging rest and limiting activities.

Administer oxygen if appropriate and elevate the head of the bed to aid in chest expansion.

Look for signs of compromised circulation and prevent edema by raising the part.

Relieve pressure to the affected part by cutting a window in the cast and padding bony areas.

Keep the patient in a comfortable position and reposition frequently to release pressure.

Utilize range-of-motion exercises to stimulate circulation.

Monitor vital signs and laboratory studies to assess for changes and improvement in status.

Discourage smoking to avoid vasoconstriction.

Remove constricting clothing and keep heavy bed linen from restricting peripheral circulation.

Tell the patient to notify the nurse if signs of compromised circulation such as discoloration, pain, swelling, or numbness of an extremity seem apparent.

Keep the patient's legs in a non-dependent position when not ambulating.

NDx: Impaired skin integrity related to the bedrest, constriction of device for immobilization, edema, and internal altered circulation

Planning: Patient outcomes

1. Patient states causes of skin breakdown and measures to prevent the occurrence or recurrence.
2. Patient relates appropriate knowledge about skin care.
3. Patient is free of skin complications.

Nursing Interventions

Teach the patient measures to prevent skin lesions from developing such as avoiding irritating sheets or garments, padding bony prominences, and maintaining cleanliness.

Have the patient inspect the skin frequently and seek medical assistance if any breakdown or soreness is noted.

Teach the patient to exercise, as tolerated, to promote good circulation and assist with range of motion exercises while on bedrest.

Turn the patient frequently and inspect pressure areas for early signs of breakdown.

Keep heavy linen from constricting the peripheral circulation by using a bed cradle.

Elevate the patient's legs when sitting in a chair.

Inspect the areas distal to constrictive devices for signs of compromised circulation.

Teach the patient and family members the proper technique for dressing areas of breakdown.

NDx: Risk for infection related to increased susceptibility secondary to bedrest, placement of internal/external fixation devices, pressure from restrictive devices or compromised circulation

Planning: Patient outcomes

1. Patient's vital signs are within normal ranges for the patient.

2. Patient is free of signs of infection such as fever, chills, tachycardia, tachypnea, pain or burning on urination, or drainage from lesions at pin sites, or under the cast.
3. Patient identifies early signs of infection and measures to prevent infections.

Nursing Interventions

Keep the patient warm and avoid extreme changes in temperature in the room.

Turn the patient as needed to stimulate circulation to prevent skin breakdown and skin infections.

Have the patient deep breathe and cough frequently to prevent respiratory infections, especially if the patient is on bedrest.

Monitor the patient's vital signs frequently, observing subtle changes that may indicate early signs of infection.

Promote good nutrition for proper healing.

Encourage a high-protein, high-vitamin, and high-fiber diet to prevent constipation.

Provide skin care frequently, especially if areas of breakdown are present.

Use aseptic technique to cleanse around pin sites as ordered.

Instruct the patient and family to continually observe for signs of developing infection and to notify the physician if such signs appear.

NDx: Risk for self-care deficit in areas of feeding, hygiene, toileting, or other activities of daily living requiring mobility related to interference from immobilization of affected part

Planning: Patient outcomes

1. Patient performs activities of daily living, using assistive devices if necessary.
2. Patient describes alternative methods to complete tasks that are restricted by musculoskeletal dysfunction.

Nursing Interventions

Assist the patient with activities of daily living as needed.
Seek alternative methods for the patient to be able to
complete the activities when restricted by a cast or
immobilization device.
Explain how to utilize other extremities to complete a task,
or how to move appropriately with the restrictive
device in place, such as how to use crutches when
the patient's leg is in a cast, immobilizer, or fixation
device.
Seek the assistance of physical therapists or occupational
therapists when necessary for consultation or teaching sessions for the patient and family.

Also refer to care of patients with a cast, patients in
traction, and patients with fixation devices in Chapter 19
in the textbook.

Gastric Cancer

All gastric cancers are adenocarcinomas and most occur
in the pyloric region. They spread by direct invasion of
adjacent tissues such as those of the lower esophagus,
pancreas, transverse colon, and peritoneum and by way of
the lymphatics to the pancreas and liver. Late in the
disease hematogenous spread occurs to the bone, brain,
and lungs. Surgery (partial or total gastrectomy, depending on the tumor) is the only curative treatment and
gastric cancers are often not diagnosed early enough for it
to be effective. Chemotherapy may be used for relief of
symptoms in advanced disease.
See Gastrectomy and Chemotherapy in Section II for
information on related nursing care.

Glomerulonephritis

Glomerulonephritis is an inflammation of the kidney
that affects the capillary loops in the glomeruli, causing

destruction of renal tissue, scarring, and hypertrophy, which impinges upon unaffected tubules. Acute glomerulonephritis is caused by an immunologic reaction that is usually the result of a beta-hemolytic streptococcus infection, often of the upper respiratory tract. It has a higher incidence in males. Treatment includes relieving symptoms, preventing complications, and diuretic and antibiotic therapy. Chronic glomerulonephritis is a progressive disorder that may have been initiated by acute glomerulonephritis, and is frequently irreversible by the time symptoms appear. It usually results in end-stage renal disease. Treatment includes supportive therapy, antihypertensives, low-sodium diet, and dialysis or renal transplantation.

ASSESSMENT

- Check the patient's history and laboratory data, especially BUN, creatinine, proteinuria, and hematuria.
- Inquire about any previous infections that may have occurred, especially a recent upper respiratory tract infection, skin infection, pericarditis, or lower urinary tract infection.
- Evaluate the current status of the patient, including signs of renal failure, respiratory distress, circulatory congestion, and systemic infection.
- Note the patient's nutritional status and current eating habits.
- Check the type and location of any pain.
- Note the color, consistency, and amount of urine.
- Check for any physical limitations brought on by the associated weakness, lethargy, and fatigue.

NURSING DIAGNOSES, PLANNING, AND NURSING INTERVENTIONS

NDx: Activity intolerance related to fatigue, fluid volume excess, and loss of energy

Planning: Patient outcomes

1. Patient follows a regimen of planned activities and rest periods each day.
2. Patient verbalizes feeling less fatigued and demonstrates signs of increased activity.

3. Patient is able to resume usual activities of daily living.

Nursing Interventions

Assist the patient in maintenance of bedrest since there is a direct relationship between physical activity and the presence of proteinuria and hematuria.

Provide patient education and encouragement to ensure compliance with this temporary, but difficult, alteration in the patient's activity level.

Instruct the patient in developing a regimen of activity, as allowed, when healing begins to occur, with frequent rest periods throughout the day.

NDx: Fluid volume excess related to decreased glomerular filtration rate

Planning: Patient outcomes

1. Patient exhibits decreased edema.
2. Patient is free of signs and symptoms of fluid overload.
3. Patient demonstrates knowledge related to therapeutic regimen to decrease fluid.

Nursing Interventions

Monitor the patient for signs and symptoms of fluid overload such as increasing blood pressure, edema, and noisy respirations.

Weigh the patient every morning and continue to monitor fluid intake and urine output.

Instruct in a low-sodium diet.

Assist patient in coping with any fluid restriction that is ordered.

Protect edematous skin from injury.

NDx: Altered nutrition: less than body requirements related to anorexia, nausea and vomiting

Planning: Patient outcomes

1. Patient increases oral intake, as evidenced by eating 75% of meals.

2. Patient describes the rationale and procedure for treatment.
3. Patient maintains desired weight.
4. Patient is free of nausea and vomiting.

Nursing Interventions

Explain to the patient the importance of consuming adequate amounts of nutrients.

Monitor intake and output, and weigh the patient daily.

Instruct the patient and family about the prescribed diet.

Teach the patient to use spices to help improve the taste of food.

Plan care so that unpleasant procedures do not take place before meals.

Medicate the patient for pain or nausea 30 to 45 minutes before meals as ordered.

Provide a pleasant, relaxed atmosphere for meals.

Assist the patient to rest or relax before meals.

Encourage small, frequent feedings, provide good oral hygiene, and allow the patient to choose food items as much as possible.

◆ Heart Failure (HF)

Congestive heart failure is the condition when cardiac output is not sufficient to meet the metabolic demands of the body, and the hemodynamics of the heart failure result in inadequate renal blood flow and increased ventricular filling pressures. *Left-sided heart failure* is the term given to the disorder when the left ventricle cannot pump its volume of blood into the systemic circulation. *Right-sided failure* occurs when the right ventricle cannot pump its blood volume into the pulmonary artery. Heart failure may involve only one side of the heart, but more frequently, there is a combination of failure on both sides. This may be the result of back-up pressure from the failed side. Management includes prescribing vasodilator drugs, afterload reducing agents, diuretics and digitalis therapy, monitoring the electrical activity of the heart and vital signs, and treating other symptoms that may appear, as well as treating any underlying medical problems.

ASSESSMENT

- Assess the patient's physical abilities since the patient with HF reports feeling fatigued to the point of exhaustion.
- Ask the patient if the fatigue is intermittent or continuous during the day.
- Ask about sleep and rest patterns, strength and endurance, and ability to complete activities of daily living.
- Assess the vital signs and note if the patient is dyspneic during activity and/or during rest.
- Ask if the patient has experienced any chest pain and, if so, get a description of the frequency, severity, duration, relief methods, and radiation.
- Auscultate the chest for rales or wheezing since left-sided failure results in adventitious lung sounds throughout the lung fields, accompanied by a productive or nonproductive cough.
- Check for tachycardia with the presence of dysrhythmias such as atrial fibrillation, premature ventricular contractions, and heart blocks.
- Assess peripheral pulses since they may be diminished with central pulses that are bounding and visible jugular, carotid, or abdominal pulsations.
- Check the blood pressure, which may be low, normal, or high, depending on the degree of failure.
- Observe for edema of the ankles and sacrum, and liver or abdominal enlargement since right-sided failure results in peripheral edema.
- Look for jugular vein distention.
- Assess capillary refill in the nailbeds, which is usually slow in congestive failure.
- Note the skin color looking for paleness, cyanosis, duskiness, or an ashen appeareance.
- Assess for fluid retention, which may cause the patient to complain of recent weight gain, loss of appetite, nausea and vomiting, and diarrhea or constipation.
- Assess the patient for gastrointestinal system problems such as abdominal pain and distention.
- Assess the patient's weight and ask about recent changes in weight.
- Observe for signs of cerebral edema such as behavior changes, confusion, and disorientation.

NURSING DIAGNOSES, PLANNING, AND NURSING INTERVENTIONS

NDx: Decreased cardiac output related to altered myocardial contractility, alterations in rate, rhythm, or electrical conduction

Planning: Patient outcomes

1. Patient's vital signs are within acceptable ranges for the patient.
2. Patient demonstrates absence or control of dysrhythmias.
3. Patient participates in activities consistent with abilities.
4. Patient is free of dyspnea.

Nursing Interventions

Monitor the patient's vital signs both at rest and with activity, auscultate the apical pulse noting the rate and rhythm, and ask about any dyspneic episodes.

Encourage the patient to rest frequently throughout the day to prevent fatigue and strain on the myocardium.

Ask if the patient is getting enough rest and sleep and prevent disturbances in the room, especially at night.

Use telemetry monitoring whenever possible, especially if the patient experiences dysrhythmias or if the patient is taking antidysrhythmic drugs.

Review the results of laboratory studies and hemodynamic monitoring.

Check the patient's intake and output, observing for adequacy and balance.

Keep the patient's legs in a nondependent position while sitting, and provide support for the extremities while lying in bed.

Pad bony prominences to prevent breakdown from pressure and poor circulation.

Prevent constriction of circulation from tight clothing or bed linen.

Teach the patient relaxation techniques and range-of-motion procedures to increase circulation while lying in bed.

NDx: Activity intolerance related to generalized weakness or an imbalance between the oxygen supply and the oxygen demand.

Planning: Patient outcomes

1. Patient increases participation in activities without intolerable dyspnea or fatigue.
2. Patient demonstrates energy-saving activities and seeks assistance as needed.
3. Patient sets a daily schedule that allows for intermittent periods of rest as needed.
4. Patient verbalizes understanding of the need for oxygen, medications, and/or supportive equipment that may increase tolerance for activity.

Nursing Interventions

Encourage the patient to do range-of-motion exercises frequently while lying in bed to maintain muscle tone and strength.

Provide supplemental oxygen as needed.

Have the patient practice deep-breathing exercises to increase oxygen and blood to the brain.

Teach the patient to practice energy-saving techniques to reduce fatigue and shortness of breath by:

Instructing the patient to develop a regimen of activity with frequent rest periods as needed.

Placing frequently used articles within the patient's reach.

Providing and encouraging frequent rest periods while delivering patient care.

Preventing interruptions during rest periods and at night whenever possible.

Reducing any disturbing noises and limiting visitors as necessary.

Encourage acceleration of activity and monitor progress as the patient moves through the rehabilitation process.

Encourage good nutrition to increase the patient's energy level.

Offer four to six meals per day since this is less tiring for the patient and will prevent gastric overdistention and prevent dyspneic episodes during meals.

NDx: Fluid volume excess related to reduced glomerular filtration rate secondary to reduced cardiac output,
increased ADH production, and sodium and water retention.

Planning: Patient outcomes

1.   Patient maintains a balanced intake and output.
2.   Patient's breath sounds are clear to auscultation.
3.   Patient's daily weight is as expected for the patient
      and edema is absent.
4.   Patient verbalizes dietary and/or fluid restrictions.

Nursing Interventions

Help the patient exercise when able to assist in the dis-
      semination of fluid.
Give prescribed diuretics and provide a bedside com-
      mode for the patient if unable to ambulate to the
      bathroom.
Teach the patient about the effects of the medications, the
      necessity for fluid intake restrictions, and the di-
      etary changes needed, such as a low-sodium meal
      plan.
Monitor the patient's intake and output carefully and
      document the results.
Weigh the patient daily and record the weight.
Inspect the skin for edematous areas and potential sites for
      skin breakdown.
Keep the patient's legs elevated and supported when
      sitting to prevent dependent edema.
Use a semi-Fowler's or high-Fowler's position for the
      patient to maximize the respiratory effort and check
      frequently for noisy respirations.

NDx: Risk for impaired skin integrity related to decreased tissue perfusion and edema

Planning: Patient outcomes

1.   Patient's skin remains intact without edema, red-
      ness, or lesions.
2.   Patient demonstrates behaviors used to prevent
      skin breakdown such as turning, keeping feet and

legs out of dependent positions, and keeping skin clean, dry, and supple.

Nursing Interventions

Inspect the skin frequently, noting skeletal prominences, presence of edema, or areas of redness that may be prone to breakdown.

Reposition the patient hourly if necessary to prevent pressure areas and to stimulate circulation.

Massage the skin to enhance circulation to prevent ischemic sites.

Keep the skin clean, dry, and supple and use lotions to prevent dry cracked skin.

NDx: Ineffective breathing pattern related to extensive pulmonary edema secondary to congestive heart failure

Planning: Patient outcomes

1.   Patient's vital signs are within normal ranges for the patient.
2.   Patient denies dyspnea, tachypnea, or productive cough.
3.   Patient is able to complete activities of daily living without breathing difficulties.

Nursing Interventions

Promote maximum respirations by positioning the patient in a semi-Fowler's or high-Fowler's position while in bed for better chest expansion.

Allow frequent rest periods while administering care so the patient does not become fatigued and dyspneic.

Teach the patient deep breathing techniques.

Tell the patient to seek assistance if activities cause more difficult breathing or extreme fatigue.

Administer oxygen as needed, observe for signs of respiratory distress — such as changes in blood gases, tachypnea, dyspnea, air hunger, noisy respirations — and administer treatments and medications as ordered.

Auscultate the chest for changes in the adventitious sounds.

Herniated Disk Disease

Herniated disk disease occurs when the intervertebral disk herniates or ruptures into the spinal canal, where it can impinge on a spinal nerve root. It is often precipitated by traumatic incidents and/or degenerative changes in supporting ligaments. Conservative management includes enforced bedrest, use of a firm mattress, avoidance of flexion of the spine, use of supportive devices such as a corset or cervical collar, use of pelvic or cervical traction, and physiotherapy. Surgery is done when other management is ineffective.

ASSESSMENT

- Check for symptoms of a herniated cervical disk: stiff neck, shoulder pain radiating down the arm, and paresthesias.
- Check for symptoms of a herniated lumbar disk: low back pain with muscle spasm, pain radiating down the leg, altered posture, limited motion of the spine, pain aggravated by sitting, standing, bending, coughing, sneezing or straining, and paresthesias.
- Assess the patient's understanding of the cause of the pain and measures that limit stress on the spine.
- Explore the patient's ability to work and participate in household activities. Assess the patient's coping mechanisms and ability to cope.

NURSING DIAGNOSES, PLANNING, AND NURSING INTERVENTIONS

NDx: Pain related to nerve irritation and muscle spasm

Planning: Patient outcomes

1. Patient restricts movements as directed.
2. Patient reports that pain is manageable and decreasing.
3. Patient performs allowed activities without exacerbated pain.

Nursing Interventions

Maintain continuous bedrest while pain is acute.

Apply traction and/or supportive devices as ordered.

Provide a firm mattress; use a bedboard if necessary.

Place the patient with a herniated lumbar disk in a supine position with HOB elevated 30° and the hips slightly flexed.

Use a pull sheet (from shoulder to mid-thigh) to move the patient with a herniated lumbar disk; place a pillow between the legs.

Instruct the patient not to move without assistance, raise self, stretch, reach for anything, write, or hold a book while lying flat.

Instruct the patient to avoid coughing and sneezing when possible.

Keep call bell and personal items within easy reach.

Administer analgesics as ordered.

Apply hot, moist packs as ordered every 1 to 2 hours for 30 minutes.

Change the patient's position to side lying with knees flexed and a pillow between the legs as permitted.

Logroll patient on and off a fracture pan to meet elimination needs.

Encourage increased water and roughage in diet to reduce straining at stool.

Administer stool softeners as ordered.

Guide the patient in the prescribed progressive exercise program.

Teach the proper method of getting out of bed, to select a straight back chair with arm rests, and to sit with the back flat against the chair and knees flexed higher than the hips.

NDx: Risk for altered tissue perfusion related to impaired venous blood flow secondary to thrombophlebitis or pulmonary embolism

Planning: Patient outcomes

1.   Patient performs foot and leg exercises as directed.
2.   Calves are free of heat, redness, and swelling.
3.   Homans' sign is negative.

Nursing Interventions

Instruct the patient regarding foot and leg exercises as soon as the acute pain subsides.

Encourage the patient to perform exercises five times with each leg every 2 to 3 hours while awake.

Apply antiembolic stockings as prescribed.

NDx: Risk for altered health maintenance related to lack of knowledge of measures to reduce stress on the lumbar spine

Planning: Patient outcomes

1. Patient explains measures to reduce stress on the lumbar spine.
2. Patient expresses willingness to comply with measures to reduce stress on the lumbar spine.
3. Patient expresses confidence in the ability to comply with measures to reduce stress on the lumbar spine.

Nursing Interventions

Instruct the patient in self-care measures to reduce stress on the lumbar spine as follows:

Maintain good posture: back straight, shoulders back, abdomen and neck tucked in. Exercise regularly during asymptomatic periods to strengthen the muscles of back and abdomen.

Perform flexion or isometric exercise routine prescribed by the physician.

Sit in a straight back chair with feet on footstool so knees are flexed above level of hips.

Avoid extended periods of sitting or driving.

Sleep on the back or side, never on stomach.

Sleep on mattress with firm support. Use bedboard if necessary, but avoid placing the mattress on the floor because getting up or down may further injure the spine.

Avoid rotating or extending the spine.

Carry objects close to the chest.

Bend at the hips and knees, not at the waist.

Face objects to be lifted directly.

Avoid lifting while bending.

Avoid lifting anything heavier than 10 pounds.
Wear lumbar corset to protect the back during strenuous
    activities.
Reduce activity at the first sign of pain.
Use a firm backrest in the car.
Stop and walk at least every 2 hours while riding.
Maintain or regain recommended body weight.

Hodgkin's Disease

Hodgkin's disease is a chronic, malignant disorder of
unknown etiology that originates in the lymph system
and spreads to other organs and structures in the later
stages. It is characterized by large atypical tumor cells or
abnormal histiocytes called Reed-Sternberg cells, which
invade the lymph nodes, spleen, and liver, causing necrosis and fibrosis. Management includes high-dose radiation therapy for Stage I and II, and radiation and chemotherapy for Stages III and IV.

ASSESSMENT

- Observe for facial and neck edema and cyanosis
  resulting from enlarged lymph nodes.
- Assess the patient's speech and swallowing for
  changes caused by pressure.
- Observe for high fever alternating with prolonged
  low-grade fever, indicative of infection.
- Check for night sweats, extreme fatigue, weight
  loss, and malaise indicative of anemia.
- Assess for dyspnea, cough, stridor, chest pain, and
  pleural effusion indicating pulmonary involvement.
- Check for complications from radiation therapy
  and chemotherapy.
- Palpate for enlargement of lymph nodes, especially
  on the sides of the neck, axillae, and groin.
- Check the patient's nutritional pattern.
- Observe for signs of malnutrition such as poor skin
  turgor, weight loss, low fluid intake, and fatigue.
- Look for edema of extremities, enlarged liver and
  spleen, and signs of vertebral compression or fractures.
- Determine the patient's emotional status and cop-
  ing ability.

NURSING DIAGNOSES, PLANNING, AND NURSING INTERVENTIONS

NDx: Ineffective breathing pattern related to tracheo-bronchial obstruction from enlarged lymph nodes and pleural effusion

Planning: Patient outcomes

1. Vital signs are within normal ranges and the patient is free of signs of cyanosis, dyspnea, tachypnea, or tachycardia.
2. Patient uses good lung expansion techniques.
3. Patient is able to perform activities of daily living without respiratory distress.
4. Patient's blood gas levels are within normal ranges for the patient.

Nursing Interventions

Have the patient turn, cough, and breathe deeply hourly while awake to help prevent respiratory infection and increase oxygen intake.

Teach the patient how to use full chest expansion.

Administer oxygen as needed.

Elevate the head of the bed to promote increased lung expansion and free movement of the diaphragm.

Review blood gas studies, observing for subtle changes indicative of complications.

Monitor vital signs frequently.

NDx: Risk for infection related to immunodeficiency, effects of chemotherapy, and the invasion of malignant cells into the viscera

Planning: Patient outcomes

1. Patient is free of evidence of cough, dyspnea, sore throat, or mouth sores.
2. Patient denies burning or pain on urination.
3. Patient identifies actions needed to prevent infections.
4. Vital signs are within normal ranges for the patient.

Nursing Interventions

Keep the patient warm and avoid extreme changes in temperature in the room.

Restrict visitors to prevent exposure to infections; use protective isolation if necessary.

Promote skin integrity by avoiding irritants to the treatment area and keep the skin clean and dry.

Monitor vital signs frequently and observe for subtle changes that may indicate early signs of infection.

Check for cough, sore throat, dyspnea, pain, or burning with urination.

Teach the patient early signs of respiratory and urinary infections and measures to prevent them.

NDx: Altered nutrition: less than body requirements related to anorexia from treatments, fatigue, and complications of disease

Planning: Patient outcomes

1. Patient chooses foods appropriate to replace dietary deficiencies.
2. Patient avoids irritating foods and fluids.

Nursing Interventions

Teach the patient to eat foods high in protein, vitamins, and calories.

Provide six to eight small meals per day to prevent irritation and distention and reduce fatigue.

Encourage the patient to avoid foods that are gas-forming, and hot, spicy, acidic foods and fluids that cause oral and gastric irritation.

Provide frequent oral hygiene to prevent infection and promote better eating habits.

Encourage increased fluid intake to prevent constipation and promote adequate hydration, and monitor fluid intake and output.

Provide analgesics as ordered and required for discomfort related to esophagitis.

NDx: Activity intolerance related to reduced energy stores, decreased oxygen from ineffective breathing pattern and inadequate nutrition

Planning: Patient outcomes

1. Patient follows a regimen of planned activities and rest periods each day.
2. Patient verbalizes feeling less fatigued and demonstrates signs of increased activity.
3. Patient is able to perform activities of daily living.
4. Patient denies shortness of breath on mild exertion.
5. Vital signs stay within normal limits for the patient.

Nursing Interventions

Instruct the patient to develop a regimen of daily activity with frequent rest periods throughout the day.

Encourage range-of-motion exercises while lying in bed to maintain muscle tone and strength.

Teach the patient to practice energy-saving techniques.

Encourage good nutrition to increase energy levels.

Have the patient practice deep breathing techniques to increase oxygen intake.

NDx: Anxiety related to inability to cope with the manifestations of the disease, fear of treatments and threat of death

Planning: Patient outcomes

1. Patient relates concerns about illness to the nurse or other appropriate member of the health care team.
2. Patient and family verbalize accurate information about the disorder, complications, and therapy.
3. Patient expresses feelings of reduced anxiety and fear.
4. Patient and family identify effective coping strategies to alleviate the anxiety and fear.
5. Patient displays physical signs of decreased anxiety such as: vital signs are within normal limits, patient appears to be resting, appears calm, and eats well.

Nursing Interventions

Allow the patient to verbalize concerns about the disease, its effect on the family, and fears about the future.

Help the patient and family members find appropriate coping strategies that are effective to deal with the anxiety level.

Seek assistance from clergy or other professional counselors if needed.
Teach the patient relaxation techniques.

◆ Hydronephrosis

Hydronephrosis is the collection of large amounts of
urine in the renal pelvis due to obstruction, resulting in
damage to the organ. If the obstruction is in a ureter the
hydronephrosis is unilateral, but if the obstruction is in
the urethra or bladder the condition usually becomes
bilateral, caused by increased pressure on the tubules.
Obstruction may cause impaired renal function secondary to renal damage. Intervention includes removal of the
obstruction and relief of the pressure from the backup of
urine through aspiration or nephrectomy. If damage is
severe from prolonged hydronephrosis, a nephrectomy
may be necessary.

NURSING CARE

Monitor fluid intake and urine output carefully.
Note the color, consistency, and amount of urine.
Administer pain medication as prescribed.
Monitor vital signs, observing for signs of increasing
        pulse and respiratory rate, which may indicate im-
        pending shock.
Review renal function studies.
Explain the condition and effects of the obstruction and
        the expected medical intervention to the patient.
Administer fluid and electrolytes per order until renal
        function improves.

◆ Hyperglycemic Hyperosmolar Non-Ketotic Syndrome (HHNKS)

HHNKS is a life-threatening emergency usually seen in
elderly non-insulin-dependent diabetic or undiagnosed
patients, who are usually hospitalized and/or dehydrated.
It is characterized by profound hyperglycemia (800 mg/

dL or greater) without ketosis, neurologic changes, and severe dehydration. Treatment goals are primarily directed toward rehydration of the patient and correction of electrolyte imbalances.

ASSESSMENT

- Check blood sugar level, serum electrolytes, serum osmolarity, and hydration status.
- Assess the patient's mental status and level of consciousness.
- Check skin turgor, mucous membranes, and urine output for signs of dehydration.

NURSING DIAGNOSES, PLANNING, AND NURSING INTERVENTIONS

NDx: Fluid volume deficit related to dehydration secondary to low fluid intake and hyperglycemia

Planning: Patient outcomes

1. Blood glucose will normalize.
2. Patient's hydration status will normalize.

Nursing Interventions

Monitor blood glucose and electrolyte levels.
Monitor the patient's hydration status: check fluid intake and urine output, mucous membranes, and skin.
Monitor intravenous fluid infusions carefully.
Encourage oral replacement fluids when appropriate.
Assess respiratory and cardiovascular status for fluid overload, observing for tachycardia, crackles, noisy respirations, and dependent edema.
Check vital signs and neurologic status frequently and document data for continued comparisons.

NDx: Altered thought processes related to electrolyte imbalance

Planning: Patient outcomes

1. Patient remains appropriately oriented and free from injury.

2. The patient's electrolyte levels are in normal ranges for the patient.

Nursing Interventions

Check neurologic status and general orientation frequently.
Maintain a hazard-free environment and assist the patient when out of bed.
Initiate therapies to correct electrolyte imbalances.
Monitor laboratory data and patient status for signs of improvement.
Provide environmental cues for orientation.
Provide a low-stimulation environment.

◆ Hypertension (Hypertensive Vascular Disease)

Hypertension is a condition in which a persistent systolic blood pressure greater than 140 mm Hg and a persistent diastolic blood pressure greater than 90 mm Hg is present. A persistent systolic blood pressure greater than 140 mm Hg with a diastolic blood pressure less than 90 mm Hg is termed *systolic hypertension.* Hypertensive vascular disease is the most common cardiovascular disorder in the Untied States. Hypertension is classified as either primary, which is usually of unknown cause but is the most common type, or secondary, which is caused by an underlying known disorder. It is managed by reducing risk factors by following a low-salt, low-cholesterol diet, relaxation exercises, a regular regimen of moderate exercise, and pharmacologic therapy. The goal of medical management is to reduce the blood pressure and maintain it within normal limits.

ASSESSMENT

- Assess the blood pressure lying, sitting, and standing, taking the measurements in both arms and legs to determine the baseline data and to note any differences bilaterally.
- Palpate the apical pulse at the midclavicular line in the fifth intercostal space and the peripheral

pulses to determine the rate, rhythm, and amplitude.

- Palpate extremities for edema.
- Auscultate for dysrhythmias, tachycardia, or abnormal breath sounds, which may indicate cardiac involvement.
- Ask about episodes of angina and get a description of the pain as to intensity, precipitating factors, duration, radiation, and relief methods.
- Examine the neck for enlarged thyroid or vein distention.
- Observe for decreased urinary output, or increased output if the patient is on diuretic therapy.
- Palpate the abdomen for masses and bruits indicative of aneurysms or stenosis of the abdominal aorta or renal arteries.
- Assess the neurologic status to detect changes associated with altered cerebral perfusion, cerebral vascular accident, or hemorrhage.
- Assess for pallor, diaphoresis, and vertigo when rising from a supine position, which may indicate orthostatic hypotension.
- Assess for skin and retinal changes indicative of progressive hypertension.
- Obtain height and weight to determine obesity.
- Review the patient's dietary pattern and check caloric levels and the amount of fat, cholesterol, and sodium regularly consumed.
- Determine food preferences and financial influences on food choices.
- Assess the patient's level of knowledge, stressors, and risk factors such as smoking, obesity, and lack of exercise.
- Determine if the patient is taking birth control pills, diet pills, cold medications, amphetamines, or alcohol, which may be associated with hypertension.
- Check the family history for hypertension, other cardiovascular diseases, or diabetes.

NURSING DIAGNOSES, PLANNING, AND NURSING INTERVENTIONS

NDx: Decreased cardiac output related to increased workload of the heart and vasoconstriction

Planning: Patient outcomes

1. Patient's vital signs are within normal ranges for the patient.
2. Patient has a balanced intake and output; is free of peripheral and central edema.
3. Patient's skin is warm, color is appropriate, no cyanosis is present, and peripheral pulses are palpable.
4. Patient maintains an adequate cardiac output as seen by the hemodynamic monitoring.

Nursing Interventions

Monitor the patient's vital signs lying, sitting, and standing.

Encourage the patient to have frequent rest throughout the day to prevent fatigue and strain on the myocardium.

Instruct the patient to stop activity if it initiates episodes of chest pain or aggravates chest discomfort, causes headache, confusion, or dizziness, indicating possible neurologic problems.

Use telemetry monitoring whenever possible, especially if the patient experiences dysrhythmias or if the patient is taking antidysrhythmic drugs.

Review the results of laboratory studies and hemodynamic monitoring.

Check the patient's intake and output, observing for adequacy and balance.

Keep the patient's legs in a nondependent position while sitting to prevent edema.

Provide support for the extremities while sitting or lying in bed.

Teach the patient relaxation techniques and range-of-motion procedures to increase circulation while lying in bed.

Prevent constriction of circulation from tight clothing or bed linen.

NDx: Altered nutrition: more than body requirements related to lifestyle resulting in obesity, atherosclerosis, and hypertension

Planning: Patient outcomes

1. Patient states accurate information about an appropriate diet plan for weight loss, including low-fat, low-cholesterol, and low-sodium foods.
2. Patient chooses food as allowed on the diet plan.
3. Patient's weight decreases.

Nursing Interventions

Teach the patient about dietary modifications needed to reduce weight.

Give the patient literature explaining the caloric content of foods, and the fat, cholesterol and sodium content.

Plan a dietary regimen for the patient, including foods of choice when able, and give sample menus to the patient and family to follow at home.

Seek dietary counseling with the dietitian as needed.

Devise an exercise regimen for the patient that will help burn calories and increase circulation, as well as make the heart more efficient and lower the blood pressure.

Encourage the family to participate with the patient in the exercise program.

NDx: Self-esteem disturbance related to hypertensive disease state, changes in lifestyle to manage disease and reduce risk factors, and/or inability to comply with the treatment plan

Planning: Patient outcomes

1. Patient states methods to cope with illness.
2. Patient denies feelings of inadequacy, helplessness, or dependency.
3. Patient appears positive, friendly, and cheerful, and actively participates in plans for discharge and patient education sessions.
4. Patient takes responsibility for self care and complies with treatment plan.

Nursing Interventions

Teach the patient self-care measures, encouraging participation and decision-making by the patient.

Explain how changes in lifestyle can benefit the patient by reducing blood pressure and risk of other disorders.

Allow time for expression of concerns, questions, and clarification of misunderstandings.

Praise the patient for knowledge gained about the disorder, for attempts at lifestyle change, and for participation in self care.

Seek assistance from clergy, family members, or other professionals when appropriate.

Make referrals for the patient upon discharge as needed.

NDx: Altered health maintenance related to lack of knowledge needed to maintain healthy lifestyle, to understand the nature of the disease, nutritional needs, treatments, and measures to reduce risk

Planning: Patient outcomes

1. Patient describes cause, effects, and risk factors associated with hypertension.
2. Patient lists symptoms and treatments for the complications of the disorder.
3. Patient relates the nutritional therapy for lowering cholesterol levels and maintaining low-fat, low-sodium meals.
4. Patient states the self care needed to prevent risk or complications of hypertension.

Nursing Interventions

Explain the cause, effects, and clinical course of hypertension to the patient.

Allow time for questions from the patient at any time.

Provide appropriate literature about hypertension for the patient and family to review.

Allow patient to verbalize concerns and fears.

Evaluate discharge needs of the patient and family.

Teach the patient or family how to take a blood pressure reading.

Alert the patient to signs and symptoms of uncontrolled hypertension and its complications, such as impaired renal function, hemorrhage, and neurologic disturbances.

Instruct the patient about dietary modifications needed to reduce risk, reduce weight, or prevent complications of the disorder.

Explain the need for decreases in dietary fats and cholesterol to prevent the effects of the disease and increases in protein and vitamins to promote good health and healing.

Instruct the patient to follow a reduced-sodium diet.

Devise a diet plan for weight reduction as needed and appropriate for the patient.

Initiate counseling with a dietitian to assist with meal planning if needed.

Teach the patient dosage, route, time, frequency, side effects, and toxic effects of any medication prescribed.

Explain the diagnostic studies completed and the need for any follow-up studies after discharge.

Include the family in any of the teaching sessions when applicable.

NDx: Noncompliance to treatment regimen related to asymptomatic disorder, side effects of medications, financial problems, inability to make lifestyle adjustments, or lack of education about disease state

Planning: Patient outcomes

1. Patient relates accurate information about the disease and the importance of following prescribed treatment plan.
2. Patient states the potential consequences or risks of not following the prescribed treatment plan.
3. Patient demonstrates compliance with the plan.
4. Vital signs, especially blood pressure, stay within normal ranges for the patient.

Nursing Interventions

Encourage the patient to comply with the prescribed treatment plan by explaining the consequences and risks of noncompliance and the benefits of compliance.

Refer the patient to a support group if applicable.

Seek assistance of social services for financial counseling and support.

Encourage the family to become involved with the
treatment regimen, especially the lifestyle
changes.
Have a family member check the patient's blood pressure and weight, if needed, weekly.
Praise the patient for compliance with the regimen.
Institute a behavior modification program using a con-
tract signed by the patient and the nurse to improve compliance.

Hyperthyroidism

Hyperthyroidism is a disorder of hypermetabolism that
results from exposure of the body tissues to excessive
quantities of circulating free thyroxine or triiodothyronine, or both. Graves' disease, the most common form of
primary hyperthyroidism, is an autoimmune disorder in
which thyroid antibodies stimulate hypersecretion of thyroid hormone. Management consists of administration of
antithyroid preparations, which inhibit thyroid hormone
synthesis; iodine preparations, which temporarily block
the release of thyroid hormone and reduce the size and
vascularity of the gland; destruction of the thyroid gland
with radioactive iodine; or removal of a portion of the
thyroid gland. Propranolol (Inderal) is often used during
treatment to alleviate the cardiovascular effects of thyroid
hormone excess.

ASSESSMENT

- Assess for exaggerated alertness, nervousness,
  tremulousness, agitation, irritability, insomnia, a
  feeling of apprehension, inability to concentrate,
  emotional lability, fatigue, and weight loss.
- Assess for tachycardia, palpitations, increased cardiac output, a bounding pulse, increased pulse pressure, systolic hypertension, atrial dysrhythmias,
  tachypnea, heat intolerance, osteoporosis, decreased
  libido, reduced fertility in women, and impotence
  in men.
- Observe for diaphoresis, cutaneous vasodilation,
  muscle weakness, fine muscle and tongue tremors,

impaired coordination, hyperreflexia, tremors of the eyelids, periorbital edema, and exophthalmos.

- Check for warm, moist skin, pruritus, nonpitting pretibial or ankle edema, orange-peel appearance of skin on pretibial or ankle areas, fine, brittle hair, hair loss, soft nails, and frequent bowel movements.
- Assess for symptoms of thyroid storm: fever (up to 106°F), severe tachycardia, profuse diaphoresis, extreme vasodilation, hypotension, atrial fibrillation, hyperreflexia, abdominal pain, nausea, vomiting, dehydration, psychosis, and coma.

NURSING DIAGNOSES, PLANNING, AND NURSING INTERVENTIONS

NDx: Anxiety related to heat intolerance and change in appearance, behavior, and activity secondary to thyroid hormone excess

Planning: Patient outcomes

1. Patient verbalizes reduction in anxiety.

Nursing Interventions

Provide factual information to the patient and significant others related to the effects of increased levels of circulating thyroid hormones.

Encourage the patient to identify and verbalize feelings.

Assist the patient in identifying relaxation techniques.

Explain procedures and maintain an unhurried manner.

Carefully select roommates and restrict visitors if necessary.

Provide a cool room with good circulation but free of drafts.

Provide lightweight bedding and sleepwear.

Provide frequent hygiene, skin care, and linen changes.

NDx: Risk for altered health maintenance related to insufficient knowledge of self-management of pharmacologic therapy during and after treatment with antithyroid, iodine, or radioactive iodine

Planning: Patient outcomes

1. Patient states name, dose, administration schedule, timetable for expected effects, and adverse and toxic effects of prescribed medications.
2. Patient demonstrates ability to monitor radial pulse.

Nursing Interventions

Teach the patient the name, dose, administration schedule, and timetable for expected effects and side effects of prescribed medications.

Instruct patients taking an iodine preparation to take it after meals, to dilute the solution with a full glass of water or juice, and to drink it through a straw.

Instruct the patient to notify the physician promptly of signs of iodine toxicity: metallic taste, stomatitis, coryza, tenderness of salivary glands, vomiting, bloody diarrhea, or abdominal pain or distention.

Instruct the patient to consult with the physician before taking over-the-counter preparations.

Teach the patient how to monitor the radial pulse for 1 full minute 2 to 3 times weekly and to record the result.

Instruct the patient to notify the physician promptly if the pulse becomes irregular or drops below 60.

NDx: Altered nutrition: less than body requirements related to hypermetabolism, hyperactivity, and increased gastrointestinal motility

Planning: Patient outcomes

1. Patient states intent to consume high-calorie, high-protein, high-carbohydrate diet until ideal weight and euthyroid state are attained.
2. Patient verbalizes understanding of the need to decrease food consumption to maintain ideal weight as metabolic rate decreases.

Nursing Interventions

Instruct the patient to weigh himself or herself 2 to 3 times weekly.

Encourage the patient to eat small, frequent high-calorie, high-protein, high-carbohydrate snacks and supplements.

Instruct the patient to avoid caffeine, spicy seasonings, and foods high in bulk or fiber.

Encourage fluids up to 4000 mL per day unless contraindicated.

Advise patient to decrease food intake as treatment becomes effective.

Additional Interventions

Plan care to allow for frequent rest periods and conservation of energy.

Provide a quiet, restful environment that is free of hazards.

Administer or teach the patient with exophthalmos proper administration of lubricating eye drops.

Monitor vital signs, pulse pressure, capillary refill, neurologic status, and renal output hourly in a patient in thyroid storm.

◆ Hypothyroidism

Hypothyroidism is a disorder characterized by deficiency of circulating thyroid hormones usually resulting from a defect in the thyroid gland itself, but may be caused by surgical removal or irradiation of the gland or dietary deficiency of iodine. Symptoms are associated with the generalized effects of slowed metabolism such as fatigue, lethargy, increased somnolence, subnormal basal temperature, bradycardia, impaired wound healing, weight gain, and slowed reflexes and mental processing. Treatment requires lifelong thyroid replacement therapy. If the hypothyroidism is due to inadequate daily intake of iodine, diet changes or supplements may be prescribed.

ASSESSMENT

- Obtain a thorough nursing history with special attention to unusual fatigue, lethargy, and somnolence.
- Obtain baseline vital signs.

- Note the presence of myxedema.
- Weigh the patient and compare to reported presymptomatic weight.
- Evaluate the patient's mental status.
- Assess the hemodynamic status if the patient is in myxedemic stupor or in a comatose state.

NURSING DIAGNOSES, PLANNING, AND NURSING INTERVENTIONS

NDx: Risk for altered tissue perfusion: systemic, related to anemia, decreased cardiac output, decreased respirations, and hypothermia secondary to decreased basal metabolism

Planning: Patient outcomes

1. Patient maintains adequate tissue perfusion as evidenced by stable vital signs, basal temperature higher than 96°F (35.5°C), pulse 60 to 100 bpm and regular, respirations 8 to 16/min, blood pressure higher than 90/60, capillary refill less than 3 seconds, urine output greater than 30 mL/h.
2. Patient is alert and oriented to person, place, and time.

Nursing Interventions

Monitor the signs of peripheral tissue perfusion and record results.
Evaluate mental and neurologic status frequently.
Maintain a warm environment.
Monitor vital signs at regular intervals.
Administer thyroid replacement as prescribed.

NDx: Activity intolerance related to fatigue, lethargy, altered sensory perception and muscular responses, and slowed mental processes

Planning: Patient outcomes

1. Patient participates in care and activities of daily living as independently as possible.
2. Patient's safety is maintained.

Nursing Interventions

Provide rest alternated with periods of activity.
Evaluate muscle strength and mobility daily.
Utilize energy-saving techniques in daily care.
Encourage range-of-motion exercises.
Remove hazards from the environment.
Reassure the patient and family that slowed behaviors,
activities, and thought processes are the result of the
disease and will reverse with treatment.

NDx: Risk for altered health maintenance related to
insufficient knowledge of self-management of the disease
with lifelong thyroid replacement

Planning: Patient outcomes

1. Patient verbalizes understanding of the effects of
the disease process, treatment modalities, and need
for follow-up care.
2. Patient maintains appropriate weight and nutritional status.
3. Patient evacuates soft, formed stool at least once
every 3 days.
4. Patient cares for skin appropriately.

Nursing Interventions

Reinforce explanation of disease and its treatment as
presented by the physician.
Teach the patient about the medication, including the
dose, expected effects, and side effects.
Advise the patient not to alter the dosage, even when
symptoms subside, without the physician's instruction.
Advise the patient to alert all health-care providers that
thyroid replacement is prescribed.
Teach the patient to monitor the pulse and to record it, and
to hold the medication and report to the physician if
greater than 100 bpm and/or irregular.
Refer the patient to the dietitian for nutritional education
assistance.
Determine normal bowel pattern and encourage
nonmethods of promotion of regularity (dietary
fiber, fluids, and exercise).

Instruct the patient to avoid excessively hot baths and
harsh soaps.
Encourage the use of topical moisturizers.

 # Increased Intracranial Pressure

Intracranial pressure (ICP) is the pressure exerted within
the cranial cavity by brain tissue, blood, and CSF. A
sustained increase in ICP may be life-threatening and can
be caused by anything that takes up space within the
intracranial compartment such as edema of the brain,
blood clots, tumors, cysts, abscesses, and hydrocephalus.
Management consists of drug therapy including osmotic
diuretics, glucocorticoids, anticonvulsants, and barbiturates; and supportive therapy including hyperventilation,
hypothermia, and maintaining the head of the bed elevated 30 to 40°. Surgical intervention includes drainage
of CSF or removal of a space occupying lesion.

ASSESSMENT

- Assess for decreasing level of consciousness, increasing blood pressure, bradycardia, pupillary
  changes, headache, and nausea.
- Observe for restlessness, irritability, drowsiness,
  confusion, apathy, and difficulty in following com-
  mands or in verbalizing appropriately.
- Observe for respiratory and motor changes, seizures, visual disturbances, and papilledema.

NURSING DIAGNOSES, PLANNING, AND NURSING INTERVENTIONS

NDx: Ineffective breathing pattern related to alteration
in level of consciousness, increased ICP

Planning: Patient outcomes

1. Respiratory rate is regular, between 12 and 24 breaths
   per minute.
2. ABG levels are within normal range.

Nursing interventions

Maintain a patent airway.

Auscultate lungs every 4 hours, document findings.
Administer O_2 as ordered.
Monitor ABG results.
Use hyperventilation techniques as ordered.
Monitor for Cheyne-Stokes respiratory pattern.

NDx: Altered tissue perfusion: cerebral, related to an increase in brain tissue, intracranial volume, or CSF volume

Planning: Patient outcomes

1. Patient maintains baseline neurologic status.
2. ICP returns to normal range.

Nursing Interventions

Document behavioral assessments every 1 to 2 hours.
Report any deviation from baseline immediately.
Maintain the head of the bed elevated 30 to 40° as ordered.
Avoid flexion of the neck.
Instruct the patient to refrain from activities that increase intrathoracic or intra-abdominal pressure such as straining at stool, isometric exercises, coughing, sneezing, blowing the nose, and sitting in a high Fowler's position.
Administer stool softeners, analgesics, diuretics, and steroids as ordered. Administer oxygen as needed and ordered.
Organize nursing care to allow for optimal rest periods.
Minimize suctioning, venipuncture, stimulation, and the use of restraints whenever possible.
Monitor temperature every 15 minutes rectally if hypothermia is used.

NDx: Risk for fluid volume deficit related to osmotic diuretic therapy or fluid restriction

Planning: Patient outcomes

1. Serum electrolytes are within normal range.
2. Serum osmolarity is within normal range.
3. Urine specific gravity is within normal range.

Nursing Interventions

Monitor and record I & O and urinary specific gravity.
Monitor serum electrolytes, osmolality, and creatine.
Check vital signs every 1 to 2 hours.
Monitor skin turgor every 4 hours.

Additional interventions

Massage bony prominences every 2 hours.
Use an air mattress.
Monitor peripheral circulation every 2 to 3 hours if hypo-
thermia is used.
Explain all procedures to family members and allow for
verbalization of feelings.

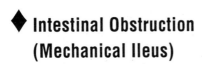

◆ Intestinal Obstruction (Mechanical Ileus)

Mechanical ileus is a condition in which movement of intestinal contents through the intestine is impaired due to a mechanical obstruction such as a tumor, adhesion, hernia, volvulus or foreign body. Management involves supportive measures such as NPO status and an NG or naso-intestinal tube to decompress the intestine and prevent vomiting, IV fluids, anti-infectives and analgesics followed by surgical correction of the underlying condition.

ASSESSMENT

- Assess for abdominal pain (type, location, severity), vomiting (amount, color, odor, consistency, frequency).
- Check bowel sounds and when the patient last had a bowel movement and passed flatus.
- Observe for signs of dehydration and hypovolemia: Check for signs of poor skin turgor and dry mucous membranes; take vital signs to check for increased temperature, rapid weak pulse, rapid respirations and hypotension; check urinary output and laboratory values of hematocrit and serum electrolytes.

- Assess for signs of peritonitis: rigid abdomen, leukocytosis, increasing pain and fever.
- Assess NG or NI tube function, amount and character of drainage, and check for irritation or discomfort from the tube in the naris.

NURSING DIAGNOSES, PLANNING, AND NURSING INTERVENTIONS

NDx: Risk for fluid volume deficit related to sequestering of ECF in the intestine, weeping of plasma into the peritoneal cavity, and vomiting

Planning: Patient outcomes

1. Blood pressure, pulse and respirations are within patient's normal range.
2. Urinary output is 50 ml or more per hour.
3. Serum electrolytes and osmolarity are within normal limits.

Nursing Interventions

Administer IV fluid and electrolytes as ordered. Typical replacement consists of isotonic NaCl alternating with 5% D & W with up to 40 mEq of potassium.
Measure and document intake and output.

NDx: Pain related to increased pressure in the intestinal lumen

Planning: Patient outcomes

1. Patient states pain is relieved.
2. Patient rests without verbal or nonverbal signs of pain.

Nursing Interventions

Give analgesics as ordered for pain.
Change patient's position frequently for comfort.
Maintain calm, restful environment.
Apply water soluble lubricant to naris to prevent irritation from the NG or NI tube.

◆ Ischemic Cardiac Disease

Ischemic cardiac disease is a generic term or category for several disorders that involve reduced blood flow to the heart. Refer to the following entries in this text for associated nursing diagnoses, planning, and nursing interventions: Angina, Myocardial Infarction, Coronary Artery Disease and Atherosclerosis.

◆ Laryngeal Cancer

Cancer of the larynx, the most common upper respiratory tract malignancy, is associated with heavy cigarette smoking and ingestion of alcohol. Intrinsic tumors develop on the true vocal cords; are well differentiated; and grow slowly. Extrinsic tumors develop above or below the true vocal cords, and grow rapidly with early lymphatic involvement. Hoarseness is a common symptom of intrinsic tumors. Management of laryngeal cancer is determined by the stage of the tumor and involves surgery or radiation therapy. Transoral cordectomy, laryngofissure, and laser surgery are performed on early intrinsic lesions. A partial, conservation, or total laryngectomy may be necessary for more advanced tumors.

See entries under Cancer, Laryngectomy, and Radiation Therapy for specific information on related nursing care.

◆ Leukemia

The term *leukemia* is used to categorize a group of disorders in which a neoplastic growth of white blood cells occurs in the bone marrow. The leukemic cells multiply while suppressing bone marrow function, resulting in a decreased production of red blood cells, platelets, and other types of cells. The cause is unknown, but leukemia has a high incidence in individuals previously exposed to excessive radiation and chemicals. It is a common cause of death among children. There are six primary categories of leukemias: acute lymphocytic leukemia (ALL), acute myelocytic leukemia (AML), acute monocytic leukemia (rare), chronic lymphocytic leukemia (CLL), chronic myelocytic leukemia (CML), and chronic monocytic leukemia (rare). See the textbook for a detailed description of each type. Management of leukemia usually involves chemotherapy, some radiotherapy, analgesics, prophylactic antibiotics, and transfusions.

ASSESSMENT

- Observe for weakness, fatigue, malaise, cyanosis, dyspnea, tachycardia, headache, and weight loss.
- Check for bleeding of the gums, petechiae, ecchymoses, purpura, bruising, and pallor.
- Observe for signs of infection such as increased temperature, cough and respiratory distress, or burning and pain with urination.
- Check for anorexia, nausea, vomiting, sore throat and mouth, and poor nutrition.
- Assess for tenderness, pain, organ enlargement, and edema.
- Ask about headaches, confusion, dizziness, and restlessness, and assess for changes in vision, papilledema, or retinal hemorrhages, indicating infiltration into the central nervous system.
- Observe for psychological and physical indicators of high stress.
- Assess patient and family's coping mechanisms for strategies that seem most functional.
- Determine the patient's emotional status and level of understanding about leukemia.

NURSING DIAGNOSES, PLANNING, AND NURSING INTERVENTIONS

NDx: Risk for infection related to the compromised immune system

Planning: Patient outcomes

1. Patient's vital signs and laboratory data are within normal limits for the patient.
2. Patient is free from infection as evidenced by the absence of sore throat, ulcerations of the mouth, chills, fever, cough, or burning on urination.

3. Patient identifies signs of infection and appropriate measures to prevent infection.
4. Patient is in protective isolation while hospitalized.

Nursing Interventions

Keep the patient warm, prevent chilling, and restrict visitors.
Use protective isolation if appropriate.
Monitor vital signs frequently and check laboratory data, observing for subtle changes that may reflect early infectious processes.
Teach the patient the signs of infections and measures to prevent them.
Promote good nutrition and encourage the patient to eat a high-protein, high-vitamin diet.
Encourage frequent mouth cleansing.
Explain the importance of preventing constipation since it can cause mucosal breakdown and infection in the rectal tissue.

NDx: Altered nutrition: less than body requirements related to anorexia secondary to sore mouth, chemotherapy, and radiotherapy

Planning: Patient outcomes

1. Patient eats well-balanced meals, choosing high-protein, high-vitamin foods.
2. Patient chooses nonirritating foods.
3. Patient eats six to eight small meals per day.
4. Patient increases amount of oral fluid intake.

Nursing Interventions

Teach the patient to eat a diet high in vitamins, protein, and calories.
Tell the patient to eat frequent small meals (six to eight per day) to prevent gastric distention and irritation.
Offer the meals in an attractive manner and encourage the patient to eat all the food offered.
Allow the patient to rest prior to eating so fatigue does not inhibit good nutritional patterns.

NDx: Pain related to enlarged lymph nodes, chemical treatments, and bone infiltration

Planning: Patient outcomes

1. Patient reports that pain is controlled with analgesics.
2. Patient states comfort measures to help relieve pain.

Nursing Interventions

Keep the patient in comfortable positions, using pillows to support bony prominences.

Help the patient find alternative methods, such as relaxation techniques, to alleviate or tolerate the pain.

Give analgesics prior to activity periods so the patient can better tolerate the movement.

NDx: Anxiety related to health status, fear of death or treatment outcomes, and complications of the disease

Planning: Patient outcomes

1. Patient's anxiety is lessened as evidenced by stable vital signs, relaxed appearance, and calm, positive attitude.
2. Patient states strategies to cope with the manifestations and treatments of the disease.
3. Patient verbalizes fears and concerns.

Nursing Interventions

Allow the patient to verbalize fears and concerns about the disease and treatment regimen.

Answer questions honestly without giving false reassurance.

Help the patient find coping strategies that are effective for reducing anxiety.

Teach relaxation techniques and encourage the patient to use them.

Explain the disease and all treatments to the patient using understandable terminology.

Provide comfort measures, both physical and emotional, to the patient and family.

NDx: Sensory/perceptual alterations: visual, auditory, and kinesthetic related to malignant infiltration into the central nervous system

Planning: Patient outcomes

1. Patient reports decrease or absence of headache, visual impairment, vertigo, nausea, and vomiting.
2. Patient requests assistance as needed when ambulatory to prevent injury.
3. Patient is alert and oriented to time, place, and person.

Nursing Interventions

Teach the patient to use safety measures at all times.
Explain to the family the need for their assistance to the patient to prevent injury.
Have the patient request assistance when getting out of bed and ambulating.
Check the patient frequently for orientation to time, place, and person.
Speak loudly if auditory problems are evident.
Decrease the external stimuli and provide periods of rest.

NDx: Activity intolerance related to weakness, poor nutrition, and depressed energy stores from anemia, complications of treatment, and stress

Planning: Patient outcomes

1. Patient reports increased ability to perform activities of daily living.
2. Patient demonstrates no shortness of breath upon mild exertion.
3. Patient reports less weakness with increased tolerance for activity.
4. Patient sleeps 6 to 10 hours per night without difficulty.

Nursing Interventions

Instruct the patient to develop a regimen of activity with frequent rest periods throughout the day.
Encourage the patient to do range-of-motion exercises frequently while lying in bed to maintain muscle tone and strength.
Tell the patient to avoid sudden movements.
Have the patient practice deep breathing exercises.

Teach the patient to practice energy-saving techniques to reduce fatigue and shortness of breath.

Provide and encourage frequent rest periods while delivering patient care.

Prevent interruptions during rest periods and at night whenever possible.

Encourage good nutrition to increase the patient's energy level. Offer four to six meals per day.

NDx: Knowledge deficit: nature of illness and complication of bleeding related to thrombocytopenia

Planning: Patient outcomes

1. Patient reports accurate information about the nature of the disease.
2. Patient states accurately the signs of bleeding and when to notify the physician.
3. Patient presents no signs or symptoms of bleeding such as petechiae, ecchymoses, epistaxis, dark stools, and so on.
4. Patient verbalizes the preventive measures necessary to prevent bleeding.

◆ Liver Cancer (Malignant Hepatic Tumors)

The liver is a major site for metastatic lesions from several other sites in the body. Cancer of the liver is rarely caused by a primary carcinoma, but if it is a primary site, there is usually linkage to hepatitis B virus infection, exposure to carcinogens, or the use of androgenic steroids. Pain and hepatomegaly are the most common physical findings. Scanning, ultrasonography, computed tomography, and magnetic resonance imaging assist in diagnosing the disease, but a biopsy is required for a definitive diagnosis. Although the prognosis is usually poor, even with treatment, management usually includes resection, transplantation, radiation, and chemotherapy.

NURSING CARE

The nursing care for the patient with cancer of the liver is similar to that for a patient with *cirrhosis*. Also refer to the entries on Cancer, Chemotherapy, and Radiation Therapy in general in this text for specific nursing diagnoses, planning, and nursing interventions.

◆ Lung Cancer

Although the exact cause is unknown, factors such as the prolonged inhalation of air pollutants, smoking, and industrial exposure to certain inorganic and organic synthetic substances, asbestos dust and radioactive substances such as radon are associated with the development of lung cancer. Squamous cell carcinomas arise centrally in the major bronchi, grow slowly, often into the lumen obstructing the airway, and tend to spread within the thorax and/or metastasize to the small bowel. Adenocarcinomas arise in the lung periphery, often spread throughout the lung in patches, and frequently invade the pleura. They metastasize early to the brain, other lung, liver, adrenal glands, and/or bone. Large-cell carcinomas are very similar to adenocarcinomas. Small-cell carcinomas (oat-cell) are the most malignant of the lung cancers. They arise centrally in the bronchus region and metastasize early to the mediastinum, liver, bone, central nervous system, and endocrine glands. Localized symptoms associated with lung cancer include cough, dyspnea, hemoptysis, stridor or wheeze, and signs of obstructive pneumonitis. Management of lung cancer varies with type of tumor, stage of disease, and general condition of the patient. It may involve surgery, chemotherapy, radiation, and general supportive measures alone or in combination.

See entries under Cancer, Bronchoscopy, Pneumonectomy, Lobectomy, Chest Drainage, Chemotherapy, and Radiation Therapy for specific nursing care that may apply to an individual patient.

◆ Mechanical Obstruction

Mechanical obstruction is a condition in which movement of intestinal contents through the intestine is impaired due to an obstruction either outside the intestine (strictures, hematomas, intramural tumors) or within the intestinal lumen (foreign bodies, intussusception, volvulus, epithelial tumors). Management involves supportive measures such as NPO status and an NG or nasointestinal (NI) tube to decompress the intestine and prevent vomiting, IV fluids, antiinfectives, and analgesics followed by surgical correction of the underlying condition.

ASSESSMENT

- Assess for abdominal pain/cramping (type, location, severity), abdominal distention, vomiting (amount, color, odor, consistency, frequency).
- Check bowel sounds and when the patient last had a bowel movement and passed flatus.
- Observe for signs of dehydration and hypovolemia: Check for signs of poor skin turgor and dry mucous membranes; take vital signs to check for increased temperature, rapid weak pulse, rapid respirations, and hypotension; check urinary output and laboratory values of hematocrit and serum electrolytes.
- Assess for signs of peritonitis: rigid abdomen, leukocytosis, increasing pain and fever.
- Assess NG or NI tube function, amount and character of drainage, and for irritation or discomfort from the tube in the naris.

NURSING DIAGNOSES, PLANNING, AND NURSING INTERVENTIONS

NDx: Risk for fluid volume deficit related to sequestering of ECF in the intestine, weeping of plasma into the peritoneal cavity, and vomiting

Planning: Patient outcomes

1. Blood pressure, pulse, and respiration are within patient's normal range.
2. Urinary output is 50 mL or more per hour.
3. Serum electrolytes and osmolarity are within normal limits.

Nursing Interventions

Administer IV fluid and electrolytes as ordered. Typical
replacement consists of isotonic NaCl alternating
with 5% D & W with up to 40 mEq of potassium.
Monitor CVP to ensure adequate replacement and prevent overload.

NDx: Pain related to increased pressure in the intestinal lumen

Planning: Patient outcomes

1. Patient states pain is relieved.
2. Patient rests without verbal or nonverbal signs of
   pain.

Nursing Interventions

Monitor function of NG tube.
Give analgesics as ordered for pain.
Change patient's position frequently for comfort.
Maintain calm, quiet environment.
Apply water soluble lubricant to naris to prevent irritation
from the NG or NI tube.

 # Meningitis

Meningitis is an inflammation of the meninges of the
brain, which may be bacterial or viral in origin. Bacterial
meningitis is often preceded by infections of the head and
upper respiratory tract, direct trauma to the head, or
invasive CNS procedures. Viral meningitis occurs secondary to a viral infection outside the CNS. Management
of the bacterial form consists of immediate IV antibiotic
therapy. Steroids, osmotic diuretics, and anticonvulsants
may also be used. Management of the viral form focuses
on supportive care and includes the use of antipyretics
and analgesics.

ASSESSMENT

- Assess for symptoms related to increased intracranial pressure such as: headache, fever, vomiting, and an altered level of consciousness (poor attention span, irritability, restlessness, slight lethargy).
- Observe for signs of meningeal irritation such as nuchal rigidity (pain when neck is flexed), Kernig's sign (inability to extend the leg from a position of 90% flexion at the hip), and Brudzinski's sign (flexion of the thighs and legs in response to passive flexion of the neck).
- Inspect the skin for petechial rash, purpuric lesions, and ecchymosis (specific to meningococcal meningitis).
- Assess for photophobia, cranial nerve dysfunction, and convulsions.

NURSING DIAGNOSES, PLANNING, AND NURSING INTERVENTIONS

See information under Encephalitis as well as that which follows:

NDX: Pain: headache and neck pain related to meningeal irritation

Planning: Patient outcomes

1. Patient exhibits ability to rest.
2. Patient states that pain is decreased.

Nursing Interventions

Consolidate nursing care activities in order to minimize unnecessary stimulation.
Maintain a quiet environment by reducing light and noise level.
Avoid startling the patient.
Administer analgesics as ordered and needed, and monitor for effectiveness.
Provide cool compresses to the head.
Change position gradually.

NDX: Risk for injury related to restlessness, disorientation, seizure activity

Planning: Patient outcomes

1.   Patient remains free from injury.

Nursing Interventions

Maintain bed in low position.
Keep side rails up.
Place pad or bumpers along side rails.
Protect all catheters (intravenous, urinary) and tubes (NG) from dislodgement.
Use restraints when necessary.
Institute seizure precautions.
Administer anticonvulsants and sedatives as ordered.

NDX: Risk for altered nutrition: less than body requirements related to anorexia, fatigue, nausea, vomiting, and inability to swallow

Planning: Patient outcomes

1.   Weight is maintained within 1 to 2 pounds of baseline.
2.   Patient is free of symptoms of dehydration.
3.   Episodes of nausea and vomiting are reduced or eliminated.

Nursing Interventions

Provide IV fluids as ordered.
Administer supplemental feedings via NG tube or total parenteral nutrition (TPN) as ordered.
Monitor I & O every 8 hours.
Weigh the patient every 3 days or more often if patient is vomiting.
Monitor laboratory values such as BUN, creatine, and albumin levels.
Administer antiemetics as ordered and needed.

◆ Mitral Valve Prolapse

A cardiac valvular abnormality in which the mitral valve is weakened and displaced upward. This results in blood flow back into the left atrium causing weakness, fatigue, dyspnea, palpitations, lightheadedness, and anxiety attacks with hyperventilation. The pathology may be the result of repeated infection and inflammation, congenital defect, trauma, or degenerative changes. It is diagnosed by physical assessment, an echocardiogram, and cardiac catheterization, and may be managed palliatively or by valve replacement.

NURSING CARE

Nursing care of the patient with mitral valve prolapse is similar to that for the patient with mitral valve stenosis.

◆ Mitral Valve Stenosis

Mitral valve stenosis is the narrowing of the mitral valve, which causes an obstruction of blood flow from the left atrium to the left ventricle. The most common cause is scarring after rheumatic endocarditis. Symptoms include weakness, fatigue, ascites, hepatomegaly, chest pain, dyspnea on exertion, and palpitations. A diastolic murmur is heard on auscultation. Mitral valve stenosis may result from congenital defects, trauma, myocardial infarction, and degenerative changes. The stenotic valve may be treated by valvotomy, commissurotomy, or valve replacement.

ASSESSMENT

- Check for dyspnea, weakness, fatigue, syncopal episodes, cough, and tachycardia.
- Assess for edema in the periphery.
- Note vital signs and observe for intermittent changes.
- Check for history of rheumatic fever, streptococcal infection, or congenital heart problems that involve the valves.

- Auscultate the heart sounds, listening carefully for a diastolic murmur.
- Assess the skin for paleness or cyanosis.
- Ask the patient about numbness or tingling in the extremities.
- Check the electrocardiogram for abnormal patterns such as atrial fibrillation or notched P waves.
- Determine the patient's anxiety level, ability to perform activities of daily living, and knowledge about cardiac disorders.

NURSING DIAGNOSES, PLANNING, AND NURSING INTERVENTIONS

NDx: Altered tissue perfusion: peripheral, related to the imbalance between oxygen supply and oxygen demand secondary to cardiac valvular disease

Planning: Patient outcomes

1. Patient demonstrates a decrease in peripheral edema.
2. Patient reports a decrease in numbness and tingling in the extremities.
3. Patient's skin remains appropriate without paleness or cyanosis.

Nursing Interventions

Conserve oxygen needs by promoting rest and assisting the patient with activities of daily living.
Elevate the head of the bed to aid in lung expansion.
Initiate oxygen therapy.
Use range-of-motion exercises to stimulate circulation.
Discourage smoking to prevent vasoconstriction.
Provide a low-sodium diet to reduce fluid retention.
Monitor vital signs and laboratory studies to assess pulmonary, circulatory, and renal function.

NDx: Knowledge deficit: Nature of cardiac valvular disorder and misconceptions about the disease process and treatment

Planning: Patient outcomes

1. Patient verbalizes understanding about the disorder.

2. Patient reports accurate information about the treatments and lifestyle changes.
3. Patient demonstrates cooperation with the treatment plan and follow-up care.

Nursing Interventions

Explain the cause, effect, and clinical course of cardiac valve disease and the resulting complications to the patient.

Allow time for questions from the patient and family.

Instruct about dietary modifications needed to reduce risk or prevent complications.

Teach the patient to participate in a moderate exercise program to increase circulation and to maintain strength and endurance.

Assist the patient to adapt to changes necessary to perform activities of daily living.

Evaluate any special discharge needs of the patient and family.

If the patient is to have surgery, explain the preoperative and postoperative course.

◆ Multiple Myeloma

Multiple myeloma is a malignant disease that is characterized by the growth of plasma cells that invade bone marrow, lymph nodes, liver, spleen, and kidneys. The cause of multiple myeloma is unknown. It develops slowly over a period of time, occurring in older adults at a median age of 60 years. Occurrence is twice as high in men as women. Bone marrow, which is usually 5% plasma cells, becomes 30 to 95% plasma cells, most of which are immature and malignant. Medical management involves chemotherapy, some radiotherapy, transfusions, and pain medication. Fewer than 10% of the patients survive more than 5 years.

ASSESSMENT

- Check vital signs, listening carefully for inspiratory crackles or absent breath sounds over involved lung areas.

- Observe for pallor, cyanosis, poor skin turgor, elevated temperature, rapid pulse, and tachypnea.
- Assess the patient's pain, noting the intensity, frequency, location, duration, and what measures are effective for relief of the discomfort.
- Check for changes in urinary output and symptoms related to the presence of renal stones.
- Monitor laboratory studies for the presence of Bence Jones protein in the urine, or above normal levels of calcium in blood or urine.
- Observe for somnolence, polydipsia, anorexia, peripheral neuropathy, and constipation, which are indicative of hypercalcemia or uremia.
- Watch for changes in activity levels and ambulation.
- Assess for changes in the pelvis, spine, and ribs, kyphosis, and symptoms of pathologic fractures.
- Check for retinal hemorrhages, papilledema, and epistaxis.
- Assess the patient's level of understanding about the disorder and emotional status.

NURSING DIAGNOSES, PLANNING, AND NURSING INTERVENTIONS

NDx: Pain related to the malignant infiltration into bone

Planning: Patient outcomes

1. Patient reports pain is controlled with analgesics.
2. Patient identifies comfort measures to help relieve pain.
3. Patient uses relaxation measures to alleviate or help tolerate the pain.

Nursing Interventions

Place the patient in comfortable positions and assist with frequent repositioning.

Give pain medications as ordered prior to activity periods so they can be better tolerated.

Help the patient find alternate measures, such as relaxation techniques, to alleviate or tolerate the pain.

Assess when the pain is most severe and allow the patient to rest during those periods.

Additional Interventions

Assist the patient in counteracting calcium overload by promoting increased oral fluid intake to as much as 4000 mL/day, unless otherwise contraindicated.

Record the consistency and amount of urine.

Prevent complications of hypercalcemia and osteoporosis by encouraging ambulation, with assistance and safety devices as needed.

Provide good skin care using skin-softening soaps, soft towels, and lotions to prevent dryness.

Myocardial Infarction (MI)

Myocardial infarction is death of myocardial tissue due to insufficient oxygen resulting from prolonged ischemia. If that portion of myocardial tissue is supplied by other nearby vessels, called collateral vessels, they may take over when there is insufficient blood supply to the myocardium, but if there are no collateral vessels, ischemia results. Prolonged ischemia leads to death of the cells in the affected area, resulting in infarction. The infarction can occur in any part of the heart but usually affects the left ventricle, either the inferior wall, the anterior and lateral walls, or the septum along with the adjoining wall. Substernal pain which may radiate to the neck, jaw, or left arm is the classic symptom of an MI. Treatment initially includes rest, analgesia, oxygen, and early detection and treatment of dysrhythmias. Pharmacologic therapy is based upon the specific dysrhythmia exhibited.

ASSESSMENT

- Assess the patient for pain immediately, determining the location, duration, severity and radiation.
- Check the patient's respiratory status, cardiac rhythm, and vital signs, and seek medical assistance as soon as possible.
- Determine the patient's ECG pattern.

NURSING DIAGNOSES, PLANNING AND NURSING INTERVENTIONS

NDx: Pain related to tissue ischemia secondary to coronary artery occlusion

Planning: Patient outcomes

1. Patient verbalizes relief or control of chest pain.
2. Patient demonstrates a relaxed manner and is able to rest quietly.
3. Patient's vital signs are within normal ranges for the patient.

Nursing Interventions

Monitor and document the characteristics of the chest pain as described by the patient.

Note nonverbal signs of pain as well as hemodynamic changes such as heart rate, respiratory rate, and blood pressure as the pain changes.

Instruct the patient to report any chest pain immediately.

Explain the medications and procedures that are used to relieve the pain.

Provide a calm, quiet environment and comfort measures to ensure effectiveness of the pain medications.

Teach the patient to use relaxation techniques for pain reduction and to relieve anxiety.

Approach the patient in a calm, confident manner.

Check vital signs prior to administering medication for pain.

Administer oxygen by nasal cannula as indicated to promote oxygen perfusion of the myocardium.

NDx: Anxiety related to change in health status, possible death, or loss of socioeconomic status

Planning: Patient outcomes

1. Patient states feelings about health status and identifies causes for the feelings.
2. Patient verbalizes a reduction in anxiety.
3. Patient demonstrates positive problem-solving skills.

4. Patient seems relaxed, less anxious and is resting well.

Nursing Interventions

Acknowledge the patient's anxiety and the perception of the threat of the situation.

Encourage expression of feelings of anger, fear or grief.

Orient the patient to routine procedures and explain all activities that take place in the patient's room.

Allow the family to express feelings and ask questions.

Keep both the patient and family apprised of changes in the patient's status or treatment plans.

Seek assistance from clergy or significant others if necessary to help allay the patient's anxiety.

Answer all questions factually and provide consistent reinforcement since the ability to understand and remember may be temporarily impaired.

Accept, but do not reinforce, the use of denial.

Support grieving behavior and let the patient know it is a normal response.

Encourage independence, self care, and decision-making.

NDx: Decreased cardiac output related to changes in cardiac rate, rhythm, or electrical conduction

Planning: Patient outcomes

1. Patient demonstrates a decrease in dysrhythmias as seen by the hemodynamic monitoring.
2. Patient demonstrates an increase in activity tolerance.
3. Patient experiences decreased episodes of dyspnea.
4. Patient's vital signs are within normal ranges for the patient.

Nursing Interventions

Treat life-threatening dysrhythmias immediately.

Provide a bedside commode to decrease expenditure of energy that is required when using a bedpan or ambulating to the bathroom.

Administer supplemental oxygen as indicated.

Elevate the head of the bed to allow for maximum lung expansion to increase oxygen intake.

Place needed utensils near the patient to save energy from
　　　excessive movement.
Feed the patient if necessary, when allowed to eat, to
　　　conserve energy.
Allow the patient time to rest between treatments and
　　　limit visitors and extra activity in the room.

NDx:　　Knowledge deficit: nature of myocardial infarction and/or coronary artery disease and treatment and
expected outcomes or potential lifestyle change

Planning: Patient outcomes

1.　　Patient verbalizes understanding of heart disease,
　　　present condition and symptoms that require im-
　　　mediate attention.
2.　　Patient verbalizes understanding of lifestyle changes
　　　such as dietary modifications, exercise, or ceasing
　　　smoking.
3.　　Patient states the purposes of prescribed medica-
　　　tions, the dose, time, frequency and side effects.

Nursing Interventions

Explain the cause, effects and clinical course of coronary
　　　artery disease and the resulting myocardial infarc-
　　　tion to the patient.
Allow time for questions from the patient at any time.
Allow patient to verbalize concerns and fears.
Evaluate discharge needs of the patient and family (see
　　　Chart 18-2).
Alert the patient to signs and symptoms of myocardial
　　　infarction for the future and the complications.
Teach the patient to use safety measures or ask for assis-
　　　tance when out of bed or when ambulating until
　　　strength and endurance improves.
Instruct the patient about dietary modifications needed to
　　　reduce risk or prevent complications of the disor-
　　　der.
Explain the need for a reduction diet if the patient is
　　　obese.
Give the patient meal plans based on the predetermined
　　　caloric limitation.

Explain the need for decreases in dietary fats and cholesterol to prevent the effects of the disease and increases in protein and vitamins to promote good health and healing.

Initiate counseling with a dietitian to assist with meal planning if needed.

Teach the patient about the effects of smoking and the importance of ceasing smoking and refer the patient to a stop smoking program.

Plan an exercise regimen for post-discharge which gradually increases the intensity and endurance of the exercise, as prescribed by the physician.

Teach the patient dosage, route, time, frequency, side effects and toxic effects of any medication prescribed.

Explain the diagnostic studies completed and the need for any follow-up studies after discharge.

Include the family in any of the teaching sessions when applicable.

Nephrotic Syndrome

A condition characterized by severe proteinuria, edema, and hypoalbuminemia. It is usually the result of glomerulonephritis, but may also follow neoplasm, metabolic disease, collegen disorders, renal thrombosis, or a pathogenic disease. Treatment includes correcting the underlying cause, protein replacement, restricted sodium diet, diuretic therapy, and antibiotics. The nephrotic syndrome may progress to chronic renal failure.

NURSING CARE

The nursing care for the patient with nephrotic syndrome is similar to that for a patient with *glomerulonephritis* and *chronic renal failure*.

ADDITIONAL INTERVENTIONS

Check vital signs, taking the blood pressure both supine and erect.

Monitor the oral intake and urine output.

Check the urine for protein content.

Instruct the patient about a low-sodium, high-protein diet.

◆ Osteoarthritis (Degenerative Joint Disease)

Osteoarthritis is a nonsystemic form of arthritis that is less destructive than rheumatoid arthritis, but causes degenerative changes in the joint surfaces of weight-bearing joints such as the spine, hips, and knees, and in the frequently used joints of the hand. It is the most common form of arthritis. Primary osteoarthritis is attributed to a genetic predisposition to deterioration of articular cartilage. Secondary osteoarthritis is the result of excessive "wear and tear" or trauma to affected joints. Treatment can slow the joint destruction. Enteric-coated aspirin and nonsteroidal anti-inflammatory agents are prescribed to relieve pain and parenteral steroids are injected into acutely inflamed joints. If the patient is obese, a weight reduction diet is recommended. Arthroplasty or joint replacement may be done to improve range of motion and reduce pain.

NURSING CARE

Nursing care for the patient with osteoarthritis is similar to that for a patient with rheumatoid arthritis. For the patient having a joint replacement for osteoarthritis, see the Total Joint Replacement entry in this text.

◆ Osteomalacia

Osteomalacia is a metabolic bone disorder that is characterized by a decrease of calcium and phosphorus deposits in new bone matrix, resulting in weak bone mass. It is caused by a lack of vitamin D, either dietary deficiency or malabsorption, which is essential for the mineralization of bone. Malabsorption of vitamin D secondary to hepatobiliary disease is the most common etiology of osteomalacia in the United States. Management of osteomalacia focuses on treating the underlying cause. Supplements of vitamin D and phosphorus may be prescribed along with a program of progressive exercises to promote recalcification of bone.

ASSESSMENT

- Observe the patient's presenting symptoms, noting deformities and areas of weakness.
- Assess for pain, noting its intensity, location, and duration.
- Observe for abnormal curvature of the spine and bowing of the long bones.
- Assess the patient's nutritional pattern.
- Determine the intake of vitamin D, calcium, and phosphorus.
- Assess the patient's level of understanding of the disorder and treatment program.

NURSING DIAGNOSES, PLANNING, AND NURSING INTERVENTIONS

NDx: Pain related to structural changes in bones and deformities in limbs

Planning: Patient outcomes

1. Patient denies discomfort or extreme pain in limbs.
2. Patient relates accurate information about analgesics prescribed.

Nursing Interventions

Give prescribed analgesics and teach the patient about the frequency, dose, side effects, and therapeutic effects.

Teach the patient relaxation strategies to reduce pain.

Tell the patient to refrain from weight bearing during painful episodes.

Pad bony prominences when the patient is in bed.
Assist with ambulation to reduce weight bearing.

NDx: Altered health maintenance related to lack of understanding about the disorder, its treatment and prevention

Planning: Patient outcomes

1. Patient states accurate information about the disorder, its prognosis, and treatment measures.
2. Patient demonstrates exercises that promote increased bone growth and performs them as prescribed.
3. Patient states accurate information on the appropriate diet and medication therapy.

Nursing Interventions

Teach the patient about the disorder, explaining its cause, symptoms, and treatment regimens.
Tell the patient about the proper use of prescribed medications.
Explain the need to take the supplements continually to help reverse the effects of the disorder and to prevent further damage.
Demonstrate the prescribed exercises and encourage the patient to practice them frequently since they will promote increased bone recalcification and formation.
Review a diet plan that contains food high in vitamins, calcium, and phosphorus with the patient.
Teach the patient how to read food labels for nutritional content.
Note which food the patient chooses from the daily hospital menu and reinforce good choices.

◆ Osteomyelitis

Osteomyelitis is an infection of the bone that may result in necrosis of bone and marrow tissue. It weakens the bone and places it at risk for spontaneous pathologic fractures or fractures with minimum trauma. It may be caused by bacteria, virus, tubercle bacilli, or the presence of foreign material. Pathogens may enter from direct contamination to an open fracture or spread from pathogens present in the blood stream. Osteomyelitis may be acute or chronic. Management consists of aggressive antibiotic therapy, wound debridement, and, if necessary, amputation.

ASSESSMENT

- Review patient's history, presenting symptoms, and diagnostic studies.
- Assess for outward signs of infection in the affected area: redness, warmth, swelling, pain.
- Ask patient about severity and duration of pain and successful relief methods.
- Check vital signs and for additional signs of fever such as flushing, night sweats, and chilling.
- Determine patient's understanding of the disease process and treatment regimen.

NURSING DIAGNOSES, PLANNING, AND NURSING INTERVENTION

NDx: Pain related to infection and inflammation

Planning: Patient outcomes

1. Patient denies pain in affected part.
2. Patient states methods to decrease pain, such as using relaxation strategies, and reduced swelling and trauma to the affected part.

Nursing Interventions

Administer prescribed analgesics and nonsteroidal anti-inflammatory drugs.

Explain the dosage, frequency, side effects, and expected therapeutic effects of the medications.

Instruct and support the patient in nonpharmacologic pain control methods.

Teach the patient to elevate and provide support to the involved body part, which will reduce swelling and pain.

Teach the patient about weight bearing if contraindicated, which might increase the pain significantly.

Teach the patient relaxation techniques.

NDx: Knowledge deficit: nature of disease, treatment, and prognosis

Planning: Patient outcomes

1. Patient states accurate information about the cause of the disease and methods to reduce complications.
2. Patient discusses concerns about the disease and states an understanding of the prognosis and treatment regimen.

Nursing Interventions

Teach the patient about the disease, the cause, methods of prevention of injury to the affected part, and appropriate treatment.

Instruct the patient that increased swelling, redness, discoloration, or decreased sensation in the affected part may be signs of complications and that the physician should be notified.

Reinforce the physician's instruction about weightlifting or weight bearing.

Teach the therapeutic effects, side effects, dosage, and frequency of the prescribed antibiotics.

Emphasize the importance of adherence to long-term antibiotic regimen and follow-up appointments.

NDx: Risk of recurrent or spreading infection related to knowledge deficit

Planning: Patient outcomes

1. Patient states local and systemic signs of infection.
2. Patient states knowledge of when to alert health care providers.

Nursing Interventions

Teach the patient about signs and symptoms of local and systematic infection and the need to inform a healthcare provider of these findings.

Provide written material for reinforcement.

Provide for continuity through referral to home or community nursing service when necessary.

◆ Osteoporosis

Osteoporosis is a metabolic bone disorder that is characterized by thinning, less dense, or porous bone mass, resulting in fragile, easy-to-fracture bones. Normal bone loss with aging is referred to as *osteopenia*. More severe bone loss that is age-related is called *primary* or *senile osteoporosis*. Factors putting individuals at high risk for osteoporosis include increasing age in white females, low dietary intake of calcium, diminished mobility, and estrogen depletion secondary to surgical or biologic menopause. The goals of management are protection from pathologic fractures and prevention of further bone loss. The use of good body mechanics decreases the risk of pathologic fractures. A back brace or corset may protect the vertebrae and help relieve back pain.

ASSESSMENT

- Assess pain, noting the intensity, location, duration, precipitating factors, and relief measures.
- Complete a musculoskeletal system assessment noting deformities, strength, range of motion, and structural changes such as diminishing height.
- Observe the patient's ability to move freely.
- Assess the patient's knowledge about the disorder, its manifestations, treatment, and prevention methods.
- Ask the patient if falls have been a problem.
- Determine the safety of the patient's environment.

NURSING DIAGNOSES, PLANNING, AND NURSING INTERVENTIONS

NDx: Risk for injury; falls, related to lack of bone integrity causing weakness and fractures

Planning: Patient outcomes

1. Patient states methods to promote safe mobility.
2. Patient uses ambulatory aids properly.

3. Patient requests assistance when needed to prevent falls.

Nursing Interventions

Teach the patient and family about injury prevention.
Help the patient and family plan strategies to make the home environment safer for the patient.
Tell the patient to ask for assistance when ambulating, if needed, to prevent a fall.
Teach the patient how to use ambulatory aid devices.
Observe the patient while using the device, checking for proper handling.
Request a referral for the patient to see a physical therapist for mobility assistance.

NDx: Impaired physical mobility related to pain, fractures and limited range of motion

Planning: Patient outcomes

1. Patient is able to perform activities of daily living.
2. Patient maintains maximum mobility of extremities.
3. Patient describes methods to compensate for limited mobility.

Nursing Interventions

Encourage maximal performance of activities of daily living to promote independence.
Assist the patient in locomotion as needed for safety.
Encourage ambulation to prevent the problems of disuse.
Utilize the assistance of the physical therapist to instruct the patient and family about the prescribed ambulatory aid and to reinforce its safe use.
Give analgesics as needed to decrease pain levels that may interfere with the patient's ability to be mobile.
Encourage participation in a daily exercise program to maintain strength and joint mobility.

NDx: Pain related to structural changes in bones and deformities in limbs

Planning: Patient outcomes

1. Patient denies discomfort or extreme pain in limbs.
2. Patient relates accurate information about analgesics prescribed.

Nursing Interventions

Give prescribed analgesics and teach the patient about the frequency, dose, side effects, and therapeutic effects.

Talk with the patient about relaxation strategies to reduce pain.

Teach the patient how to apply the back brace and when to use it.

Tell the patient to refrain from weight bearing during painful episodes.

Pad bony prominences when the patient is in bed.

Assist with ambulation to reduce weight bearing.

NDx: Altered health maintenance related to lack of understanding about the disorder, its treatment, and prevention

Planning: Patient outcomes

1. Patient states accurate information about the disorder, its prognosis, and treatment measures.
2. Patient demonstrates exercises that promote increased bone growth and performs them as prescribed.
3. Patient states accurate information on the appropriate diet and medication therapy.

Nursing Interventions

Teach the patient about the disorder, explaining its cause, symptoms, and treatment regimens.

Tell the patient about the proper use of prescribed medications.

Explain the need to take the calcium supplements continually to help reverse the effects of the disorder and to prevent further damage.

Demonstrate the prescribed exercises and encourage the patient to practice them frequently.

Review a diet plan with the patient that contains food high in calcium, vitamin D, and phosphorus.

Teach the patient how to interpret food labels for nutritional content.

Teach the patient safety measures and how to create a safe environment in the home.

Demonstrate the use of ambulatory aids if needed.

 Pancreatic Cancer

Pancreatic cancers are usually adenomas arising from the epithelial lining of the duct system. Most originate in the head of the pancreas. As the tumor grows, it blocks the ducts and frequently extends into nearby structures such as the stomach, liver, and intestines as well as into the lymph nodes. The tumor tends to grow quickly and rapidly metastasizes to the liver, lungs or bones. Management of pancreatic cancer is usually surgical. If the head of the pancreas is involved and there is no metastasis, a radical pancreatoduodenectomy (Whipple procedure) is done. The treatment goal for all other pancreatic cancers is palliation of symptoms through a combination of a simple surgical procedure such as cholecystojejunostomy, radiation, and chemotherapy.

See entries under Chemotherapy and Radiation Therapy in Section II for information on related nursing care.

 Pancreatitis

Acute pancreatitis is a diffuse inflammation of the pancreas caused by activation of pancreatic enzymes within the organ itself, which precipitates a process of pancreatic autodigestion. The precise reason for pancreatic enzyme activation is unknown; however, obstruction of the pancreatic ducts and reflux of duodenal contents into the pancreas are considered etiologic factors. Acute pancreatitis is associated with the excessive use of alcohol, thiazide diuretics, steroids, acetaminophen, and oral contraceptives; biliary tract disease; and abdominal surgery or other trauma. The cause of chronic pancreatitis is similar to that of the acute form except it does not occur in association with biliary tract disease. Management of acute pancreatitis includes keeping the patient NPO; administering anticholinergic and analgesic drugs, antibiotics, and insulin as necessary; instituting nasogastric suction; and administering Ringer's lactate, blood, and oxygen therapy as needed. Management of chronic pancreatitis includes a low-fat, high-carbohydrate, high-protein, bland diet with abstention from alcohol and caffeine; as well as oral pancreatic enzymes, anticholinergic drugs, antacids, gastric acid inhibitors, and parenteral vitamin B12.

ASSESSMENT

- Assess for intense left upper quadrant abdominal pain radiating to the midback or left shoulder, nausea, and vomiting.
- Check vital signs, hemodynamic status, and urinary output.
- Observe for ascites and signs of electrolyte imbalance.
- Inspect the oral and nasal mucosa for dryness and cracking.
- Assess for signs of respiratory infection.
- Auscultate for bowel sounds every 4 hours.
- Assess for weight loss and frothy, foul-smelling stools.

NURSING DIAGNOSES, PLANNING, AND NURSING INTERVENTIONS

NDx: Pain related to the inflammatory process in abdomen

Planning: Patient outcomes

1. Patient states pain is diminished.
2. Patient assumes a high Fowler's position without discomfort.

Nursing Interventions

Administer medications as ordered.
Maintain a calm, quiet environment.
Institute comfort measures.
Guide the patient in relaxation exercises.

NDx: Risk for fluid volume deficit related to vomiting, gastric suction, and activation of pancreatic enzymes

Planning: Patient outcomes

1. Skin turgor is normal.
2. Mucous membranes are moist.
3. Vital signs are within patient's baseline range.
4. Capillary refill is within normal limits.
5. Fluid intake approximates fluid output.

Nursing Interventions

Monitor vital signs hourly.
Monitor the amount of nasogastric tube drainage and check it and the stool for signs of bleeding.
Measure urinary output hourly.
Administer IV fluids as ordered.
Monitor laboratory data related to fluid and electrolyte status.

NDx: Altered oral mucous membrane related to drying effects of NPO status and anticholinergic drugs

Planning: Patient outcomes

1. Oral mucous membranes are moist and supple.
2. Oral mucous membranes are free of cracks.

Nursing Interventions

Encourage the patient to rinse the mouth every 1 to 2 hours while awake.
Avoid the use of glycerin and commercial mouthwashes that contain drying agents.
Apply water-soluble lubricant to the lips as needed.

NDx: Risk for altered health maintenance related to insufficient knowledge of self care after discharge

Planning: Patient outcomes

1. Patient describes dietary and other lifestyle adjustments to be followed after discharge.
2. Patient verbalizes intent to comply with lifestyle adjustments.

Nursing Interventions

Explain to the patient and family that the recovery period is extended.

Reinforce to the patient and family the need to avoid alcohol completely and refer to Alcoholics Anonymous as necessary.

Instruct the patient in therapeutic diet and medications as follows:

- Avoid large meals.
- Eat small amounts of food high in carbohydrates (450 g) and proteins (120 g).
- Eat only small amounts of fats (30 g) until there is no evidence of steatorrhea.
- Limit fiber intake because this may increase steatorrhea.
- Eliminate coffee, tea, and spices from the diet because they stimulate pancreatic secretion.
- Avoid alcohol completely because it can stimulate the pancreas and can precipitate acute attacks of pancreatitis.
- Report as directed for vitamin B12 injections.
- Take prescribed enzyme replacements with or immediately after meals, being certain to swallow them whole and not disrupt their protective coating with hot foods or liquids.

Additional Interventions

Maintain the patient in Fowler's position to promote respiratory expansion.

Turn the patient and encourage coughing and deep breathing every 2 hours while awake.

Apply water-soluble lubricant to naris to lessen irritation from NG tube.

Give small, frequent feedings as ordered once bowel sounds have returned.

◆ Parkinson's Disease

Parkinson's disease is a progressive neurologic disorder that is characterized by degenerative changes in the basal ganglia that result in decreased levels of dopamine. Its cause is unknown, but viral agents, genetic predisposition, and premature aging are considered possible etiologic factors. Management consists primarily of drug therapy and includes the use of amantadine (Symmetrel), bromocriptine, levodopa and carbidopa (Sinemet), anticholinergics, and selegiline (Eldepryl). Alternative treatments are currently under investigation.

ASSESSMENT

- Observe for resting tremors (a pill-rolling motion of the hands when at rest), muscle rigidity, bradykinesia, flexion posture, "stooped" appearance, shuffling, propulsive gait, and loss of automatic, coordinated movement.
- Assess for fatigue, expressionless, mask-like face with fixed gaze, drooling, oily skin, dysphagia, urinary hesitancy, depression, irritability, heat insensitivity, dysarthria, and a whispering monotone voice.
- Determine the patient's ability to communicate.
- Explore the patient's current medication regimen.
- Assess the patient's ability to perform ADL.
- Assess the social and emotional impact of the disease on the lifestyle and self-concept of the patient.

NURSING DIAGNOSES, PLANNING, AND NURSING INTERVENTIONS

NDx: Impaired physical mobility related to muscular rigidity, bradykinesia, muscle tremors, and loss of postural reflexes

Planning: Patient outcomes

1. Patient performs ADL.
2. Patient maintains current level of mobility with or without assistance.
3. Patient remains free from accidental injury.

Nursing Interventions

Encourage the patient to be as physically independent in ADL as possible.
Provide active and passive range of motion exercises at least every 6 hours.

Allow sufficient time to perform ADL.

Provide for periods of activity and rest.

Administer medications as prescribed to reduce and control symptoms.

Evaluate the patient's response to the medications, including the degree of symptom relief and side effects.

Instruct patient to reduce the intake of vitamin B_6 and high protein foods that decrease the level of available dopamine.

Consult with the physical and occupational therapists to assist the patient in mobility and to provide assistive devices.

Instruct the patient regarding safety hazards and maintenance of a safe environment.

Instruct the patient to walk erect, use a wide base marching gait, and swing arms

Advise that warm baths help to relieve rigidity.

NDx: Self-esteem disturbance related to physical limitations and changes in appearance

Planning: Patient outcomes

1. Patient verbalizes positive feelings about self.
2. Patient maintains social interactions with family and friends.

Nursing Interventions

Allow the patient to verbalize fears and feelings about loss of function.

Inform the patient about the resources and support groups available.

Explore strengths, weaknesses, and effective coping and defense mechanisms.

Assist the patient in setting realistic short-term goals.

Discuss the impact of symptoms on self-image.

Support physical and social activities within physical limitations.

Instruct the patient in the use of self-help devices for feeding and dressing.

NDx: Impaired verbal communication related to dysarthria, and whispering monotone speech

Planning: Patient outcomes

1. Patient communicates without frustration.
2. Patient uses alternate methods of communication as necessary.

Nursing Interventions

Provide an accepting, unrushed environment for the patient to communicate.

Decrease noise and move in close proximity when communicating with the patient.

Ask questions that require a yes or no answer.

Recognize the patient's frustration when communication is unsuccessful.

Instruct the patient to perform face and tongue exercises to maintain optimal muscle strength.

Consult with the speech therapist.

Encourage the patient to clearly convey feelings.

NDx: Risk for altered health maintenance related to insufficient knowledge of self care

Planning: Patient outcomes

1. Patient and family describe self-care measures presented below.
2. Patient and family verbalize willingness and ability to follow guidelines presented below.

Nursing Interventions

Instruct the patient and family in self-care measures as follows:

- Provide good lighting in all living areas.
- Remove all loose or scattered rugs.
- Remove doorsills that are easily stumbled over.
- Place sharp-cornered tables or other objects out of the traffic pattern, so that if the patient should fall, the likelihood of injury from striking a sharp object is decreased.
- Arrange patient's living quarters on one floor if possible.
- Install sturdy stair rails on both sides if stairs are unavoidable.

- Install handles on walls adjacent to doorknobs to provide the patient with a secure source of support while he or she opens doors.
- Facilitate getting in and out of chairs by using a chair with sturdy arms and a slightly forward tip. The forward tip can be arranged by having a carpenter lengthen the back legs or by placing secure 2- to 4-inch blocks under them.
- Facilitate getting in and out of bed by placing a heavy piece of furniture next to the bed for support or by tying a rope or a sheet with a knot in the end to the bottom of the bed to use to pull self into a sitting position.
- Install bars on either side of the toilet to facilitate getting on and off the toilet. Buy or make a toilet seat that is elevated 2 inches above the bowl to allow patient to remain seated while wiping self.
- Keep home temperature slightly above normal to eliminate need for layers of clothing that are difficult for the patient to put on and that increase the difficulty of moving.
- Use elastic shoelaces or wear shoes with Velcro fasteners to avoid having to tie the shoes or tripping on untied laces.
- Use Velcro patches to fasten clothing; maintain proper appearance by sewing buttons on the top surface.
- Leave neckties knotted; slip over head and tighten to wear.
- Choose raglan rather than set-in sleeves.
- Contact rehabilitation center or support group for information about companies in your area that carry specially designed "easy to get into and out of" clothes.
- Perform daily home exercises as taught.
- Participate in a formal exercise program once or twice a week; this may be an individual session or a group session offered through a Parkinson patient self-help group.
- Remember that overdoing exercises can be counterproductive, so follow physician's guidelines carefully.
- Remain involved in family and social activities.

- Drive if able, but consider staying in low-traffic areas and having another driver with you to allow breaks if needed.
- Be aware that there is no need to restrict travel, although having a companion along is desirable.
- Eat 1500 to 2000 calories per day.
- Eat small, frequent meals because problems chewing, swallowing, and handling food items makes eating a slow, difficult process.
- Reduce dietary protein moderately because proteins reduce the absorption of levodopa; do not drastically reduce protein unless specified by your physician.
- Use an electric warming tray to keep foods warm and palatable during the time it takes to eat.
- Select foods that are easy to handle, chew, and swallow, such as mashed potatoes and other vegetables, meat loaf, and stew.
- Remember that semi-solid foods are easier to swallow than liquids or solids and that a commercial product (Thick-It) is available that can be used to thicken fruit juices and carbonated beverages.
- Keep a light on at night.
- Keep a radio playing softly.
- Consult a physician if serious sleep pattern disturbances persist, because a change in medication may be helpful.

◆ Peptic Ulcer Disease

Peptic ulcer refers to a sharply defined break in the muscularis mucosa in any part of the GI tract that is exposed to gastric juice containing acid and pepsin. Thus a peptic ulcer can occur in the distal esophagus, the stomach, the duodenum, or any part of the stomach that has been surgically connected to the stomach. When referring to an ulcer it is necessary to identify it by location; for example, a gastric ulcer or a duodenal ulcer, because there are differences in incidence and etiology. Gastric ulcers apparently result from decreased mucosal resistance to gastric acid whereas duodenal ulcers result from increased exposure to gastric acid secondary to an increase in its volume and more rapid entering into the duodenum. Management is similar for both gastric and duodenal ulcers. It consists of dietary modifications, rest, antacids to neutralize gastric acid and provide an environment conducive to healing the ulcer and histamine H_2-receptor antagonists to decrease secretion of gastric acid. Other drugs used include sucralfate and the proton pump inhibitors as well as antibiotic therapy. Surgery such as gastric resection or subtotal gastrectomy, vagotomy, and pyloroplasty is used when conservative measures are ineffective or when required by complications.

ASSESSMENT

- Assess for pain (type, location, time of onset, precipitating factors), nausea, vomiting, and change in appetite or weight.
- Explore dietary habits, use of prescription and nonprescription drugs, use of tobacco and alcohol, patient's perceived level of stress, and methods of coping.
- Assess the probability of the patient's complying with therapy.
- Assess for symptoms of complications:
- Perforation—sudden, sharp colicky pain beginning in the midepigastric area and spreading over the abdomen, rigid boardlike abdomen, nausea, occasionally vomiting, decreased to absent bowel sounds, rapid, shallow respirations, tachycardia, cold, clammy skin, and hypotension.
- Obstruction—sensation of fullness followed by vomiting of partially digested gastric contents; abdominal distention.
- Hemorrhage—hematemesis, coffee ground material in emesis or NG drainage, melena.

NURSING DIAGNOSES, PLANNING, AND NURSING INTERVENTIONS

NDx: Pain related to the irritating effects of gastric acid on injured tissue

Planning: Patient outcomes

1. Patient describes dietary modifications conducive to pain reduction.
2. Patient selects or plans nutritionally balanced meals that exclude pain-producing foods.
3. Patient listed prescribed medications aimed at reducing pain, stating dose, route, and frequency of each.
4. Patient reports that pain is relieved.
5. Patient sleeps through the night without pain.

Nursing Interventions

Teach self-administration of antacids, histamine antagonists, or other medications, adhering strictly to prescribed schedule. For antacids this is usually 1 to 3 hours after meals and at bedtime. If pain occurs at a regular time during the night antacids may be routinely taken 1 hour earlier.

Encourage patient to avoid foods that exacerbate pain.

Explain that foods that cause pain vary from one person to another but usually include highly spiced foods, cola, tea, coffee, and chocolate.

Instruct patient to keep daily log of foods eaten and pain experienced to identify foods to be avoided.

Assist the patient to plan a daily diet that is well tolerated.

Instruct the patient to eat several small meals per day, eat slowly, chew thoroughly, and drink 6 to 8 glasses of water per day.

Maintain a restful environment.

NDx: Risk for altered health maintenance related to insufficient knowledge of disease process, aggravating factors, promotion of physical and psychological rest, and need for follow-up care

Planning: Patient outcomes

1. Patient describes the relationship among gastric acidity, mucosal damage, and symptomatology.
2. Patient lists substances known to aggravate the disease process.

3. Patient describes the relationship of stress to the disease process.
4. Patient describes a plan to reduce stress and promote physical rest.
5. Patient lists symptoms to be reported.

Nursing Interventions

Explain the relationship among gastric acidity, mucosal damage, and symptoms as well as the effects of smoking, caffeine, and drugs containing aspirin.

Discuss importance of physical and psychological rest and explore with the patient strategies for reducing stress and organizing activities to allow for rest period.

Instruct the patient in the importance of follow-up care.

Instruct patient to report severe abdominal pain, nausea, vomiting; abdominal distention or persistence of original symptoms despite compliance with treatment.

NDx: Risk for noncompliance related to dietary modifications, reduction of smoking, or medication regimen

Planning: Patient outcomes

1. Patient reduces smoking.
2. Patient adheres to dietary and medication regime.
3. Complications are absent.

Nursing Interventions

Allow the patient to express feelings about limitations on diet, need to avoid smoking, and the need for daily medications.

Stress that patient is taking control of his or her life when lifestyle changes are made to promote healing of the ulcer.

Assist the patient to identify factors seen as interfering with compliance and to explore ways of dealing with them.

Involve family or significant others in planning for self care.

◆ Peripheral Vascular Disease (PVD)

Peripheral vascular disease is a generic term or category for several disorders that involve reduced blood through peripheral arteries and veins of the extremities. Refer to the following entries in this text for peripheral vascular disorders and associated nursing diagnoses, planning, and nursing interventions: Atherosclerosis, Chronic Arterial Occlusive Disease, and Varicose Veins.

◆ Peritonitis

Peritonitis is an inflammation of the peritoneum due to 1) bacterial infection secondary to escape of organisms through an abnormal opening in the GI tract or to extension of an infection through the wall of a hollow organ, or 2) chemical irritation from GI secretions, e.g., due to leakage of an internal suture line. Management includes IV antibiotics, NG suction, and fluid and electrolyte replacement as well as treatment of the underlying disorder.

ASSESSMENT

- Observe for symptoms of peritonitis: severe, localized abdominal pain intensified by movement; rigid abdomen; nausea and vomiting; sudden spike in temperature and diminished or absent bowel sounds.
- Assess fluid balance: measure intake and output, including NG drainage, and check skin turgor, mucous membranes, and urine specific gravity.
- Monitor for signs of shock: oliguria, tachycardia, hypotension, sweating, and pallor.
- Check vital signs and bowel sounds every 2 to 4 hours.
- Observe for abdominal distention.
- Check for proper functioning of the NG tube.

NURSING DIAGNOSES, PLANNING, AND NURSING INTERVENTIONS

NDx: Pain related to inflammation of the peritoneum.

Planning: Patient outcomes

1. Patient states abdominal pain is relieved.
2. Signs of severe pain, such as knees pulled up, are absent.
3. Patient rests quietly.

Nursing Interventions

Maintain patient on bedrest in semi-Fowler's position to minimize discomfort and promote localization of infection in abdomen.

Use nonpharmacologic measures to promote comfort, since analgesics are used sparingly as they can mask symptoms.

NDx: Risk for altered mucous membrane related to mouth breathing and NPO status.

Planning: Patient outcomes

1. Oral mucous membranes are pink and moist.
2. Lips are smooth and free of cracks.

Nursing Interventions

Brush teeth and rinse mouth frequently, avoiding use of lemon and glycerine swabs and alcohol-containing commercial mouthwashes, which are drying.

Apply water-soluble lubricant to lips to prevent drying and cracking.

Additional Interventions

Administer IV fluids, electrolytes, and antibiotics as ordered.

Keep NG tube taped securely to nose and maintain its function.

Apply water-soluble lubricant to naris to prevent irritation and discomfort.

Give clear fluids as ordered when peristalsis returns and progress diet as tolerated.

◆ Pheochromocytoma

A pheochromocytoma is a catecholamine-producing tumor arising from chromaffin cells of the sympathetic nervous system. It is characterized by unregulated hypersecretion of catecholamines. Most pheochromocytomas occur in the adrenal medulla and are benign tumors. Treatment is surgical excision of the tumor(s).

ASSESSMENT

- Obtain a detailed nursing history.
- Evaluate the blood pressure carefully, observing for paroxysmal malignant hypertensive episodes.
- Collect appropriate urine specimens for urinary catecholamines and their metabolites (VMA).
- Assess the patient's emotional status and knowledge level of the disorder and planned treatment to determine the teaching needs.
- Assess the patient's weight history, present weight, and nutritional status.

NURSING DIAGNOSES, PLANNING, AND NURSING INTERVENTIONS

NDx: Risk for altered tissue perfusion; cardiopulmonary, cerebral, and renal, related to rapid fluctuations in cardiovascular status

Planning: Patient outcomes

1. Patient avoids activities that precipitate hypertensive episodes.
2. Patient notifies the nurse immediately of the onset of hypertensive episode.
3. Patient maintains adequate tissue perfusion preoperatively and postoperatively as evidenced by stable

vital signs within normal ranges, normal neurologic responses, urine output greater than 30 mL/h, and lungs clear upon auscultation.

Nursing Interventions

Monitor vital signs and neurologic signs every 15 minutes for 4 hours during/following a hypertensive crisis.

Admisister catecholamine-blocking agents as prescribed.

Monitor the urine output frequently and weigh the patient daily.

Auscultate heart and lung sounds and report any abnormalities.

Elevate the head of the bed to a semi-Fowler's position and keep the side rails up.

Provide a physically and emotionally restful environment.

NDx: Risk for altered nutrition: Less than body requirements related to increased metabolism, abdominal pain, nausea, vomiting, and/or constipation secondary to prolonged catecholamine hypersecretion

Planning: Patient outcomes

1. Patient maintains a stable weight within the recommended norms.
2. Patient defecates soft, formed stool at least every third day.
3. Patient eats well-balanced, high-fiber, high-calorie meals.

Nursing Interventions

Weigh the patient and compare the results with the acceptable weight norms for the patient.

Monitor the patient's blood glucose levels.

Provide frequent, small well-balanced, high-fiber, high-calorie meals in accordance with the patient's preferences.

Instruct the patient to avoid stimulating foods and beverages.

Administer stool softeners, as needed, to relieve constipation.

NDx: Anxiety related to nervous system overstimulation by excessive levels of catecholamines and knowledge deficit about the disorder

Planning: Patient outcomes

1. Patient identifies the disease process as one cause of the feelings of anxiety.
2. Patient uses relaxation exercises to reduce anxiety.
3. Patient verbalizes knowledge of disorder and its complications and treatment regimen.

Nursing Interventions

Provide factual information to the patient about the effect of increased catecholamine levels on the nervous system.

Encourage the patient to identify and describe feelings and concerns.

Teach the patient relaxation techniques and encourage their use.

Provide emotional support during a hypertensive crisis.

Explain the disorder, its treatment, and complications using terminology understandable to the patient.

Encourage the patient to utilize support systems.

◆ Pneumonia

Pneumonia is an acute inflammation of the respiratory bronchioles, alveolar ducts, alveolar sacs, and alveoli. Pneumonia most often refers to an acute infectious process; however, it can also result from noninfectious causes such as aspiration of gastric contents or a foreign body. In these cases it is referred to as aspiration pneumonia. Infectious pneumonia is classified by its etiology as community acquired, nosocomial (hospital acquired), or opportunistic and may be divided into typical and atypical pneumonia. The majority of community acquired pneumonias (CAP) are viral in origin. Community acquired bacterial pneumonias occur less frequently, are more serious, and commonly require hospitalization among older adults. Nosocomial pneumonias, most often caused by gram-negative organisms, and pneumonias due to other opportunistic organisms have high mortality rates. Management includes adequate hydration, supportive nutrition, supplemental oxygen, bedrest, analgesics, and antibiotics as appropriate. Bronchodilators, chest physiotherapy, and expectorants may be prescribed.

ASSESSMENT

- Assess respiratory status noting respiratory rate, depth, lung sounds, use of accessory muscles, splinting of chest, nasal flaring, dyspnea, and cyanosis.
- Observe for fever, chills, productive cough, chest wall discomfort, and general malaise. Determine the type and location of chest pain and its relationship to inspiration or expiration.
- Note characteristics of the cough (shallow, deep, dry, loose) and sputum (color, odor, consistency, and amount).
- Assess I & O, skin turgor, electrolyte levels, and caloric intake.
- Monitor for signs of complications such as lung abscess, empyema, pulmonary edema, and pleural effusion.
- Monitor oxygenation via pulse oximetry and ABGs.
- Assess the patient's understanding of general health measures.

NURSING DIAGNOSES, PLANNING, AND NURSING INTERVENTIONS

NDx: Ineffective airway clearance related to retained secretions.

Planning: Patient outcomes

1. Patient demonstrates effective coughing and deep breathing techniques.
2. Secretions are thin, white, and watery.
3. Patient coughs and expectorates easily.

Nursing Interventions

Encourage coughing and deep breathing every 2 hours.
Maintain fluid intake at 3 to 4 L per day unless contraindicated.
Suction as necessary and coordinate timing with bronchodilator treatments and postural drainage.
Teach the patient and family breathing techniques and exercises to raise secretions.

NDx: Impaired gas exchange related to ventilation/ perfusion mismatching and increased intrapulmonary shunt

Planning: Patient outcomes

1. Patient states dyspnea is absent.
2. Respiratory rate and depth are within normal limits.
3. Lungs are clear on auscultation.
4. ABG values are within normal limits.

Nursing Interventions

Position the patient to maximize oxygenation by placing the good lung down.
Administer O_2 therapy as prescribed.
Monitor oxygenation via pulse oximetry or ABGs.

NDx: Pain related to chest and lung expansion secondary to infection in the lung

Planning: Patient outcomes

1. Patient demonstrates splinting techniques to reduce discomfort associated with coughing.
2. Patient states pain is diminished or relieved.
3. Patient remains pain free for periods of 4 to 6 hours.

Nursing Interventions

Administer analgesics as needed and ordered.
Assess patient for evidence of cerebral hypoxemia (e.g., restlessness, confusion, aggression) prior to administering an analgesic with a CNS depressant.

Assist the patient to splint the chest during coughing and
deep breathing.

Additional Interventions

Limit the patient's activity while temperature is elevated.
Monitor and record I & O.
Collect sputum specimens as ordered.
Provide time for the patient to ask questions and express
concerns.
Explain expected symptoms and procedures, and reas-
sure the patient as appropriate.
Teach high-risk patients about the benefits of the influ-
enza and pneumococcal vaccine.
Inform the patient who smokes about smoking cessation
programs.
Meet the patient's nutritional needs as follows:
• Provide an intake of at least 1500 calories daily.
• Ensure diet rich in protein.
• Aim for a positive nitrogen balance.
• Provide a liquid or blenderized diet if better toler-
ated.
Instruct the patient in self care after discharge as follows:
• Increase activities gradually to avoid fatigue.
• Obtain sufficient rest and avoid getting chilled.
• Avoid exposure to people with colds and flu.
• Report change or worsening of cough, change in
color of sputum, shortness of breath, or recurrence
of fever.

◆ Pneumothorax and Hemothorax

Pneumothorax is a condition in which there is air or gas
in the pleural space. An open pneumothorax is one in
which a hole in the chest allows atmospheric air to flow
into the pleural space. In a closed (spontaneous) pneumothorax, air enters the pleural space from the lung. In
both types of pneumothorax, the air in the pleural space
causes increased intrapleural pressure resulting in partial
or total collapse of the lung. A tension pneumothorax
occurs when air leaks into the pleural space during inspiration, but is prevented from leaking out during expira-

tion. In addition to collapse of the lung, this results in a mediastinal shift. Hemothorax is an accumulation of blood in the pleural space caused by bleeding of the pulmonary parenchyma, the heart, or blood vessels. Management of both pneumothorax and hemothorax consists of insertion of a chest tube to reestablish the intrapleural pressure. Immediate intervention for a tension pneumothorax includes the insertion of a large bore needle to relieve the tension. An open pneumothorax is covered and taped on three sides.

ASSESSMENT

- Observe for dyspnea, tachypnea, retractions, labored breathing, nasal flaring, cyanosis, asymmetry of the chest wall, cough, restlessness, and contusion.
- Auscultate the chest for distant or diminished breath sounds and for vocal fremitus or hyperresonance on affected side.
- Palpate for tracheal deviation and subcutaneous emphysema.
- Note the characteristics of any cough or sputum.
- Check blood pressure, pulses, patient's color, and I & O.

NURSING DIAGNOSES, PLANNING, AND NURSING INTERVENTIONS

NDx: Impaired gas exchange related to collapse of an area of the lung

Planning: Patient outcomes

1. Respiratory rate and depth are within normal limits.
2. Arterial blood gases are within normal range.

Nursing Interventions

Place the patient in a semi-Fowler's position to facilitate breathing.
Encourage coughing and deep breathing to remove secretions and enhance ventilation.
Administer supplemental oxygen and medications as ordered.

Monitor ABGs, electrolytes, and blood counts.

Provide care as described under Chest Drainage in Section II.

NDx: Anxiety related to dyspnea/treatment

Planning: Patient outcomes

1. Patient states rationale for treatment and procedures.
2. Patient rests without behavioral signs of excessive anxiety.

Nursing Interventions

Explain all procedures as well as overall treatment plan. Be calm and provide the patient with appropriate reassurance.

◆ Prostate Cancer

The cause of prostate cancer is unknown although hormones are generally believed to play a role. Genetic, viral, environmental, and dietary factors may also be involved. Most prostate cancers are adenocarcinomas. Because symptoms generally do not occur until late in the disease, metastasis to the lymph nodes, bone, lung, and liver is common. Central nervous system involvement usually comes after bone involvement. Preferred treatment for cancer of the prostate gland is radical prostatectomy performed via a perineal or retropubic approach. Complications of this procedure include urinary incontinence, stricture of the surgical vesicourethral anastomosis, rectal injury, thromboembolic phenomena, lymphocele, lymphedema, wound infection, bladder neck contracture, and erectile impotence.

Radiation therapy is used for palliation in patients with extensive local prostatic cancer who, because of age or other medical problems, are not appropriate candidates for radical surgery and for those who refuse surgery. In some cases, radiation therapy may be prescribed as adjunction therapy following radical prostatectomy to decrease the likelihood of tumor recurrence. Radiation therapy is also used to control pain in patients with bone metastasis.

Endocrine therapy in the form of bilateral orchiectomy or administration of LHRH analogue and antiandrogen drugs may also be used. Chemotherapy may be used as an adjunctive therapy.

See entries under Prostatectomy, Chemotherapy and Radiation Therapy in Section II for information on related nursing care.

Pulmonary Embolism

Pulmonary embolism is an occlusion of the pulmonary artery or one or more of its branches by matter carried by the blood stream from a vein or the right side of the heart to the lung. Most pulmonary emboli are detached portions of venous thrombi originating in the deep veins of the lower extremities or pelvis (DVT). Predisposing factors include damaged vein endothelium, venous stasis, and hypercoagulability of blood (Virchow's triad). Immobilized patients, including those with cardiac disease, long bone fractures, and pelvic or abdominal surgery, are at greatest risk. Additional risk factors include pregnancy, use of oral contraceptives, varicose veins, and obesity. The best management is prevention through the use of aspirin or low-dose heparin therapy and oral anticoagulants; early ambulation, leg elevation, physiotherapy, elastic stockings, and pneumatic calf compression to prevent stasis; and good hydration. If embolism occurs, management is aimed at stabilization of cardiorespiratory status and institution of anticoagulant therapy to prevent recurrence. Thrombolytic agents and occasionally surgical intervention may also be used.

NURSING CARE

- Check at-risk patients for a positive Homans' sign.
- Assess for tachypnea, tachycardia, dyspnea, chest pain, cough, hemoptysis, pleural friction rub, cyanosis, fever, apprehension, hypotension, and shock.

- Place the patient in semi-Fowler's position to facilitate breathing, administer oxygen, and establish an IV line as ordered.
- Give analgesics as ordered to foster good ventilation because pain is usually pleuritic.
- Implement the prescribed medical regimen of anticoagulant or thrombolytic therapy. Monitor cardiorespiratory status, including ECGs, lung sounds, arterial blood gases, prothrombin time, partial thromboplastin time, oxygen saturation with pulse oximetry, and hemodynamic measurements.
- Check the patient for signs of bleeding.
- Keep the patient informed about his or her condition and reassure the patient that someone will respond quickly if called.
- Institute measures to protect skin from pressure breakdown.
- Instruct patient prior to discharge on self-administration of prescribed anticoagulants, related precautions, and prevention of recurrences.

◆ Rheumatoid Arthritis

Rheumatoid arthritis is a chronic systemic disease that is characterized by inflammation of the joints and extra-articular manifestations. The cause of rheumatoid arthritis is unknown, but it is believed to be an autoimmune disorder. Antibodies produced by the immune system, that usually protect the body, become destructive agents that attack and destroy joint structures. The antibodies first attack the synovium of the joint, causing inflammation and swelling with excess synovial fluid. Eventually, through several degenerative changes, the joint becomes ankylosed or fused. The patient is left with a joint that is painful, deformed, and has very limited or no range of motion. Early management involves education about the disease process, providing adequate nutrition, having the patient maintain good general health while avoiding physical stress, instruction in stress control techniques, and administration of drug therapy to decrease the inflammatory reaction. Long-term care involves several health care professionals to assist the patient in coping with lifestyle changes, maintaining some mobility, and managing self care. Surgical intervention includes synovectomy, arthrodesis, and arthroplasty.

ASSESSMENT

- Assess the patient's pain tolerance, debilitating effects of the disease, and which joints are most affected.
- Determine the patient's perception of the pain experienced, what time of day it is most severe, and what precipitates it.
- Ask the patient which, if any, medications have been beneficial in relieving pain, stiffness, or inflammatory reactions.
- Examine the affected joints, observing for redness, edema, crepitation, deformity, subluxation, dislocation, ankylosis, and muscle contractions.
- Look at the affected limbs, noting atrophy, decreased subcutaneous fat, and the presence of subcutaneous nodules.
- Note mobility problems and difficulties with hand motions.
- Determine the patient's and family's understanding of the disease and its progression.
- Determine if there is need for a referral to rehabilitation therapy services.
- Ask the patient about effective coping mechanisms used in the past and what personal support systems are available.

NURSING DIAGNOSES, PLANNING, AND NURSING INTERVENTIONS

NDx: Pain related to joint or muscle deformity and inflammation

Planning: Patient outcomes

1. Patient reports an absence or tolerable level of pain.
2. Patient identifies methods to decrease pain such as rest and relaxation therapies.
3. Patient describes appropriate use of analgesics or anti-inflammatory agents, and the TENS unit, if prescribed.

Nursing Interventions

Give analgesics and anti-inflammatory agents as prescribed, and explain the dosage, side effects, frequency, and expected therapeutic effects of the medications.

Teach the patient deep breathing, imagery, and distraction techniques, and other full body relaxation strategies.

Move the patient carefully while in bed.

Apply prescribed heat or cold packs to decrease muscle spasms and promote pain relief.

Advise the patient that a warm shower may be helpful to relieve morning pain and stiffness.

Reinforce instructions from the therapist in the use of the TENS unit, as ordered.

Maintain rest and support of affected inflamed joints.

NDx: Impaired physical mobility related to the rheumatoid disease process and pain

Planning: Patient outcomes

1. Patient moves in bed with assistance and an overhead trapeze.
2. Patient performs or is assisted with range-of-motion exercises to maintain strength and joint movement during periods of immobility.
3. Patient maintains mobility with the assistance of an ambulatory aid.

Nursing Interventions

Teach the patient how to use the overhead trapeze while still on bedrest to prevent complications of immobility.

Assist the patient in reducing joint use during acute inflammation.

Reposition the patient frequently to stimulate circulation.

Assist in locomotion to reinforce and promote safe use of ambulatory aids.

Utilize the assistance of a physical therapist to instruct the patient about the ambulatory device.

Encourage the patient to continue to be as mobile as possible.

NDx: Self-esteem disturbance related to change in appearance from deformities and inability to move freely

Planning: Patient outcomes

1. Patient relates feelings of self-worth.
2. Patient maintains social activity.
3. Patient is able to look at self with understanding and acceptance.

Nursing Interventions

Allow the patient to vent feelings about the disorder and provide information about self-help groups.

Assist the patient in the organization of daily tasks to promote the accomplishment of goals.

Encourage the patient to continue to maintain as much independence as possible.

Seek assistance from clergy or professional counseling services to assist the patient in coping with the disease.

Assist the patient to find positive aspects of life to focus on during periods of depression.

Assist the patient and family to utilize effective coping mechanisms.

NDx: Self-care deficit: bathing, dressing, or grooming, related to decrease in strength and deformities of joints with restricted movement

Planning: Patient outcomes

1. Patient cares for self with little assistance from others.
2. Patient utilizes assistive devices to provide support for self-care.
3. Patient practices exercises to maintain joint mobility and, therefore, independence.

Nursing Interventions

Provide assistance with bathing and grooming as needed, while promoting independence.

Teach the patient methods to complete hygiene tasks that use alternatives to the standard techniques, and accommodate the patient's limited joint function.

Explain to the family that Velcro fasteners on garments may be easier for the patient to use than standard snaps and zippers.

NDx: Risk for trauma; falls, related to mobility problems secondary to joint deformity and pain, and improper use of ambulatory aids

Planning: Patient outcomes

1. Patient remains free from injury.
2. Patient demonstrates safe use of ambulatory aid device.
3. Patient states accurate information about the causes of injuries and methods to prevent injury.

Nursing Interventions

Provide assistance with locomotion, as needed, until the patient becomes skillful with the use of the ambulatory aid.

Reinforce the information about the device as presented by the therapist, and teach the family how to assist the patient.

Explain how to make the home environment safer for the patient.

Tell the patient that proper fitting shoes with gripper soles should be worn while ambulating.

◆ Shock

Shock is a syndrome that is characterized by hypoperfusion of body tissues, resulting in hypotension, tachycardia, cool, pale skin, anxiety, diaphoresis, and, potentially, loss of consciousness or death. The various types of shock may be classified as follows:

Hypovolemic shock — characterized by reduction of volume in the vascular compartment by 15 to 25%. It may be due to blood loss as occurs in hemorrhage, fluid losses as occur in heat exhaustion, or fluid shifts as occur in burns. Treatment usually includes administering blood, blood products, intravenous solutions, and plasma expanders.

Cardiogenic shock — characterized by the inability of the heart to pump sufficient blood to perfuse the cells of the body. Treatment includes positive inotropic/contractility medications and interventions to promote optimum preload and afterload reduction.

Vasogenic shock — characterized by massive dilation of blood vessels throughout the body. Specific types of vasogenic shock include neurogenic shock, anaphylactic shock, and septic shock. Treatment includes administering antibiotics, antihistamines, and epinephrine.

ASSESSMENT

- Check the following :
    1. blood pressure, temperature, pulse, and respiratory rate.
    2. arterial blood gases.
    3. central venous pressure, pulmonary arterial pressure, pulmonary capillary wedge pressure, and cardiac output, if appropriate vascular lines are in place.
    4. oral intake and urine output.
    5. body weight.
    6. laboratory data, especially the CBC and electrolytes.
    7. general mental status and orientation.
- Question the patient about the precipitating factors.
- Determine the patient's emotional status.

NURSING DIAGNOSES, PLANNING, AND NURSING INTERVENTIONS

NDx: Altered tissue perfusion, cerebral, cardiopulmonary, renal, gastrointestinal, and peripheral, related to circulatory failure secondary to loss of circulatory control or fluid loss

Planning: Patient outcomes

1. Patient tolerates care interventions without evidence of tissue/organ hypoperfusion.
2. Patient's vital signs remain stable.
3. Patient's intravascular volume, cardiac function, and vascular tone are within normal ranges as evidenced by the hemodynamic monitoring, blood gases, and physical assessment.

Nursing Interventions

Provide emergency equipment and interventions as indicated by the type of shock.

Limit activities and stimulation to reduce oxygen demand on vital organs.

Evaluate the effects of therapy.

Monitor vital signs and hemodynamic changes.

Inform the patient and family of the cause of the shock and treatments to be instituted.

Spinal Cord Injury

Causative factors of traumatic spinal cord injury include vehicular accidents, falls, sports injuries, and gunshot wounds. Trauma to the spinal cord is produced by compression of the spinal cord, can occur at any point along the spinal column, and can range from concussion to complete transection of the cord.

Injuries involving:

*   C3 and above are generally fatal
*   C4 and above are prone to respiratory failure and result in paralysis of all four extremities
*   T6 or above result in quadriplegia
*   T7 or below result in paraplegia (lower extremities)

Injuries to the spinal cord are usually the result of a force exerted on the vertebral column, which in turn affects the spinal cord. These injuries most often affect cervical and lumbar areas of the vertebral column and include hyperflexion, hyperextension, subluxation, and compression injuries. Spinal cord syndromes associated with these injuries include Anterior Cord Syndrome, Brown-Séquard Syndrome (Lateral Cord Syndrome), Central Cord Syndrome, and Homer's Syndrome. Gunshot and stab wounds result in open or direct injuries to the spinal column. Direct injury to the spinal cord causes a loss of function below the level of the area injured. Management of a spinal cord injury may be surgical, nonsurgical, or a combination of both. Nonsurgical treatment includes the use of immobilization and traction. Cervical fractures require skeletal traction or skeletal fixation. Cervical tongs or the halo device are used.

ASSESSMENT

- Assess the patency of airway, rate and depth of respirations, and vital signs.
- Observe motor strength, sensation, and reflexes.
- Assess for symptoms of spinal shock including flaccid paralysis and absence of sensation and perspiration below the level of the lesion, urinary and fecal retention, hypotension, and priapism in males.
- Assess for symptoms of autonomic dysreflexia including hypertension, bradycardia, profuse sweating above the level of the injury, and cyanosis below the level of the injury; and for possible causes such as bowel or bladder distention.

NURSING DIAGNOSES, PLANNING, AND NURSING INTERVENTIONS

NDx: Risk for ineffective breathing pattern related to impaired function of the diaphragm secondary to spinal cord edema

Planning: Patient outcomes

1. Patient has clear bilateral breath sounds.
2. ABG values remain within normal limits for the patient.
3. Patient remains free from pulmonary complications.

Nursing Interventions

Maintain a patent airway with proper positioning and suctioning as needed.

Auscultate breath sounds every 2 to 4 hours.
Encourage the patient to perform coughing and deep-breathing exercises every 2 hours.
Instruct the patient to use an incentive spirometer.
Obtain vital capacity measurements every 6 to 8 hours.
Provide humidity with air mister/vaporizer.
Administer O_2 as ordered.
Obtain ABG values and pulse oximetry readings.

NDx: Risk for injury related to unstable vertebral column

Planning: Patient outcomes

1. Baseline neurologic function is maintained.
2. Immobilization device is correctly maintained.

Nursing Interventions

Maintain traction weights at the ordered level.
Ensure that weights are free-hanging and not lying on the floor or headboard.
Logroll the patient and use adequate help to maintain proper alignment of the head and neck.
Report any deterioration in motor or sensory function immediately.
Notify the physician if looseness of pins, bolts, and/or vest structure (with halo traction) occurs.
If ambulatory, caution the patient in a halo vest regarding limited flexibility of the trunk of the body; provide rubber-soled shoes and a walker until a steady gait develops.

NDx: Impaired physical mobility related to motor and sensory deficits, spine instability

Planning: Patient outcomes

1. Joint flexibility is maintained.

Nursing Interventions

Maintain patient in proper alignment at all times.
Use supports such as hand and trochanter rolls.
Provide passive range of motion exercises every 4 hours.

Instruct the patient in active range of motion exercises as appropriate.

Apply antiembolic hose; remove every 8 hours to assess skin integrity and circulatory status.

Apply posterior splints or high-top sneakers.

Instruct the patient to avoid stimuli that trigger spasms such as fatigue, anxiety, extremes in temperatures, and emotional stress.

Additional Interventions

Inspect skin around the pins of the cervical traction device or halo device every 8 hours.

Cleanse pin area daily as ordered.

Measure input and output.

Force fluids to 3000 mL per 24 hours.

Provide catheter care BID.

Monitor the patient's temperature every 8 hours.

Encourage high-fiber foods.

Administer stool softeners and bulk producers as ordered.

Encourage the patient to express feelings of fear and anger.

Testicular Cancer

Seminomas that grow slowly and are usually localized are the most common type of testicular cancer. Less common nonseminomas tend to be invasive and metastasize quickly via the blood and lymph. Management consists of obtaining baseline serum levels of tumor markers, confirming biopsy with immediate orchiectomy (removal of the testis), diagnostic tests to determine extent of disease, and periodic monitoring of tumor marker levels. Depending on type of tumor and clinical stage of disease, chemotherapy, radiation therapy, and/or more extensive surgery, e.g., radical orchiectomy or retroperitoneal lymphadenectomy, may be done.

INGUINAL ORCHIECTOMY

Preoperative Care

Provide basic care as described under the Preoperative Care entry in this text. Although the diagnosis of cancer is not confirmed until surgery, do not give false hope.

Postoperative Care

Assessment

- Make usual postoperative assessments related to physiologic stabilization.
- Observe for scrotal edema, bleeding, and pain.
- Note time and amount of voiding.
- Assess emotional response to surgery and understanding of any further treatment.

Nursing Diagnoses, Planning, and Nursing Interventions

NDx: Pain (inguinal and scrotal) related to surgical trauma and edema of scrotum

Planning: Patient outcomes

1. Patient reports pain is decreased or no longer present.
2. Patient moves in bed and ambulates without major discomfort.

Nursing Interventions

Elevate scrotum using a Bellevue bridge or athletic support.
Apply ice pack to scrotum as ordered.
Splint incision when patient coughs and changes position.
Use comfort measures to promote relaxation.
Administer analgesics as ordered and needed.

NDx: Risk for body image disturbance related to removal of the testis

Planning: Patient outcomes

1. Patient describes realistically the effects of the surgery on appearance and function.

2. Patient expresses feelings of self-worth and sexual adequacy.
3. Patient resumes self-care activities.

Nursing Interventions

Encourage the patient to express feelings about self in light of the surgery.

Provide time and privacy for the patient and his significant other to share feelings about the impact of the surgery on their relationship.

Describe the wound during wound care and allow patient to view it when desired.

Suggest discussion of scrotal implant with the surgeon if the patient expresses concern about appearance.

NDx: Risk for altered health maintenance related to insufficient knowledge of diagnosis, plan of further treatment, postdischarge care, and TSE

Planning: Patient outcomes

1. Patient states signs and symptoms of wound complications to be reported.
2. Patient demonstrates TSE, describing its importance in the early detection of cancer in the remaining testis.

Nursing Interventions

Instruct the patient to report signs of wound complications: increased erythema, bloody or purulent drainage, dehiscence, and fever.

Instruct the patient in TSE as follows, explaining its importance since cancer can develop in the remaining testis.

- Perform TSE once a month. Do it after a warm bath or shower because the heat relaxes the scrotal skin and makes it easier to feel anything unusual.
- Stand naked in front of mirror. Look for any swelling on the skin of the scrotum.
- Examine each testicle gently with both hands. The index and middle fingers should be placed underneath the testicle while the thumbs are placed on the top. Roll the testicle gently between the thumbs and fingers. One testicle may be larger that the other.

- Find the epididymis (a cord-like structure on the top and back of the testicle that stores and transports the sperm). Do not confuse the epididymis with an abnormal lump.
- Feel for a small lump about the size of a pea on the front or the side of the testicle. These lumps are usually painless.
- Contact the doctor right away if a lump is found.

Adopted from: *Male Self-Exam for Testicular Cancer*
U.S. Department of Health and Human Services
Public Health Service
National Institutes of Health Publication
No. 85 - 2636, June 1985

Thromboangiitis Obliterans (Buerger's Disease)

Thromboangiitis obliterans is a chronic inflammatory process that leads to arterial occlusion. It involves the medium-size arteries and veins, with arteries more commonly and severely affected. Although the cause is unknown, it most often affects male smokers between 20 and 45 years of age, with the greatest incidence among Asian and Jewish populations. Peripheral vascular ischemia results in cold painful extremities with frequent numbness, tingling, and spasms. Specific exercises are prescribed along with vasodilators, analgesics, and nicotine restriction.

ASSESSMENT

- Palpate distal pulses bilaterally, noting the rate, regularity, and intensity.
- Check the extremities for temperature, cyanosis, dependent rubor, and sensation.
- Assess for pain, noting the frequency, duration, intensity, location, and relief methods.
- Check for edema, lesions, or gangrene of the extremities.
- Note if the patient is taking medication or uses tobacco in any form.

NURSING DIAGNOSES, PLANNING, AND NURSING INTERVENTIONS

NDx: Pain related to the inflammation and ischemia secondary to the disease state

Planning: Patient outcomes

1.   Patient reports an absence or reduction in pain.
2.   Patient states methods of relaxation to reduce pain and coping strategies to deal with the presence of pain.
3.   Patient displays behaviors that may reduce painful effects of the disease such as ceasing smoking or other tobacco use.
4.   Patient describes and practices Buerger-Allen exercises to increase circulation to prevent ischemic pain.

Nursing Interventions

Instruct the patient to cease smoking or use of other tobacco products since it increases ischemia and exacerbates the disorder.

Use diversional activities to decrease the patient's awareness of pain.

Teach relaxation strategies and encourage frequent use of the techniques.

Teach the Buerger-Allen exercises to the patient (See Highlight 10-2 in textbook).

Tell the patient to avoid wearing constricting clothing or shoes that interfere with circulation in the extremities.

Have the patient wear warm clothing to protect the extremities against extreme temperatures.

Administer pain medication as prescribed, and teach the patient about the dosage, frequency of use, and potential side effects.

NDx: Knowledge deficit: nature of disease, factors contributing to manifestations of disease, and preventive measures

Planning: Patient outcomes

1.   Patient states accurate information about the disease process and the manifestations of the disorder.

2. Patient relates measures to decrease the effects of the disease.
3. Patient complies with behavioral changes necessary to reduce manifestations of the disease.

Nursing Interventions

Explain the disease process to the patient in understandable terms.

Allow time for questions and concerns.

Give the patient and family appropriate literature about the disease.

Tell the patient and family about the manifestations of the disorder and preventive measures to protect the patient from complications, such as keeping warm, exercising to increase circulation, preventing stress, and avoiding injury to extremities.

◆ Thrombocytopenic Purpura

Thrombocytopenic purpura is a condition resulting from platelet deficiency, causing spontaneous bleeding into surrounding tissue when platelet counts are less than $100,000/mm^3$. There are two types of thrombocytopenic purpura: idiopathic thrombocytopenic purpura (ITP) and secondary thrombocytopenic purpura. In ITP the platelets are destroyed prematurely by antiplatelet antibodies. The cause is unknown but it is thought to be an autoimmune reaction directed against the surface of the platelets. In children, ITP usually follows a viral infection and is self-limiting. Secondary thrombocytopenic purpura results from drug sensitivity or from a primary disorder. Management includes removing the cause, platelet transfusions, steroid therapy, or splenectomy.

ASSESSMENT

- Observe for joint pain and edema, indicative of bleeding into the joints.
- Assess for other signs of bleeding such as ecchymoses, petechiae, or epistaxis.
- Check the urine and stools for blood.

- Review laboratory studies for abnormal bleeding times and low platelet counts.
- Observe for weakness, tachycardia, hypotension, and air hunger, and monitor vital signs.
- Check the peripheral pulses.
- Ask the patient about recent use of anticoagulants, aspirin, NSAIDs, or drugs that suppress bone marrow function.
- Ask about any history of bleeding episodes or familial bleeding tendencies.
- Determine the patient's level of understanding about the disorder, especially about observing for bleeding tendencies.

NURSING DIAGNOSES, PLANNING, AND NURSING INTERVENTIONS

NDx: Altered tissue perfusion, cardiopulmonary, peripheral, and cerebral, related to destruction of platelets causing excessive bleeding

Planning: Patient outcomes

1. Patient's extremities are warm, color is adequate, and pulses are present.
2. Patient's laboratory studies are within normal ranges for the patient.
3. Patient denies headache, confusion, or nausea.
4. Patient is able to perform activities of daily living without tachycardia, tachypnea, and dyspnea.

Nursing Interventions

Help the patient conserve oxygen needs by encouraging rest, limiting activities, and assisting the patient with self care.

Administer oxygen as needed and elevate the head of the bed to aid in chest expansion.

Monitor vital signs and laboratory studies, noting abnormal values.

Check the patient's orientation to time and place, and ask about episodes of dizziness or weakness.

Discourage smoking to avoid vasoconstriction. Assist the patient when ambulating because decreased cerebral circulation may cause disorientation and vertigo.

NDx: Risk for altered health maintenance related to insufficient or inadequate knowledge about the disorder and the signs and symptoms of bleeding

Planning: Patient outcomes

1. Patient relates accurate information about the bleeding disorder, its clinical course, and the complication of hemorrhage.
2. Patient accurately states the signs of bleeding and when to notify the physician.
3. Patient verbalizes the measures to prevent bleeding.

Nursing Interventions

Explain the need for avoiding sharp objects, contact sports, injections, and venipuncture whenever possible.

Instruct the patient about the clinical course of the disorder and the complication of hemorrhage.

Explain the signs and symptoms of bleeding and when to seek medical intervention.

Tell the patient to carry an identification card listing the blood disorder, patient's name, address, blood type, a family member to call in case of an emergency, and the physician's name.

Teach the patient measures to prevent bleeding as listed in the textbook Highlight 13-5.

◆ Thrombophlebitis (Venous Thrombosis)

Thrombophlebitis is the development of a clot in the vein wall with inflammation of the vessel causing partial or complete occlusion of the vein. This results in pain, fever, chills, edema, and cyanosis along the affected vein if in deep veins, or minor symptoms if in superficial veins. The vein feels hard and thready when palpated. The primary cause of thrombophlebitis is venous stasis, but injury to a vessel wall, increased blood coagulation, oral contraceptives, and some blood dyscrasias may predispose the patient to increased risk of clot formation. The treatment includes bed rest with elevation of the affected extremity, application of warm compresses, analgesics for pain, and anticoagulant therapy. Heparin is used for initial and short-term therapy, but oral anticoagulants are usually used for long-term anticoagulation.

ASSESSMENT

- Check lower extremities for edema, discoloration, pulses, and tenderness.
- Ask about pain, noting its location, duration, and intensity
- Check for the presence of Homans' sign (calf pain with dorsiflexion of the foot).
- Observe for signs of pulmonary embolism, such as sudden chest pain, dyspnea, restlessness, diaphoresis, and cyanosis.
- Auscultate breath sounds to check for wheezes or crackles indicative of respiratory complications such as infection or embolus.
- Observe for complications of immobility such as skin breakdown, infection, and pressure areas.

NURSING DIAGNOSES, PLANNING, AND NURSING INTERVENTIONS

NDx: Pain in extremities related to venous inflammation

Planning: Patient outcomes

1. Patient reports absence of pain or decrease in pain to tolerable level.
2. Patient states comfort measures to help relieve pain such as positioning, relaxation techniques.

Nursing Interventions

Instruct the patient to cease smoking since it causes an increased demand for blood and oxygen to tissues, and vasoconstriction, which increases the ischemia and thus, the pain.

Tell the patient to avoid wearing constricting clothing and anything that interferes with circulation.

Apply warm, moist compresses to decrease edema and relieve spasms.

187

Give analgesics as ordered.

Teach relaxation techniques and encourage their use during painful episodes.

NDx: Altered tissue perfusion, peripheral, related to impaired venous flow from thrombus formation

Planning: Patient outcomes

1. Patient demonstrates increased perfusion as noted by warm, dry skin and absence of edema and cyanosis in the extremities.
2. Patient's vital signs are within normal ranges for the patient.

Nursing Interventions

Help the patient conserve energy and decrease oxygen demand by providing frequest rest periods and assisting the patient with activities as needed.

Monitor vital signs, checking peripheral pulses frequently.

Encourage ambulation when allowed to increase circulation.

Discourage smoking to reduce vasoconstriction and remove tight clothing.

Tell the patient not to cross legs in bed or to allow legs to hang in a dependent position while sitting.

NDx: Impaired physical mobility related to extended bed rest and pain secondary to disease state

Planning: Patient outcomes

1. Patient reports increased mobility, strength and endurance.
2. Patient is able to perform activities of daily living.

Nursing Interventions

Assist the patient when ambulating since weakness may be severe at first.

Use durable medical equipment to assist the patient with repositioning and exercising while in bed.

Teach the patient to perform range-of-motion exercises while in bed to maintain strength and endurance.

Start the patient on a mild daily activity regimen, when
 allowed, and encourage the patient to continue to
 improve strength and endurance at a moderate rate.

NDx: Impaired skin integrity in the extremities related
to effects of immobility

Planning: Patient outcomes

1. Patient's skin remains intact without evidence of
   shearing, infection, ulceration or gangrene.
2. Patient states appropriate skin care measures to
   prevent impairment of skin integrity.

Nursing Interventions

Handle the patient's legs and feet with care, especially if
 the skin is not intact.
Use aseptic technique when bathing and dressing areas
 where skin breakdown is present to prevent infection.
Keep linen off the extremities with the use of a bed cradle.
Instruct the patient to avoid wearing constricting clothing.
Keep the extremities warm and dry.
Check for early signs of complications and compromised
 skin integrity.

◆ Thyroid Cancer

Neoplasms of the thyroid gland are relatively rare.
They are divide into several types:
- Papillary carcinoma—the most common type, with
  excellent prognosis if diagnosed and treated prior
  to metastasis.
- Follicular carcinoma—a more aggressive type, but
  responds well to radioactive iodine.
- Medullary carcinoma—a highly aggressive type,
  especially locally; treated by total thyroidectomy
  with lymph node dissection.

- Undifferential (anaplastic, giant cell, or small cell) carcinoma—a highly aggressive type that is resistant to treatment; generally palliative treatment efforts only are made.

The etiology of thyroid cancer is unknown but the thyroid carcinomas are more common in persons receiving irradiation to the neck. Other risk factors include familial disposition, prolonged thyroid-stimulating hormone stimulation, and goiter. Cancer of the thyroid is treated by a subtotal or total thyroidectomy with or without radical neck incision, radiation, chemotherapy, and thyroid suppression therapy.

NURSING CARE

The nursing care for the patient with cancer of the thyroid is similar to that for a patient with *hyperthyroidism*. Also refer to the entry on Cancer in general and Thyroidectomy in this text for specific nursing diagnoses, planning, and nursing interventions.

◆ Tuberculosis

Tuberculosis is an infectious disease caused by the bacillus *Mycobacterium tuberculosis* (TB) and spread primarily by the airborne route. Although the most common site of TB is the lungs, it can occur at any site in the body or as disseminated disease. Infection occurs when droplet nuclei containing the tubercle bacilli are inhaled into the alveolar surfaces of the lung. Clinically evident active disease occurs in 5 to 10% of those infected, and may be manifested by progression of the original infection (primary infection) or reactivation of the disease months or years after the initial infection (post-primary infection). Management consists primarily of chemotherapy. Four-drug therapy with isoniazid, rifampin, pyrazinamide, and either ethambutol or streptomycin is the initial regimen (2 months) for treating TB in most patients in order to prevent the emergence of resistant organisms. The regimen can be adjusted when susceptibility studies become available. For multidrug resistant TB, consultation with the Infectious Disease Department is recommended. In the acute care setting, patients are isolated in a negative-pressure room. Individually fitted disposable particulate respirators are worn by health care providers when delivering direct patient care or when high-risk procedures are performed.

ASSESSMENT

- Observe for low-grade fever, pallor, chills, night sweats, cough, easy fatigability, anorexia, weight loss, dyspnea, and chest pain.
- Assess lung sounds and eating habits.
- Assess the patient's understanding of the disease, its prognosis, the course of therapy, disease transmission, and methods for preventing its spread.
- Determine the patient's understanding of self-administration of drugs and need for consistent long-term therapy.
- Determine the patient's willingness and ability to comply with therapy.
- Assess the patient's and family's reaction and emotional response to the diagnosis.

NURSING DIAGNOSES, PLANNING, AND NURSING INTERVENTIONS

NDX: Knowledge deficit: mechanism of spread and precautionary measures

Planning: Patient outcomes

1. Patient explains how tuberculosis is spread.
2. Patient describes measures to prevent the spread of TB to others.
3. Patient's contacts remain free of TB as evidenced by a negative tuberculin test.

Nursing Interventions

Instruct the patient and family about how to prevent the transmission of TB:
- Explain that the most important way to prevent the spread of TB is to cover the mouth and nose with double thickness tissue when coughing or sneezing, and to take the prescribed medication.

- Emphasize the importance of good handwashing after using tissues and their proper disposal.
- Provide specific instruction for preventing transmission of TB in the home setting such as keeping the door to the patient's room closed, ventilating the room, limiting visitors during the first 2 weeks of therapy, arranging for direct observation of medication administration (DOT), and testing family members with PPD and treating positive results prophylactically.

If hospitalization is required:
- Maintain the patient in isolation.
- Wear the prescribed respirator during all direct patient care.
- Assist other health care providers and visitors to comply with isolation requirements.
- Provide diversional activities such as TV, radio, books, or tapes.

NDx: Risk for altered health maintenance related to nonadherence to drug therapy secondary to duration, cost, or lack of perceived importance.

Planning: Patient outcomes

1. Patient describes a plan for remembering to take the medication.
2. Patient states how and where one is able to obtain the medication.
3. Patient verbalizes importance of taking medication as prescribed and intent to comply.
4. On follow-up examination sputum cultures are negative and chest x-rays improved.

Nursing Interventions

Stress to the patient and family that cure depends upon strict adherence to the medication schedule.

Assist the patient to devise a method for remembering to take the medication, e.g., a monthly check-off chart of scheduled doses to be hung in a corner of the bathroom mirror.

Inform the patient that antituberculosis drugs are available free of charge from most health departments.

Instruct the patient in the importance of returning for follow-up tests as scheduled to protect both self and others.

NDx: Risk for altered health maintenance related to insufficient knowledge of disease and follow-up care

Planning: Patient outcomes

1. Patient describes cause, treatment, and prognosis of TB.
2. Patient states name, dose, route, and frequency of prescribed medications.
3. Patient explains importance of taking medication consistently for as long as ordered.
4. Patient describes supportive self-care measures, need for medical follow-up, and symptoms that require prompt reporting.
5. Patient identifies community support services to assist with medication, necessary laboratory work, transportation, and follow-up care.

Nursing Interventions

Learn as much as possible about the patient: past medical history, beliefs and attitudes, social supports, and whether there are any barriers to adherence to the treatment plan.

Assess knowledge of the disease process—reinforce accurate information, correct misconceptions.

Explain what TB is, who gets it, and how it is spread using simple, nonmedical terms, handouts, and written instructions.

Teach the patient about the prescribed medications: name, dose, route, frequency, and expected action.

Instruct the patient to report side effects from medications so that the regimen can be adjusted appropriately, and never to discontinue the prescribed medications unless directed to do so by the health care provider.

Explain the importance of follow-up sputum cultures to determine the effectiveness of the medication regimen.

Counsel the patient on the importance of plenty of rest and a nutritious diet high in protein and vitamins.

Instruct the patient to report the recurrence of symptoms or the development of hemoptysis or pleuritic pain immediately.

Provide the patient with information related to available community resources.

Additional Interventions

Collect sputum specimens as follows:

- Collect specimens in the morning, preferably when the patient first awakens.
- Have the patient cleanse the mouth and deeply cough up at least 1 teaspoon of mucus into a sterile, wide-mouthed cup.
- Replace the lid, seal in a plastic bag, and refrigerate if necessary.

Provide opportunity and encouragement for the patient to discuss feelings and ask questions about the diagnosis.

◆ Ulcerative Colitis

Ulcerative colitis is a form of inflammatory bowel disease (IBD) most often beginning in the rectum and spreading to the sigmoid and descending colon. Its cause is unknown but immunologic dysfunction, food allergy, infection, and heredity are considered possible etiologic factors. Management of mild to moderate disease includes a low-roughage diet free of milk or milk products, anticholinergics to decrease peristalsis and GI secretion, antidiarrheal agents, antiinfectives, and, in some cases, corticosteroids and immunosuppressive drugs. Total colectomy (or protocolectomy) with ileostomy is done for severe cases and is considered curative.

NURSING CARE

Nursing care is similar to that for the patient with Crohn's disease. If the patient is treated surgically, see care under Ileostomy in Section II.

♦ Urinary Tract Infections

An infection exists in the urinary tract when specific microorganisms can be identified through urine culture. To meet the definition of urinary tract infection (UTI) there must be more than 10^5 (100,000) organisms per milliliter in a clean catch urine specimen. UTIs are described in relation to the anatomic area involved: cystitis, urethritis, or pyelonephritis. Most urinary tract infections are treated with antibiotics, antimicrobials, antispasmodics, and analgesics.

Cystitis is the inflammation of the bladder that usually results from the invasion of bacteria into the urinary tract. In the female patient, bacteria that enter the urinary tract usually originate from either the rectum or vagina and ascend upward via the urethra. In the male patient, cystitis is usually the result of an existing problem in the urinary tract, such as prostatitis or benign prostatic hypertrophy.

Urethritis is an inflammation of the urethra that may be acute or chronic. In males the most common cause is gonorrhea. Some of the organisms more commonly associated with urethritis are *Ureaplasma*, *Chlamydia*, and *Trichomonas vaginalis*. Urethritis can also be caused by irritants, such as soaps, perfumed toilet paper and sanitary napkins, and bubble baths.

Pyelonephritis is an infection of the upper urinary tract that produces pain and edema in the kidney, renal pelvis, and surrounding structures. It can become chronic, resulting in hypertension and uremia in some patients. Pyelonephritis is the original diagnosis in one-third of renal failure patients. The most common cause of pyelonephritis is the reflux of infected urine from the bladder to the upper urinary tract. The source of bacteria contaminating the urinary tract is usually fecal flora. An *E. coli* infection is the most common, though pyelonephritis due to *Proteus*, *Pseudomonas*, *Enterobacter*, *Klebsiella*, *Enterococcus*, *Serratia*, *Morganella*, and *Staphylococcus* is not uncommon.

ASSESSMENT

- Check the patient's voiding patterns:
  - Assess for uropenia, hesitancy, frequency, and dysuria.

195

- Obtain information about the color and odor of the urine.
- Observe for any blood or mucus in the urine.
- Ask the patient to describe any pain or discomfort that has occurred with voiding.
- Ask if the patient is able to empty the bladder at regular intervals, or if voiding is often delayed for several hours.
- Assess the patient for malaise, fatigue, chills, and fever.
- Inspect the area of the costovertebral angle (CVA) for asymmetry or swelling that would indicate inflammation.
- Inspect the lower abdomen and the urethral meatus to determine if tissues are inflamed. Palpate the urinary bladder for distention or pain.
- Review the patient's daily hygiene and dietary practices as well as asking about activities that may predispose the patient to urinary tract infections such as frequently taking bubble baths or wearing tight-fitting blue jeans.
- Assess the patient's level of knowledge about the disorder, treatment, and care needed.

NURSING DIAGNOSES, PLANNING, AND NURSING INTERVENTIONS

NDx: Altered patterns of urinary elimination related to inflammation and irritation

Planning: Patient outcomes

1. Patient adheres to established voiding schedule.
2. Patient reports relief of irritative voiding symptoms.
3. Patient resumes normal voiding pattern.

Nursing Interventions

Administer antimicrobial medications as ordered to sterilize the urine, and antispasmodics or analgesics as ordered to relieve the accompanying suprapubic discomfort brought on by bladder spasms.

Encourage an increased oral fluid intake of up to 3000
    mL/d (unless contraindicated for other medical
    reasons) since a more dilute urine lessens the irrita-
    tion to the bladder mucosa.
Encourage voiding at regular intervals since frequent
    bladder emptying decreases intravesical irritation
    and prevents stasis of urine.

NDx: Pain related to inflammation and irritation

Planning: Patient outcomes

1.   Patient verbalizes comfort and pain relief.
2.   Patient voids without pain or burning.

Nursing Interventions

Administer analgesics and antispasmodics as ordered.
Offer a warm sitz bath 2 to 3 times per day to relieve
    perineal or suprapubic discomfort.
Encourage the patient to drink 2 to 3 L/d.

NDx: Knowledge deficit related to factors that may
predispose the patient to urinary infections and/or treatment regimen

Planning: Patient outcomes

1.   Patient lists factors that predispose the patient to
     infections.
2.   Patient describes medical and dietary regimen.
3.   Patient verbalizes measures to prevent urinary tract
     infections.

Nursing Interventions

Teach the patient to recognize symptoms of UTI and
    report them to the physician.
Review the practice of proper hygiene with the patient.
Teach the patient activities that may be performed to
    prevent a recurrence of the UTI such as: if the pa-
    tient's bladder infection occurred following sexual
    intercourse, then teach the patient the practice of
    voiding immediately after coitus; similarly, if the
    patient experiences irritating voiding symptoms

after taking a tub bath, then encourage showering to prevent the ascent of bacteria into the urinary tract from the bath water.

Incorporate information about the dosage and potential side effects of the medication prescribed and a reminder to complete the entire course of therapy, even though symptoms have subsided.

Teach the patient to drink 2 to 3 L/d, obtain adequate rest, and follow a good nutritional pattern.

Explain the diagnostic studies completed and the need for any follow-up studies after discharge.

Include the family in any of the teaching sessions when applicable.

Varicose Veins

Varicosities are the result of abnormal dilation of the veins caused by venous insufficiency with valvular malfunction. This may be due to congenital malformations of the vein walls and valves, repeated episodes of thrombophlebitis, or conditions that cause venous stasis such as pregnancies or prolonged standing or sitting. Heavy lifting, obesity, deep vein thrombosis, obstruction, or inflammation may cause high venous pressure resulting in varicosities. A genetic predisposition to varicose veins is also common. Elastic stockings are prescribed to give support and to promote venous return. Severe varicose veins may be treated by sclerotherapy or by surgical transection, ligation and stripping.

NURSING CARE

Teach the patient about the proper care of the extremities and preventive measures similar to those for thrombophlebitis.

Postoperative care includes routine care as described under the Postoperative Care entry in this text.

Apply elastic stockings, check the dressing sites, and assess for bleeding, decreased sensation, pulses, and edema.

Encourage ambulation as soon as the patient is able to decrease edema and increase venous return, but elevate the patient's legs while in bed.

◆ Vasospastic Disorder (Raynaud's Disease)

Vasospastic disorder is a vascular disorder that is characterized by paroxysmal, bilateral digit ischemia resulting from vasospasms induced by cold and dampness or emotional stress. The cause of the disorder is unknown but it frequently accompanies other diseases. It is more common in women than in men. The characteristic vasospastic episodes usually affect the fingers, last just a few minutes to hours, and may occur several times per day, or may not occur for weeks at a time. It is usually treated palliatively by avoidance of precipitating factors, but may require pharmacotherapeutic intervention with the use of vasodilators.

NURSING CARE

The nursing care for a patient with vasospastic disorder is similar to that for a patient with *thromboangiitis obliterans*.

◆ Venous Stasis Ulcers

Venous stasis ulcers (leg ulcers) associated with chronic venous insufficiency occur from extensive damage to the integrity of the skin and subcutaneous tissues. This is the result of edema, decreased venous circulation leading to inadequate supply of oxygen and nutrients to the area, and accumulation of toxic wastes. These changes usually occur in the lower leg near the ankle. Venous stasis ulcers are more common in the elderly. Management involves treatment with compresses of isotonic saline solution, Burrow's solution, or Silvadene. Whirlpool therapy may be utilized, as well as use of systemic antibiotics and debridement or skin grafting.

ASSESSMENT

- Assess the affected area for discoloration, warmth, drainage, and edema.
- Ask the patient about pain, tenderness, or sensation in the affected limb.
- Note the color and amount of drainage.
- Assess the patient's knowledge level regarding the disorder, the medications prescribed, and measures to prevent recurrence of the ulcerations.
- Observe the patient's activity level, and note whether mobility is impaired as a result of the leg ulcerations.
- Review the patient's typical meal plan, and check for vitamin and protein content of the food choices.

NURSING DIAGNOSES, PLANNING, AND NURSING INTERVENTIONS

NDx: Impaired physical mobility, strength, and endurance

Planning: Patient outcomes

1. Patient reports increased mobility, strength, and endurance.
2. Patient is able to perform activities of daily living.

Nursing Interventions

Assist the patient when he or she is allowed out of bed.
Use durable medical equipment accessories, when appropriate, to assist the patient in maintaining mobility.
Teach the patient to perform range-of-motion exercises to increase circulation and to maintain or improve strength and endurance.
Prepare a daily exercise schedule for the patient as soon as he or she is allowed to be mobile again, increasing the level as tolerable.

NDx: Impaired skin integrity in the extremities related to immobility

Planning: Patient outcomes

1. Patient's skin remains intact without evidence of infection, ulcerations, or gangrene.
2. Patient states appropriate skin care measures to prevent impairment of skin integrity.

Nursing Interventions

Maintain the patient on bedrest during the acute phase.

Elevate the legs to decrease venous pressure.

Culture any drainage from the ulcerations if ordered.

Teach the patient to perform dorsiflexion while on bedrest to promote blood flow.

Cleanse the ulcerations daily with prescribed solution and technique to prevent infection.

Apply lotion to the surrounding skin to prevent dryness.

Reposition the patient frequently to prevent pressure areas.

Teach the patient measures to prevent recurrence of the ulcers such as wearing graduated compression elastic hose and elevating the legs periodically to promote venous flow.

Discourage standing in place or sitting with the legs in a dependent position for long periods of time.

Encourage leg exercises such as walking to increase circulation to the distal limbs.

Instruct the patient to avoid wearing constrictive clothing and extreme hot or cold temperatures.

Encourage the patient to eat a diet high in vitamin C, protein, and minerals to enhance healing and maintain tissue integrity.

NDx: Knowledge deficit: Nature of the disease, its complications, treatments, and measures to reduce risk

Planning: Patient outcomes

1. Patient describes cause, effects, and risk factors associated with venous stasis ulcers.

2. Patient lists symptoms and treatments for the complications of the disorder, including how and when to apply graduated compression elastic hose and care of the ulcerations at home.
3. Patient states the self care needed to prevent risk or complications of venous stasis ulcers.
4. Patient chooses foods that promote health and healing.

Nursing Interventions

Explain to the patient the cause, effects, and treatments for venous stasis ulcers.

Allow the patient to verbalize concerns and fears.

Evaluate discharge needs of the patient and family and obtain referrals as required.

Alert the patient to the complications of ulcerations such as impaired mobility, pain, and infection of the extremities.

Teach the patient how to achieve comfort by frequent repositioning and the padding of bony prominences.

Explain the use of a bed cradle to prevent pressure on joints and sensitive areas.

Teach the patient how to apply the graduated compression elastic hose, which compresses superficial veins to enhance circulation to deep veins and decreases the chance of recurrence of the venous ulceration.

Teach the patient the dosage, route, time, frequency, side effects, and toxic effects of any medication prescribed.

Explain the benefit of a diet high in vitamins and protein, and give the patient lists of appropriate foods.

◆ Viral Hepatitis

Viral hepatitis is an inflammation of the liver with spotty liver cell necrosis and regeneration. The types of hepatitis are classified as follows:

- Hepatitis A (HAV)—the most common type; transmitted by fecal-oral route.
- Hepatitis B (HBV)—a common type that is on the rise, especially in AIDS cases; transmitted parenterally as well as through sexual contact and by perinatal route.
- Hepatitis C (HCV), — viral hepatitis without evidence of HAV, HBV, or HDV; often posttransfusion hepatitis; formerly known as non-A, non-B hepatitis (NANB).
- Hepatitis D (HDV) — a complication of HBV.
- Hepatitis E (HEV) — formerly known as enterically transmitted non-A, non-B hepatitis.

Incubation periods and the severity of hepatitis depend on the causative organism and type. All types of hepatitis are characterized by three phases: *preicteric, icteric,* and *posticteric,* which usually follow similar patterns of symptomatology and time frames. Diagnosis is based on physical findings including enlarged liver and spleen, and laboratory data including serologic tests, liver enzymes, serum bilirubin, coagulation studies, and leukocyte count. There is no specific treatment for viral hepatitis, but rest, a well-balanced diet, and abstinence from alcohol are usual interventions. Complications include chronic hepatitis (persistent or actual) and fulminant hepatitis.

ASSESSMENT

- Question the patient regarding known or possible exposure to hepatitis.
- Palpate and percuss the liver for enlargement, tenderness, and pain.
- Ask about episodes of extreme fatigue, anorexia, nausea, or vomiting.
- Assess the patient's urine for color, consistency, and amount.
- Observe for any bleeding tendencies such as petechiae or ecchymoses.
- Check with the patient about potential exposure to others in the home or work environment.

NURSING DIAGNOSES, PLANNING, AND NURSING INTERVENTIONS

NDx: Risk for altered health maintenance related to insufficient knowledge of viral hepatitis disease process and transmission

Planning: Patient outcomes

1. Patient relates cause and usual progression of viral hepatitis.
2. Patient verbalizes precautions to prevent transmission of the disease.

Nursing Interventions

Explain the types of hepatitis and modes of transmission of the disease and its usual progression.

Tell the patient about the importance of correct handwashing to prevent spread of the disease.

Demonstrate the handwashing technique to the patient and family.

Explain enteric precautions to the patient and all visitors.

Caution the patient to refrain from alcohol ingestion, and to check with the physician prior to taking any medications (prescription or over-the-counter).

Tell the patient that blood, tissue, and organs may not be donated.

NDx: Activity intolerance related to fatigue secondary to the disease process

Planning: Patient outcomes

1. Patient participates in activities of daily living without complaints of fatigue.
2. Patient increases ambulation distance daily.

Nursing Interventions

Alternate activity and rest periods throughout the day.

Encourage the patient to increase the amount of self-care activities and other physical activities completed in gradual increments.

Increase the patient's ambulation distance by 10 to 20 feet daily, assisting the patient when needed.

Monitor the effects of the activity on the cardiovascular system.

Encourage the patient to follow the prescribed regimen of activity, but to set limits based on personal tolerance.

Section II

Diagnostic and Therapeutic Procedures

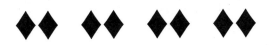

◆ Amputation

An amputation of a body part may occur as a result of trauma, or may be completed as a therapeutic surgical intervention. A traumatic amputation refers to any type of injury that cuts off an appendage or body projection. The body part, if it can be recovered, is saved for possible reattachment by microvascular anastomosis. If reimplantation is not possible, debridement and closure of the residual part are completed. Prognosis depends on the time since the injury, access to an institution performing microsurgery, degree of damage of the part, and the patient's stability, age, and health status prior to the incident. Therapeutic surgical amputations may be done for severe peripheral vascular disease, acute vascular occlusion, osteomyelitis, bone tumors, or necrosis secondary to other diseases.

PREOPERATIVE NURSING CARE

If the amputation is a therapeutic surgical intervention for a preexisting condition, the preoperative care is similar to that for a patient with a peripheral vascular disease, such as varicosities, who is having surgery. In cases of traumatic amputation the time between the presentation of the patient to the hospital and the initiation of surgical intervention is extremely limited. Most nursing interventions, other than the initial emergency care, occur in the postoperative period.

Assessment

- Assess the patient's awareness of the situation and knowledge of the impending surgery.
- Check vital signs, noting peripheral pulses in affected area.
- Assess the patient's pain, noting the intensity, whether analgesics have been given, and the patient's response.
- Determine if the patient has significant others available for assistance and emotional support.
- Complete the preoperative assessments as detailed in the Preoperative Care entry in this handbook.

POSTOPERATIVE NURSING CARE

Assessment

- Assess the patient's neurovascular status proximal and distal to the surgical site.
- Palpate pulses, check color, sensation, and edema of the part, and ask the patient about sensation in the area.
- If the entire limb is bandaged, assess the bandages for tightness and for signs of circulatory compromise.
- Check for drainage on the bandages, noting the margins and time checked.
- Assess the patient's anxiety level, coping ability, and understanding of the incident and the treatment regimen.
- Assess pain and general discomfort.
- Check if the patient is able to rest and sleep comfortably at intervals.

NURSING DIAGNOSES, PLANNING, AND NURSING INTERVENTIONS

NDx: Anxiety related to traumatic injury, potential loss of limb (even if reattached), or loss due to preexisting condition, and pain

Planning: Patient outcomes

1. Patient denies anxiety, fear or nervousness about the outcome of the surgery.
2. Patient appears relaxed, is able to rest at intervals and to sleep well.
3. Signs of increased anxiety such as twitching, nervousness, increased respirations, and pulse are absent.

Nursing Interventions

Explain the purpose of all treatments to the patient.
Teach the patient how to reposition in the bed.
Allow the patient time to ask questions and relay concerns.
Reinforce information from the physician to the patient.

Give support without offering unrealistic reassurances and seek assistance from clergy or other professional therapists.

Check vital signs and watch for changes indicating increased anxiety.

Teach the patient relaxation methods and strategies to cope with the fears of hospitalization and necessary medical interventions.

Have the patient practice range-of-motion exercises to help relieve discomfort from the static position and to maintain muscle tone and joint motion of unaffected extremities, as allowed.

Provide diversional activity for the patient to relieve the boredom and anxiety of bedrest.

NDx: Pain related to trauma or preexisting condition, manipulation during surgery, usual postoperative physiologic events, and phantom limb sensations

Planning: Patient outcomes

1. Patient denies pressure, pain, discomfort, or alteration in sensation.
2. Patient is able to exercise and tolerate mobility (of unaffected body parts) without interferences from acute pain episodes.

Nursing Interventions

Utilize a pain-rating scale for assessing pain and discuss pain management objectives with the patient and family utilizing the AHCPR guidelines.

Place the patient in comfortable positions and reposition frequently.

Check the affected extremity to ensure proper alignment and positioning.

Use pillows to support bony prominences.

Assess when the pain is most severe and allow the patient to rest during those periods.

Give pain medications prior to activity periods so the patient can better tolerate the movement.

Help the patient find alternate methods to alleviate or be able to tolerate the pain.

Inspect the skin and palpate pulses in distal areas for signs
of compromised circulation or skin breakdown due
to constrictive bandages or positioning, which may
be the cause of the pain.

Tell the patient to report any signs of pain, numbness, or
change in temperature immediately.

NDx: Risk for infection related to original injury and
surgical intervention

Planning: Patient outcomes

1. Patient's vital signs are within normal ranges for the
   patient.
2. Signs of infection such as fever, chills, tachycardia,
   tachypnea, pain or burning on urination, or drainage from suture lines or at IV site are absent.
3. Patient will identify early signs of infection and
   measures to prevent infections.

Nursing Interventions

Keep the patient warm and avoid extreme changes in
temperature in the room.

Turn the patient as needed to stimulate circulation to
prevent skin breakdown and skin infections, and
massage bony prominences.

Have the patient deep breathe and cough frequently to
prevent respiratory infections, especially while the
patient is on bedrest.

Monitor the patient's vital signs frequently, observing
subtle changes that may indicate early signs of
infection.

Promote good nutrition for proper healing by serving
meals the patient will eat, in a relaxed, supportive
atmosphere.

Encourage a diet high in proteins, vitamins, and minerals
with generous fluid intake.

Use aseptic technique when changing bandages and cleansing suture line, as ordered.

Check the IV site for signs of infection and use aseptic
technique when cleansing around insertion site.

Teach the patient and family to continually observe for
signs of developing infection and to notify the physician if such signs appear.

Stress the importance of taking antibiotics as prescribed.

NDx: Knowledge deficit: Nature of postoperative expectations, potential for rehabilitation and ability to manage self care, and resources available for assistance

Planning: Patient outcomes

1. Patient states accurate information about the surgical intervention and expected postoperative course as explained by the physician.
2. Patient demonstrates adapted methods for providing self care.
3. Patient demonstrates exercises for maintenance of mobility of nonaffected extremities and any exercises prescribed for the affected area.
4. Patient recalls resources available for assistance if necessary.

Nursing Interventions

Explain all interventions to the patient.
Tell the patient about the postoperative expectations.
Reinforce the physician's information about recovery and the rehabilitation process.
Teach the patient about the prescribed medications—dosage, side effects, and therapeutic effects.
Explain the correct dosage, frequency, side effects, and therapeutic effects.
Tell the patient when to notify the physician if any problems become evident.
Instruct the patient about the signs of complications such as extreme pain, discoloration, intense swelling, temperature change, or decreased sensation after the normal sensation has returned to the affected part.
Assist the patient with activities of daily living (ADLs) as needed and discuss the need for modifications in the home environment to accommodate the patient and provide safety.
Seek alternative methods for the patient to be able to complete the ADLs when restricted by the affected extremity.

Teach the patient how to maneuver with the assistance of supportive aids, if the affected part was a lower extremity.

Explain how to utilize other extremities to complete a task, or how to move appropriately when unassisted.

Seek the assistance of physical therapists or occupational therapists, when necessary, for consultation or teaching sessions for the patient and family.

Provide a list of possible resources for assistance in the community to the patient and family, and make appropriate referrals prior to the patient's discharge.

◆ Arterial Blood Gases

ABG analysis determines the actual levels of oxygen and carbon dioxide circulating in a sample of arterial blood. It includes determination of the partial pressure of oxygen (PaO_2), the oxygen saturation level of hemoglobin (SaO_2), the partial pressure of carbon dioxide ($PaCO_2$), the degree to which arterial blood is acid or alkaline (pH), and the level of bicarbonate (HCO_3^-) present.

ABGs are used to evaluate respiratory functioning and help determine the need for, and the effectiveness of, therapeutic interventions such as the administration of supplemental oxygen.

ABG assessment can indicate the presence of hypoxemia (inadequate oxygen in the arterial blood as measured by PaO_2), hypoxia (inadequate oxygenation at the cellular level), hypercapnia (excessive carbon dioxide in the arterial blood as measured by $PaCO_2$), acidosis or alkalosis (as measured by the pH), and the presence of the body's compensatory efforts to reduce an acid-base imbalance.

NURSING IMPLICATIONS

Use a heparinized syringe to collect the blood specimen from an arterial catheter or via percutaneous puncture of the femoral, radial, or brachial artery.

Place specimen on ice and label with time, patient's temperature, whether patient was breathing room air or receiving oxygen, whether on mechanical ventilation, and if yes, the settings.

Apply manual pressure for at least 5 minutes over a percutaneous puncture site.

Cover with a sterile dressing.

Monitor for bleeding and hematoma formation.

Check peripheral circulation in affected extremity.

Interpret ABGs in relationship to acid-base balance as shown below.

1. First examine the pH and determine whether it is normal, above normal, or below normal.
   a. If it falls between 7.35 and 7.45, the patient is within normal limits.
   b. If it is below 7.35, the patient is acidotic.
   c. If it is above 7.45, the patient is alkalotic.

2. Next, determine the origin of the imbalance by examining the partial pressure of the arterial carbon dioxide ($PaCO_2$).
   a. If the patient is acidotic and the $PaCO_2$ is below normal (above 45 mm Hg), the origin of the acidosis is respiratory. If the $PaCO_2$ is normal or below 35 mm Hg, the lungs could not possibly be be the source of the excess acid; the origin must therefore be metabolic.
   b. If the patient is alkalotic and the $PaCO_2$ is below normal (below 35 mm Hg), the origin of the alkalosis is respiratory. If the $PaCO_2$ is normal or above 45 mm Hg, the lungs could not possibly be responsible for the deficiency of acid; the origin must therefore be metabolic.

3. Finally, look for evidence of compensation by examining the bicarbonate ion HCO_3- along with the $PaCO_2$. When compensation has occurred, the value that is causing the imbalance and the value that is compensating for the imbalance will both be abnormal in the same direction (i.e., both will be elevated or both will be below normal levels).
   a. A patient with respiratory acidosis with compensatory efforts will have elevated $PaCO_2$ levels and elevated HCO_3- levels as well.
   b. A patient with respiratory alkalosis with compensatory efforts will have decreased $PaCO_2$ levels and decreased HCO_3- levels as well.

c. A patient with metabolic acidosis with compensatory efforts will have decreased HCO_3 levels and decreased $PaCO_2$ levels as well.

d. A patient with metabolic alkalosis with compensatory efforts will have elevated HCO_3 levels and elevated $PaCO_2$ levels as well.

Hint: When arrows are used to reflect the direction of deviation for each value including pH, $PaCO_2$, and HCO_3, the following rules apply:

a. Examine the pH to determine whether the patient is acidotic or alkalotic.

b. When the pH and $PaCO_2$ point in the opposite directions, the origin of the imbalance is respiratory.

c. When the pH and $PaCO_2$ point in the same direction, the origin of the imbalance metabolic.

d. When compensatory efforts are present, the $PaCO_2$ and the HCO_3 will always point in the same direction.

pH $\Downarrow$	$PaCO_2$ $\Uparrow$	HCO_3 $\Uparrow$ =	respiratory acidosis
pH $\Uparrow$	$PaCO_2$ $\Downarrow$	HCO_3 $\Downarrow$ =	respiratory alkalosis
pH $\Downarrow$	$PaCO_2$ $\Downarrow$	HCO_3 $\Downarrow$ =	metabolic acidosis
pH $\Uparrow$	$PaCO_2$ $\Uparrow$	HCO_3 $\Uparrow$ =	metabolic alkalosis

◆ Arterial Lines

Arterial blood pressure monitoring, pulmonary artery pressure monitoring, and pulmonary wedge pressure monitoring provide a more accurate picture of the critically ill patient's status than such measurements as the standard cuff blood pressure or the central venous pressure measurement. The central line catheter is usually placed into the radial, brachial, or axillary artery, or, if measuring pulmonary artery pressures, is threaded through the heart to the pulmonary artery. The catheter is attached to a transducer that converts the pressures to electrical impulses on an oscilloscope and into numerical terms. An arterial line may also be used to obtain blood samples for laboratory tests such as blood gases.

NURSING CARE

Observe the catheter for patency, and flush after use as ordered.

Observe for signs of inflammation or bleeding at the insertion site.

Evaluate the pulse, color, and temperature of the patient's extremities every 2 hours.

Observe and document the data about the pressures as ordered.

Arteriography (Angiography)

Arteriography is an x-ray of specific arterial systems using a contrast dye to diagnose pathologic conditions of the lower extremities. It is particularly useful for locating peripheral arterial occlusions. Radiopaque dye is injected into a femoral artery catheter and sequential x-ray films are taken of the arterial system as the dye perfuses to the distal areas of the extremity.

PREPROCEDURE CARE

Note baseline vital signs, especially peripheral pulses.

Check for signed informed consent.

Assess for signs of coagulation problems, such as petechiae, bruising, and prolonged bleeding times.

Check that NPO status has been maintained for 8 hours prior to testing.

Determine the patient's emotional response and level of understanding about the procedure.

POSTPROCEDURE CARE

Monitor vital signs as described under Postoperative Care entry in this text.

Maintain pressure on the arterial puncture site.

Check the catheter insertion site frequently for signs of bleeding.

Keep the patient on bedrest for 6 to 8 hours to prevent site bleeding.

Observe for signs of reaction to the contrast dye.
Check the extremities for color, pulses, discomfort, or decreased sensation.

◆ Arthroscopy

Arthroscopy is an endoscopic examination of a joint for diagnostic or corrective purposes. It is performed under local or general anesthesia and is most commonly used for knee disorders.

NURSING CARE

Observe for pain, bleeding, drainage, and edema following the procedure.
Check dressing or wrap before patient is discharged.
Reinforce the physician's instructions for self care at home.

◆ Biopsy

A biopsy is a procedure performed to obtain a piece of tissue to definitively diagnose the type of tissue or cells within the specimen by microscopic examination. Three types of biopsies include:
Incisional biopsy — surgical removal of a section of a tumor.
Excisional biopsy — surgical removal of the entire tumor.
Aspiration biopsy — removal of a small piece of a tumor using a needle or syringe
Biopsies may be performed on any neoplasm or on any body tissue. Examples of frequently performed biopsies to diagnose cancer of the organ include the liver biopsy, breast biopsy, cervical biopsy, lymph node biopsy, and bone biopsy. Nursing care may depend on the location of the neoplasm from which the specimen is taken, and the invasiveness of the procedure.

ASSESSMENT

- Evaluate the patient's emotional status and knowledge about the biopsy and potential findings.
- Determine the patient's support systems and coping ability.

NURSING DIAGNOSES, PLANNING, AND NURSING INTERVENTIONS

NDx: Anxiety related to knowledge deficit about the procedure and fear of potential findings

Planning: Patient outcomes

1. Patient and significant others express concerns about the procedure and outcome.
2. Patient verbalizes feeling less anxious.
3. Patient describes the procedure as presented by the physician.

Nursing Interventions

Explain the procedure in detail to the patient and significant others.

Allow time for expression of concerns and questions.

Answer questions factually without giving false reassurances.

Tell the patient the biopsy does not lead to a spread of the cancer.

Have the patient relate the information given by the physician and correct any misunderstandings.

Seek assistance from clergy or other support resources the patient identifies.

Explain the postprocedure routine to the patient and any follow-up care needed.

Additional Nursing Interventions

Refer to the entries in this text on the organ-specific types of neoplasms (liver cancer, cervical cancer, prostate cancer, etc.) for more information on biopsies and related nursing care, to the entry on Cancer for nursing care in general related to the diagnosis of cancer if the biopsy is positive, and to the sections on Preoperative and Postoperative Care for nursing care related to surgical management.

♦ Blood Transfusions

A patient may receive various types of blood and blood components such as whole blood, packed red blood cells, frozen red blood cells, platelets, granulocytes, plasma, albumin, coagulation factor concentrates, cryoprecipitate, or immune serum globulins. The type of blood component used is dictated by the clinical situation and its particular requirement for volume expansion, increased oxygen-carrying capacity, control of bleeding, or treatment of clotting disorders. Blood for transfusions may be collected from donors (homologous blood), from the intended recipient (autologous blood), or from a donor designated by the recipient (designated [directed] blood). Blood collected from a donor for transfusion to another individual is the most frequently used blood. Some risks associated with blood transfusions include hemolytic and anaphylactic reactions, and development of malaria, hepatitis, syphilis, and AIDS.

PRETRANSFUSION NURSING CARE

Assessment

- Check baseline vital signs and record them.
- Check for a signed informed consent.
- Notify the physician if the temperature is elevated.
- Ask the patient about a history of transfusion reactions.
- Assess the patient's level of understanding about the procedure.

Nursing Diagnoses, Planning, and Nursing Interventions

NDx:　Knowledge deficit: Nature of procedure and signs of potential complications

Planning: Patient outcomes

1. Patient relates accurate information about transfusions and the symptoms of a reaction.
2. Patient reports any unusual symptoms immediately.

Nursing Interventions

Describe the procedure, length of transfusion, and expected outcome in terms that are understandable to the patient.

Explain the symptoms of a transfusion reaction and instruct the patient to report any unusual feeling immediately.

Additional Interventions

Follow the institutional policy for administration of blood or blood components.

Check the blood for type and crossmatch, and match with the patient's chart and blood band prior to administration.

Document this information and have another RN confirm the check.

Observe for abnormal color or cloudiness, indicating hemolysis, and for gas bubbles, indicating bacterial growth.

Follow body substance precautions when performing the venipuncture or handling the blood products.

Observe for an immediate reaction to the blood product and check vital signs after starting the transfusion.

NURSING CARE DURING TRANSFUSION

Continue to assess the patient for signs of a reaction to the blood products.

Check vital signs at frequent intervals (per institutional policy) and record the data.

Check the flow rate frequently during the infusion.

Tell the patient to notify the nurse if any untoward symptoms become evident.

Check the unconscious patient and take vital signs at least every 15 minutes since the patient cannot report symptoms of a reaction.

Check for a weak pulse, tachycardia or bradycardia, wheezing, rashes, hypotension, oliguria, chills, increased temperature, chest pain, muscle aching, headache, tingling, and numbness.

POST-TRANSFUSION NURSING CARE

Assessment

- Document all pertinent information per institutional policy.
- Check vital signs.
- Observe for signs of a latent reaction.
- Determine the patient's level of understanding about the signs and symptoms of a delayed blood reaction and when to seek medical attention.

Nursing Diagnoses, Planning, and Nursing Interventions

NDx: Knowledge deficit: Nature of delayed transfusion reaction, signs and symptoms, and when to seek medical intervention

Planning: Patient outcomes

1. Patient relates accurate information about delayed transfusion reactions, the signs and symptoms, and when to seek medical intervention.
2. Patient observes for signs and symptoms of a blood reaction after discharge and seeks medical assistance if symptoms are evident.

Nursing Interventions

Teach the patient to observe for signs of infection such as chills, fever, cough, respiratory distress, or circulatory changes.

Explain that symptoms of respiratory distress should be reported immediately.

Tell the patient the signs of a mild delayed reaction may include just a rash, itching, low-grade fever, or headache.

Inform the patient that a reaction can occur as long as 2 weeks posttransfusion.

Allow the patient to ask questions and voice concerns.

TRANSFUSION REACTIONS

There are various types of transfusion reactions that may occur, including acute hemolytic, febrile, non-hemolytic, anaphylactic, septic, mild allergic, delayed reaction, and circulatory overload. Treatment depends upon the severity of the reaction. The blood infusion is discontinued in all but very mild reaction cases. In life-threatening cases, emergency treatment is instituted immediately. Drugs such as vasoconstrictors and mannitol are given, while life support techniques may also be necessary. Antihistamines and antipyretics may be used in mild reactions.

Nursing Care

Perform the following actions in the event of a transfusion reaction (per institutional policy):
- Stop the transfusion immediately.
- Keep the vein open with the primary solution.
- Take vital signs, have a nurse stay with the patient, and document the symptoms.
- Institute appropriate interventions if life-threatening symptoms appear.
- Report the reaction to the physician and the blood bank.
- Institute medical orders.
- Send the blood container with attached labels to the blood bank.
- Collect urine and blood samples and send to the laboratory.
- Document the treatment instituted, patient reaction, and follow-up care.
- Explain the situation to the patient and family, reassure them, make the patient comfortable, and continue to observe for further symptoms.

◆ Bronchoscopy

Bronchoscopy is the direct visualization of the walls of the trachea, the main-stem bronchus, and the major subdivisions of the bronchial tubes by means of a bronchoscope. It may be done for diagnosis, treatment, or evaluation of disease progression or effectiveness of therapy. Prior to the procedure, the patient is NPO for 6 hours; signed consent is obtained; dental prostheses are removed; and the patient is premedicated with atropine and either a sedative or a narcotic. After an anesthetic is sprayed on the patient's pharynx to suppress the cough and gag reflexes, the bronchoscope is then inserted through the mouth into the airways.

NURSING CARE

Assess the patient's anxiety level, understanding of the procedure, and ability to comply with instructions.

Tell the patient what to expect before, during, and after the procedure.

Allow the patient to verbalize concerns and encourage the use of relaxation techniques.

Monitor the pulse during the procedure.

Check for return of the swallow and cough reflexes following the procedure.

Observe for signs of complications: cyanosis, dyspnea, stridor, hemoptysis, hypotension, tachycardia, and dysrhythmias.

Position the patient who is not fully conscious in a flat side lying position.

Position the conscious patient in a flat or semi-Fowler's side lying position and instruct him or her to let saliva drain out of the corner of the mouth into a basin or tissues.

Keep the patient NPO until swallow and cough reflexes return (2-8 hours), then give warm liquids, gargles, and throat lozenges for sore throat.

Discourage talking, clearing the throat, coughing, and smoking to avoid further throat irritation.

Apply an ice collar for throat discomfort.

Expect blood-streaked sputum for several hours if a biopsy was done, but report frank red blood.

◆ Cardiac Catheterization

A cardiac catheterization is an invasive procedure using contrast dye to diagnose pathologic conditions of the heart, coronary arteries, and great vessels. It is also used to determine and evaluate the effects of prior medical or surgical interventions. Catheter insertion is through a peripheral vessel into the heart, where pressures are recorded and contrast dye is injected for radiography of the structures.

PREPROCEDURE CARE

Assessment

- Note the baseline vital signs.
- Determine the patient's level of understanding about the procedure and emotional status.
- Check for allergies to iodinated dye.
- Assess for signs of increased anxiety such as restlessness and changes in vital signs.
- Confirm that an informed consent has been obtained.
- Assess all preoperative requirements (as identified by the institution).
- Check that NPO status has been maintained for 4 to 8 hours prior to the procedure.

NURSING DIAGNOSES, PLANNING, AND NURSING INTERVENTIONS

NDx: Knowledge deficit: Nature of the invasive procedure, potential findings, and follow-up medical management necessary

Planning: Patient outcomes

1. Patient verbalizes the necessity for the procedure.
2. Patient describes the procedure as presented by the physician, radiologist, or nurse.

Nursing Interventions

Describe the procedure and the diagnostic equipment using terminology that is easily understandable to the patient.

Explain that some hot flashes may occur during the injection of the contrast dye.

Tell the patient that some discomfort may be experienced from lying on the hard table for 1 hour or more, and some mild nausea may occur from the dye.

Ask the patient to reiterate the information given by the physician and radiologist to check for understanding and to correct misconceptions.

Explain what care will be initiated during the postprocedure time period.

NDx: Anxiety related to fear of the test findings, and the discomfort associated with the testing procedure

Planning: Patient outcomes

1. Patient verbalizes a decrease in anxiety.
2. Patient's vital signs are within normal ranges.
3. Patient rests well prior to the procedure.

Nursing Interventions

Reassure the patient about the necessity for the procedure.

Use comfort measures to promote relaxation.

Allow the patient to verbalize concerns about the potential findings and necessary treatment.

Answer questions honestly, but refrain from giving false reassurance.

Administer a mild sedative (if PRN order available) prior to the testing.

Explain that the discomforts associated with the procedure are usually minimal such as slight stiffness, some minor hot flashes, and mild nausea.

Provide an emesis basin at the patient's side.

POSTPROCEDURE CARE

Monitor vital signs and compare to the previously established baseline data.

Assess for pain.

Palpate pulses distal to the catheter insertion site and compare to the opposite side.

Apply pressure to the peripheral insertion site and continually assess for bleeding at the site.

Assess for dyspnea, tachycardia, flushing, rashes, or wheals, which may indicate a reaction to the contrast dye.

Keep the patient on bedrest for 4 to 8 hours (as specified) to reduce bleeding and to observe for untoward effects from the procedure.

◆ Casts

A cast provides circumferential support and protection of an involved body part without prohibiting movement of the entire body. Usually the cast encompasses the joint just above and below the bone to be immobilized, but it may also be applied to the entire trunk or part of the trunk of the body. The body part to be immobilized, corrected, or rested determines the type of cast applied. The cast should correctly fit the specific body part.

ASSESSMENT

- Prior to the casting:
  — Assess the skin for lesions and areas of redness, swelling, or irritation.
  — Check and document proximal and distal neurovascular function to establish a baseline.
- After the casting:
  — Check for proper cast fit by assessing neurovascular status of the area involved every hour for 48 hours and every 8 hours thereafter.
  — If distal pulses are covered by the cast, check capillary refill, color, and warmth of the distal part.
  — Observe for skin irritation under and around the cast edge and on bony prominences.
  — Assess for any drainage or foul odors, which may indicate lesions or infection of lesions under the cast.
  — Assess the patient's knowledge about self care and the care of the cast prior to discharge.
  — If the patient is in a body cast:
    a. observe for signs and symptoms of cast syndrome, anorexia, nausea, vomiting, abdominal discomfort, or distention.
    b. observe for restricted chest expansion and auscultate breath sounds in exposed areas of the chest, if applicable, for early signs of respiratory problems.
    c. observe the perineal area, noting any problems with fecal matter or urine on the cast.
- After cast removal:

— Observe the skin for dryness, irritation, or the presence of breakdown. (Expect the skin to be somewhat dry, pale, and slightly irritated.)
— Inspect the limb for atrophy, weakness, and loss of range of motion.

NURSING DIAGNOSES, PLANNING, AND NURSING INTERVENTIONS

NDx: Risk for altered tissue perfusion; peripheral, related to constriction of circulation and possible nerve/vascular damage from the cast

Planning: Patient outcomes

1. Patient's extremities are warm, color is adequate, and pulses are present.
2. Evidence of complications from compromised circulation is absent.
3. Patient denies pain or decreased sensation in affected extremities.

Nursing Interventions

Perform neurovascular assessment of casted extremity to determine peripheral circulation.

Keep the patient in a comfortable position and reposition frequently to release pressure.

Utilize range-of-motion exercises to stimulate circulation and maintain joint mobility.

Monitor vital signs and laboratory studies to assess for changes and improvements in status.

Encourage ambulation as allowed, but provide for frequent rest periods to decrease cardiac workload and prevent further compromised peripheral circulation.

Discourage smoking to avoid vasoconstriction.

Remove constricting clothing and keep heavy bed linen from restricting peripheral circulation.

Tell the patient to notify the nurse if signs of compromised circulation from the cast seem apparent, such as discoloration, pain, swelling, or numbness of an extremity.

Keep the patient's legs in a nondependent position when not ambulating.

NDx: Impaired skin integrity related to insufficient peripheral circulation and/or irritation from the cast over the skin and bony prominences

Planning: Patient outcomes

1. Patient verbalizes factors associated with irritation and skin lesions, and measures to prevent the occurrence or recurrence.
2. Patient relates appropriate knowledge about skin care.
3. Patient is free of skin complications.

Nursing Interventions

Teach the patient measures to prevent skin breakdown from developing.

Have the patient inspect the skin frequently around the edges of the cast and to seek medical assistance if any breakdown or soreness is noted.

Teach the patient to exercise, as tolerated, to promote good circulation to the skin.

Encourage range-of-motion exercises while on bedrest to maintain joint mobility.

Turn the patient frequently and inspect pressure areas for early signs of breakdown.

Inspect the areas distal to the cast for signs of compromised circulation.

Use aseptic technique to cleanse any lesions.

Teach the patient and family members the proper technique for dressing areas of breakdown.

Keep the cast and skin around the cast clean and dry.

Clean the patient thoroughly after urination or bowel movements if the patient is in a body cast.

Teach the patient or family to do the same cleansing process at home to prevent breakdown of the skin in the perineal area.

NDx: Self-care deficit, feeding, hygiene, toileting, or other activities of daily living related to interference with mobility due to cast

Planning: Patient outcomes

1. Patient performs activities of daily living (ADL), using assistive devices as necessary.

2. Patient states alternative methods to complete tasks that are restricted by musculoskeletal dysfunction and cast therapy.

Nursing Interventions

Assist the patient with ADLs as needed while encouraging independence.

Seek alternative methods for the patient to be able to complete the ADLs when restricted by the cast.

Assist the patient as needed to clean the perineal area.

Position the patient for maximum comfort for urination.

Develop an exercise regimen to increase strength and endurance.

Teach the patient how to maneuver with the assistance of supportive aids such as an overhead trapeze or the side rails.

Explain how to utilize other extremities to complete a task, or how to move appropriately with the cast in place, such as how to use crutches when the patient's leg is in a cast.

Seek the assistance of physical therapists or occupational therapists when necessary for consultation or teaching sessions for the patient and family.

NDx: Pain related to pressure of the cast, itching or inability to move freely

Planning: Patient outcomes

1. Patient denies feelings of discomfort, itching, or other irritation from the cast.
2. Patient rests and sleeps well, appears relaxed and able to cope with wearing the cast.

Nursing Interventions

Assist with the changes in balance or weight bearing, if applicable, when allowed to be mobile.

Help the patient change positions frequently to relieve pressure areas.

Give pain medications as prescribed to reduce discomfort.

Relieve pressure areas from the cast by valving or cutting windows, if ordered.

NDx: Altered health maintenance related to knowledge deficit and lack of understanding about self care needed and care of the cast

Planning: Patient outcomes

1. Patient states accurate information about self care and cast care after discharge.
2. Patient states the signs of complications of cast therapy and when to seek medical intervention.
3. Patient relates the measures necessary to lessen the risk of complications.
4. Patient shows no evidence of complications of cast therapy such as inability to complete ADLs, deformities, skin breakdown, or infection.

Nursing Interventions

Instruct the patient about the effects of immobility if the patient is in a full body cast and the effects of disuse of the affected extremity in the case of an arm or leg cast.

Teach the patient and family the signs of complications such as elimination difficulty, discoloration of the skin, skin breakdown, diminished pulses, numbness, and the symptoms of infections.

Tell the patient when to seek medical assistance if symptoms appear.

Explain the need for and initiate safety measures if locomotion is a problem.

Teach the patient about cast-care management as described in the textbook in Highlight 19- 3.

Explain proper methods necessary to prevent further irritation and ulceration of skin where pressure has occurred from the cast.

Allow the patient to ask questions as needed.

Include the family in the education sessions when appropriate.

Additional Interventions

Provide firm support for the entire cast once it has been applied and until it is dry.

Cleanse any excess casting material from the skin.

Have a cast cutter available in case the cast needs to be removed quickly in case of extreme swelling, or just bivalved to release minor pressure from edema.

Reposition the patient frequently, maintaining body and cast alignment.

Initiate measures to promote comfort and combat itching such as massaging the skin around the edges of the cast, directing cool air under the cast, or encouraging isometric exercises of the casted body part to increase blood flow and decrease itching, unless contraindicated.

Provide proper care of the body part after removal of the cast by washing the skin gently with a mild soap and water.

Apply lotion with lanolin as a protective emollient to the dry areas.

If the patient is in a spica or body cast:

- Assess for abdominal distention, nausea and vomiting, which are symptoms of pressure on the mesenteric artery or abdomen.
- Place the patient in a prone or side-lying position if any abdominal symptoms occur and notify the attending physician.
- Encourage good nutrition to promote healing and to help maintain proper elimination patterns.
- Prepare the patient with a cast for the appearance of dry, scaly skin and lack of muscle strength and tone in the affected part upon the removal of the cast.
- Prepare patient for rehabilitation process if indicated.

Refer to Patient Education Highlight 19-3 in the textbook.

◆ Chemotherapy

Chemotherapy is the use of drugs to kill cancer cells. As with radiation, chemotherapeutic drugs affect both normal and malignant cells. Depending on characteristics of the tumor and stage of disease, one or several drugs may be prescribed and chemotherapy may be used alone or in combination with surgery, radiation, or immunotherapy.

ASSESSMENT

Assess patient's understanding of the goals of chemotherapy and the treatment schedule.
Assess for toxic effects:

- Hematologic Toxicity
  — Observe for signs of infection.
  — Check VS and WBC.
  — Obtain cultures if indicated.
  — Check hemoglobin, hematocrit, and platelet
    count.
  — Assess patient for signs and symptoms of bleed-
    ing.
    • Inspect skin for petechiae, ecchymoses, and
      hematomas.
    • Observe neurologic status for changes associ-
      ated with intracranial bleeding.
    • Monitor for bleeding into joints.
    • Measure abdominal girth.
    • Inspect and test all body secretions and fluids
      for blood.
  — Check blood pressure in reclining, sitting, and
    standing positions to assess for postural hypoten-
    sion.
  — Ask about symptoms of syncope, drowsiness,
    dyspnea, diaphoresis, chest pain, and fatigue.
- GI Toxicity
  — Check for nausea and vomiting (time, frequency,
    amount), diarrhea or constipation (frequency and
    character of bowel movement), and signs of de-
    hydration and electrolyte imbalance.
  — Review serum electrolytes.
  — Inspect mouth for moisture, color, ulceration,
    inflammation, and infection.
  — Note quality, color, and amount of saliva.
  — Assess for symptoms such as pain, dysphagia,
    inability to open the mouth, eat or take fluids,
    taste changes, and voice changes.
- Neurotoxicity
  — Assess for symptoms of peripheral neuropathy:
    • Paresthesias of hands and feet
    • Numbness and tingling sensation in extremi-
      ties
    • Muscle pain
    • Loss of Achilles' tendon reflex

- Falls, loss of balance
- Bone and joint pain
- Changes in gait
— Assess effect of symptoms present on physical activity.
- Skin Toxicity
— Assess for photosensitivity, alopecia, and hyper-pigmentation.
— Observe for erythema, blisters, and rashes.
- Pulmonary Toxicity
— Observe for cough, fever, tachycardia, dyspnea on exertion, and weakness.
— Check lung sounds and blood gas values.
- Cardiotoxicity
— Observe for signs of HF: tachycardia, moist cough, shortness of breath, dyspnea on exertion, distended neck veins, pedal edema, orthopnea.
- Renal Toxicity
— Check for hematuria and symptoms of dysuria.
— Review results of urinalysis and renal function studies.
- Sexual Dysfunction
— Explore concerns related to sexuality.
— Determine current method of birth control.

NURSING DIAGNOSES, PLANNING, AND NURSING INTERVENTIONS

NDx: Risk for infection related to chemotherapy-induced leukopenia

Planning: Patient outcomes

1. Patient is afebrile.
2. Signs of specific localized infections are absent.
3. Patient describes measures to reduce the risk of infection.

Nursing Interventions

Restrict visitors.
Protect patient from people with known infections.
Provide a private room.
Instruct the patient, family, and visitors in handwashing technique.

Encourage fluids if not contraindicated by other medical
   disorders.
Suggest a low bacteria diet.
Avoid fresh fruits and vegetables.
Cook all foods.
Bathe daily with antiseptic soap; include nail care.
Change intravenous tubing every 24 hours.
Avoid injections.
Institute measures to prevent skin breakdown.
Monitor exit sites of central venous catheters, intravenous
   lines or other venous access devices.
Encourage ambulation, coughing, and deep breathing.
Avoid indwelling urinary catheters.
Encourage good hygienic measures after bowel move-
   ments.

NDx: Risk for decreased cardiac output related to bleeding secondary to chemotherapy-induced thrombocytopenia

Planning: Patient outcomes

1.   Signs and symptoms of bleeding are absent.
2.   Patient describes self-care measures to decrease the
     risk of bleeding.

Nursing Interventions

Limit injections and venipunctures.
Use small gauge needles, and apply pressure after all skin
   punctures.
Avoid:
   • Shaving with a straight-edged razor.
   • Straining during bowel movements.
   • Taking any medication that contains aspirin.
   • Nasotracheal suctioning.
   • Vomiting.
Eliminate objects in patient's environment that may cause
   bruising due to falls.
Suggest:
   • Use sponges or gauze for mouth care; do not use
     toothbrush or floss.
   • Eat a soft diet high in fiber and protein.
   • Limit physical activity.

- If indicated, pad side rails and take precautions to prevent falls.

Use humidifier if oxygen therapy is indicated to prevent mucosal drying.

NDx: Fatigue related to chemotherapy-induced anemia

Planning: Patient outcomes

1. Patient identifies a plan for limiting activity and providing frequent rest periods.
2. Patient reports that he or she is able to carry out basic activities of daily living.

Nursing Interventions

Instruct patient to:
- Report symptoms.
- Limit physical activity.
- Plan frequent rest periods.
- Take soft diet high in protein, vitamins, and iron.

Administer red blood cell transfusion as ordered by physician.

NDx: Risk for fluid volume deficit related to inadequate fluid intake and excessive fluid loss secondary to nausea and vomiting

Planning: Patient outcomes

1. Skin turgor is firm.
2. Mucous membranes are moist.
3. Fluid intake approximates output.

Nursing Interventions

Instruct in measures that provide relief.
Advise patient to:
- Eat salty foods.
- Try dry foods such as toast or crackers.
- Drink clear, cool liquids.
- Eat small portions of low-fat foods.
- Report symptoms and severity.
- Limit physical activity after meals.

Administer antiemetics as prescribed. Suggest taking
     antiemetics before receiving chemotherapy and us-
     ing antiemetics in suppository form.
Offer support by:

- Explaining that nausea and vomiting are expected
  side effects.
- Suggesting diversionary activity.
- Being available for questions and follow-up.

NDx: Altered oral mucous membranes related to effects of chemotherapeutic agents on the mucosal cells

Planning: Patient outcomes

1. Oral mucous membranes are intact.
2. Oral mucous membranes are pink and moist.
3. Patient is able to ingest foods and fluids without
   oral discomfort.

Nursing Interventions

Encourage and assist with mouth care.
Rinse mouth with alkaline solutions every hour (1 tsp. of
     baking soda in 8 oz. of warm water).
Use soft sponge or gauze instead of toothbrush.
Remove thick saliva with gauze; irrigate mouth with
     sodium bicarbonate solution or dilute solution of
     hydrogen peroxide.
Remove dentures for cleaning, keep dentures in place
     only if comfortable and not causing irritation.
Use and evaluate effects of topical analgesics, artificial
     saliva, and lip lubricant.
Instruct patient to avoid alcohol, smoking, commercial
     mouthwashes, and hot, spicy, acidic foods and flu-
     ids.
Encourage:

- Fluids
- Ice popsicles
- Soft bland diet
- Using a straw to sip soups and beverages
- Frequent oral irrigation

NDx: Diarrhea related to side effects of chemotherapeutic agents on the intestinal mucosa

Planning: Patient outcomes

1. Stool is formed.
2. Stool is evacuated at intervals normal for the individual patient.

Nursing Interventions

Implement measures to control and prevent diarrhea:
Avoid:
- Bowel-irritating foods
- Gas forming foods
- Fatty foods
- Lactose and caffeine-containing products
- Smoking

Suggest:
- Diet low in residue, high in protein and carbohydrates
- Small frequent meals

Teach perianal hygiene:
- Cleanse with water and mild soap after bowel movement.
- Use sitz baths, if indicated.
- Apply topical anesthetics to rectal area, if indicated.

Administer and monitor the effects of medications to control diarrhea.
- Antidiarrheal agents
- Antispasmodics
- Opiates and opiate substitutes

NDx: Constipation related to side effects of chemotherapeutic agents on the bowel

Planning: Patient Outcomes

1. Stool is soft and formed.
2. Stool is evacuated at regular intervals without straining.

Nursing Interventions

Implement measures to prevent and alleviate constipation:
Suggest:
- Diet high in fiber, roughage, and fluid

- Drinking warm fluids to stimulate intestinal motility
- Increase in physical activity to increase intestinal motility
- Using toilet or bedside commode instead of bedpan

If patient has past history of constipation and will receive vinca alkaloid agents, suggest all the above to start after the first chemotherapy dose.

Instruct patient to avoid using enemas or suppositories without consulting physician.

Administer and monitor the effects of medications prescribed to relieve constipation.

- Stool softeners: dioctyl sodium sulfosuccinate, mineral oil
- Bulk producers: psyllium, calcium, polycarbophil
- Osmotic and saline laxatives: sodium, potassium, and magnesium salts
- Lactulose is especially effective for constipation caused by vinca alkaloids
- Cathartics: castor oil, senna, cascara, bisacodyl

NDx: Risk for injury related to paresthesias, loss of balance, or other symptoms of peripheral neuropathy

Planning: Patient outcome

1.   Patient remains free of injury.

Nursing Interventions

Explain to the patient that:
- Symptoms may be related to chemotherapy.
- Reporting the symptoms is important.

Instruct the patient to:
- Avoid use of heating pads to areas with reduced feeling.
- Test bath water temperature to avoid scalding.
- Use gloves for washing dishes and gardening, and protect hands when cooking.

Assist with and teach range of joint motion exercises.

Use foot board if indicated for foot drop.

Use pillows to correct body alignment.

Refer patient to visiting nurse service for follow-up care if indicated.

NDx: Risk for impaired skin integrity related to sun-burn

Planning: Patient outcomes

1. Skin is intact.
2. Skin is free of erythema and lesions.

Nursing Interventions

Teach patient to:
- Avoid the rays of the sun by wearing protective clothing and applying sunscreen (SPF 15) if exposed to the sun.
- Report signs and symptoms.
- Follow topical medication schedules if ordered.

Explain:
- Skin reactions are expected and related to the chemotherapy
- Nail growth may be slowed
- Skin changes and vein and nail darkening are usually temporary.

NDx: Risk for body image disturbance related to loss of hair and skin hyperpigmentation

Planning: Patient outcomes

1. Patient verbalizes acceptance of self with skin and hair changes.
2. Patient identifies positive aspects of self.
3. Patient expresses pleasure at visits from family and friends.

Nursing Interventions

Implement measures to assist the patient in adapting to a change in physical appearance.

Explain:
- Hair loss is almost always temporary (except in high doses of radiotherapy to the scalp).
- Timing of hair loss — will start approximately 14 days after treatment.
- Hair sometimes grows back while the patient is still receiving treatment and it can fall out again.

- Hair will start to permanently grow after treatment is withdrawn.
- New hair may be different in color and texture.
- Facial and body hair can also be affected.
- The scalp may become irritated with skin flaking.
  — Inform the patient that the cost of wigs and hairpieces is covered by most third party health insurance companies. Local units of the American Cancer Society will lend patients wigs free of charge.

Suggest:
- Purchasing a wig or hairpiece before alopecia begins.
- Cutting long hair to decrease the anxiety associated with losing large amounts of hair.
- Using a mild shampoo to alleviate scalp irritation.
- Using hats and scarves.
- Methods to reduce the rate of hair loss:
  — Limit hair brushing.
  — Avoid using harsh shampoos.
  — Wear a hair net to sleep at night.
  — Review hypothermia technique if indicated and with physician approval.

NDx: Risk for ineffective breathing pattern related to inflammation and decreased lung expansion

Planning: Patient outcomes

1. Lung sounds are normal.
2. Arterial blood gases are within the patient's normal range.

Nursing Interventions

Medicate with antibiotics, steroids, and bronchodilators as prescribed.

Adjust patient to comfortable sitting position.

Administer and teach use of respiratory therapy measures as ordered.

Administer and monitor effects of oxygen therapy if indicated.

Refer patient to visiting nurse service for continued home follow-up.

Provide support by explaining all procedures and interventions to patient.

NDx: Risk for decreased cardiac output related to toxic effects of chemotherapeutic agents on the heart

Planning: Patient outcome

1. Signs and symptoms of heart failure are absent.

Nursing Interventions

Teach signs and symptoms of heart failure, and encourage the patient to report all symptoms.
Record cumulative doses of doxorubicin and daunorubicin.
Monitor and report changes in interval physical assessments and interval cardiac test results to physician.

NDx: Sexual dysfunction related to physiologic and psychological effects of chemotherapy

Planning: Patient outcomes

1. Patient describes potential effects of chemotherapy on sexual function.
2. Patient verbalizes concerns about sex role and desirability as a sexual partner.
3. Patient identifies measures supportive of sexual function.

Nursing Interventions

Inform females about:
- Possible amenorrhea
- Possible onset of early menopause with symptoms of "hot flashes," vaginal dryness, and dyspareunia
- Birth control methods if premenopausal
- Possible dyspareunia related to decreased lubrication of vaginal walls. Use of water-soluble lubricant or steroid cream if indicated.

Inform males about:
- Possible temporary or permanent sterility
- Possible impotence related to therapy, anxiety, and fatigue

Provide information about penile prosthesis implantation, if indicated.

Suggest sperm banking before therapy begins, if indicated.

Refer patients and partners to appropriate professionals, if indicated.

Allow time for discussion of sexual dysfunction.

Provide written information regarding contraception methods.

Chest Drainage

Chest drainage is used to remove air or fluid from the chest, thus restoring negative pressure and reexpanding the lung. A chest drainage system consists of a chest tube attached to a valve mechanism designed to allow air or fluid to drain out of, but not into, the chest cavity. A single chest tube is placed in the pleural space to remove air. Two tubes are placed to remove both air and fluid — one anteriorly through the second intercostal space to remove air and the other posteriorly through the eighth or ninth intercostal space in the midaxillary line to drain blood or other fluid.

ASSESSMENT

- Assess respiratory status: auscultate lungs q2h; check VS q4h; observe for abnormal chest movements and cyanosis.
- Be alert for signs of extended pneumothorax (increased area of absent breath sounds and hyperresonant percussion note, increased tachycardia, increased respiratory distress, cyanosis, restlessness, sudden sharp chest pain, confusion) or hemothorax (diminished or absent breath sounds, dyspnea, cyanosis).
- Assess function of the chest drainage system q1h:
  — Check that the drainage system is below the level of the patient's chest.
  — Check that the tube is free of kinks, dependent loops, or other external obstruction.
  — Check that all connections are secure.
  — Note color and amount of drainage.

— Observe for fluctuation of the fluid level in the water-seal chamber, as it indicates a patent system.
— Observe the water-seal chamber for constant bubbling, which is suggestive of an air leak.
• Assess the patient's anxiety level and his or her understanding of chest drainage.

NURSING DIAGNOSES, PLANNING, AND NURSING INTERVENTIONS

NDx: Ineffective breathing pattern related to decreased lung expansion

Planning: Patient outcomes

1. Breath sounds are normal.
2. Respirations are unlabored and occur at a rate of 16 to 20 per minute.
3. ABG values are approaching normal.
4. Lung reexpansion is seen on chest x-ray film.

Nursing Interventions

Maintain an airtight, patent, functioning chest-drainage system.

Retape all connections as needed.

Retape chest-tube dressing if tape is loose. If the dressing becomes saturated with drainage, reinforce and tape securely or, if allowed, remove and replace wet gauze, being certain not to disrupt the petrolatum gauze seal.

Keep the tubing free of loops, kinks, or other external pressure that could interfere with drainage.

Place a rolled towel under the chest to protect tubing from the body's weight.

Encourage the patient to cough and deep breathe frequently.

Change the patient's position frequently to promote both drainage and ventilation.

Ask the patient to cough or change position immediately if fluctuation in the water-seal chamber ceases and the tubing is not kinked or otherwise obstructed.

Clamp the tube or place the end of the tube in a bottle of sterile saline held below the level of the chest and immediately replace the system if the drainage system is broken or interrupted. Remember that a chest tube can be clamped only momentarily if air can enter the pleural cavity with inspiration.

Keep an occlusive petrolatum jelly dressing at the bedside.

If the chest tube is accidentally dislodged, immediately cover the opening in the chest wall with an occlusive, petrolatum jelly dressing. Tape this dressing in place on three sides. Leave the fourth side untaped.

Additional Interventions

a. Mark the amount of chest drainage in the collection container at 1- to 4-hour intervals by placing a piece of tape vertically on the container and drawing a line with date and hour noted each time the drainage is checked.

b. Notify the physician if there is constant bubbling in the water-seal chamber or if drainage becomes bright red or increases suddenly.

c. Provide the patient with basic information about the chest-drainage system to allay anxiety.

d. Reassure the patient that a staff member is nearby and provide easy access to the call bell or intercom.

e. After chest tube removal, monitor the patient for respiratory distress and check the airtight dressing over the wound for drainage.

◆ Cholecystectomy

Cholecystectomy is the surgical removal of the gallbladder through a high right subcostal incision. A laparoscopic cholecystectomy is performed through a 1-cm incision located in the lower umbilical area of the abdomen while a conventional open cholecystectomy is through a high right subcostal incision. Following open cholecystectomy a Penrose drain is inserted to prevent accumulation of drainage in the operative area. It exits through a stab wound on the abdominal wall near the incision. If a choledocholithotomy (incision into the common bile duct to remove stones from the bile duct) is performed, a T-tube is placed in the duct to ensure its patency until the edema subsides and to prevent narrowing secondary to healing. Bile flows both to the duodenum and to the drainage collection system.

PREOPERATIVE CARE

Provide basic preoperative care as described under that entry.

Assess for the clinical manifestations of cholecystitis: intolerance to fatty foods, nausea with or without vomiting, flatulence, elevated temperature, right upper quadrant discomfort or pain radiating to the right scapula and shoulder, jaundice, clay colored stool, and dark colored urine.

Monitor serum prothrombin time in patients with obstructive jaundice and administer vitamin K before surgery as ordered.

Assess respiratory status and carefully teach prophylactic measures such as coughing and deep breathing.

POSTOPERATIVE CARE

Assessments

- Make usual postoperative assessments related to physiologic stabilization.
- Check vital signs and I & O.
- Auscultate the lungs for decreased or adventitious sounds.
- Observe for shallow or guarded breathing and weak cough.
- Check for displacement and patency of the T-tube.
- Observe the amount, color, consistency, and odor of the drainage from the T-tube, Penrose drain, and NG tube if in place.
- Inspect the suture line for signs of infection and the skin for signs of irritation.
- Inspect the sclerae for jaundice.
- Auscultate for bowel sounds and palpate the abdomen for distention.
- Review WBC counts and note any elevation.

Nursing Diagnoses, Planning, and Nursing Interventions

NDx: Risk for impaired gas exchange related to shallow breathing secondary to pain on deep breathing

Planning: Patient outcomes

1. Rate and depth of respirations are within patient's normal range.
2. Lungs are clear to auscultation.
3. ABG values are within patient's normal limits.

Nursing Interventions

Administer analgesics every 3 to 4 hours for the first 24 to 48 hours postoperatively as ordered to facilitate deep respiratory excursion.

Splint the incision site while encouraging the patient to cough and deep breathe every hour in the early postoperative period.

Place the patient in a low Fowler's position when in bed to reduce pressure on the diaphragm.

Turn the patient every 2 hours and ambulate as soon as allowed.

NDx: Risk for impaired skin integrity related to copious drainage from the surgical site

Planning: Patient outcomes

1. Skin is free from excoriation.
2. Dressing remains dry and intact.

Nursing Interventions

Avoid altering position of T-tube during dressing changes.

Change the dressing frequently for the first 24 hours if a Penrose drain is in place.

Use Montgomery straps to minimize skin irritation.

Cleanse the suture line with sterile normal saline or an antiseptic at each dressing change.

NDx: Risk for altered health maintenance related to insufficient knowledge of self care after discharge

Planning: Patient outcomes

1. Patient lists signs and symptoms that should be reported to a health care professional.
2. Patient demonstrates care of the wound.
3. Patient states date of follow-up appointment.

Nursing Interventions

Instruct the patient in self care after discharge as follows:

- Keep the T-tube drainage bag below the level of the T-tube.
- Prevent pull on the tube by coiling the drainage tubing and securing to the abdomen with tape or other fastener.
- Avoid tight fitting clothing, which can irritate the wound or put pressure on the T-tube.
- Expect possible bile leakage; select clothing that can be washed in a solution of detergent, bleach, and baking soda if staining occurs.
- Open the drain spout and empty the T-tube drainage bag each day at the same time. Be sure to note the amount of drainage in the bag so that changes in the amount of drainage can be identified.
- Never irrigate, aspirate, or clamp the T-tube.
- Change the dressing around the T-tube daily. While holding the tube in place, remove the old dressing, wipe skin area around the tube with an antiseptic, apply a clean precut dressing, and tape in place.
- Take showers, not tub baths, to help prevent bacteria from entering the wound.
- Avoid strenuous activities, which could place strain on the wound.
- Report increased, purulent, or foul-smelling drainage; redness, swelling, warmth, or pain at the incision line; oral temperature greater then 100°F; abdominal pain; nausea or vomiting.
- Return for follow-up cholangiogram on (specify date, time, and place).

Additional Interventions

Apply antiembolic stockings as ordered.
Instruct the patient to do foot and leg exercises every hour while awake.

Encourage early ambulation and avoidance of sitting or standing in one position for a long time.

Attach the T-tube to the patient's gown to prevent pull on the tube from the drainage bag.

Keep the drainage tubing free of kinks and below the level of the suture line to prevent reflux of bile.

Never irrigate, aspirate, or clamp the T-tube.

Return excess bile to the patient via NG tube as ordered.

When peristalsis is reestablished and the NG tube is removed, give clear liquids as tolerated and progress gradually to a full diet.

Colonoscopy

Colonoscopy is the direct visualization of the lining of the large intestine all the way to the ileocecal valve by means of a colonoscope passed through the anus. It is used to help distinguish inflammatory from malignant disease in patients with constipation and diarrhea, anorexia, persistent rectal bleeding, or lower abdominal pain and to check for recurring polyps or malignant tumors. The bowel is cleansed and the patient may be kept NPO for 8 hours. A sedative may be given IV; a digital rectal examination is done; and the colonoscope is inserted, slowly advanced to the ileocecal valve, then slowly withdrawn to allow detailed visualization. Biopsy and cytology specimens may be obtained, polyps excised, and photographs taken if required. Infrequent but possible complications are bleeding and perforation of the bowel wall. If either of these occur, surgical intervention may be necessary.

NURSING CARE

Assess the patient's understanding of the procedure and the preparation for it.

Explain that a sensation of cramping or needing to have a bowel movement is not uncommon.

Following the procedure, assess for signs of perforation: sudden temperature spike, tachycardia, abdominal pain.

Encourage rest for 30 to 60 minutes.

Give fluids and foods when patient has passed flatus.

Observe stool for red blood.

Make certain someone is available to escort the patient
home after any sedation has worn off if the procedure was done on an outpatient basis.

◆ Colostomy

A colostomy is a surgically created opening between the
colon and the abdominal wall through which fecal matter
is expelled. Consistency of stool varies with location of the
colostomy: liquid stool from an ascending colostomy,
mushy from a transverse, semi-formed from a descending, and essentially normal from a sigmoid colostomy.

Preparation for the procedure is similar to that for any
intestinal resection with the addition that the stoma site
may be marked on the abdomen preoperatively by the
surgeon or enterostomal therapist.

PREOPERATIVE CARE

Provide basic care as described under Preoperative and
Postoperative Care in this text.
Assess patient's ability to accept and care for a colostomy:
previous experience with an ostomy, perception of
its effects on his/her lifestyle, and available sources
of support.
Reinforce information regarding the location and function of the colostomy as well as meaning of terms
such as *stoma* and *appliance*.
Orient patient to equipment to be used after surgery.
Provide significant others with an opportunity to ask
questions and express concerns, as they are often as
upset as the patient.
Offer to arrange a visit from an Ostomate.

POSTOPERATIVE CARE

Assessment

- Make basic assessments required by an intestinal
  resection (see entry).
- Assess stoma for shape, color (normally deep pink
  to red, shiny, and moist), and consistency (soft or
  slightly firm to touch).

- Observe stoma for more than the normal amounts of pinpoint bleeding expected and for edema that is significant but decreases over 4 to 6 weeks.
- Observe pouch to determine amount and character of discharge, which should consist of mucus and serosanguineous drainage for 24 to 72 hours.
- Assess for return of bowel function: listen for bowel sounds, check for passage of flatus.
- Note color, consistency, and amount of fecal drainage when colostomy begins to function.
- Check peristomal skin for signs of impaired circulation, irritation, and separation from the stoma.
- Assess patient's coping.

Nursing Diagnoses, Planning, and Nursing Interventions

NDx: Bowel incontinence related to the formation of a colostomy and loss of rectal functioning

Planning: Patient outcomes

1. Patient uses the selected pouching system effectively to collect fecal drainage.
2. Patient identifies factors such as change in diet and times of eating that affect pattern of colostomy function.

Nursing Interventions

Monitor collection pouch applied at time of surgery for accumulation of flatus and drainage and change at about one-third full as back pressure can disrupt suture line.

Assist patient in selection of a collection system that is best suited to individual needs.

Use collection system selected by patient consistently to avoid confusion.

Stress that appliances need to be fitted to the stoma and that size should be checked 3 weeks after surgery and finally at 12 to 16 weeks to allow for the progressive decrease in edema.

Explain to patients with a descending sigmoid colostomy that control may be attained and the need for a pouch eliminated through a pattern of regular diet and exercise.

NDx: Risk for impaired skin integrity related to irritation of the peristomal skin from contact with ostomy output, from removal of adherent appliances, or from sensitivity to adhesives and other materials

Planning: Patient outcomes

1. Peristomal skin is free of erythema and blisters.
2. Peristomal skin is intact.

Nursing Interventions

Remove mucus or feces with a tissue.

Wash the peristomal skin thoroughly to remove all traces of intestinal discharge.

Rinse carefully to remove all soap residue; dry gently and completely.

Omit soap and wash with warm water only if the patient is an elderly person whose skin tends to be dry.

Do not use oily soaps or emollients because they interfere with the adherence of the collection pouch.

Use a skin barrier to protect the eighth of an inch of exposed skin between the stoma and the pouch opening from exposure to fecal drainage.

Warm pectin based wafers by placing under the patient's upper back or between the hands to increase adhesiveness to the skin.

Use pastes in conjunction with wafers to fill in creases and folds to obtain a better and longer lasting pouch seal for patients whose colostomy is in a difficult location.

Apply a skin sealant to peristomal skin area where adhesive will be applied to hold the collection pouch in place.

Apply the pouch snugly and monitor routinely for leaking.

Change the pouch immediately if leaking occurs.

Use an electric or straight razor to remove hair from peristomal skin if needed; avoid depilatories because of the risk of sensitivity to them.

If the skin around stoma is reddened:

- Change the appliance every 1 to 2 days.

- Wash the area with warm water, pat dry, and then expose to a heat lamp with a 60-watt bulb positioned 12 to 16 inches from the stoma for 20 minutes.
- Place gauze wet with saline over the stoma to protect it.
- Apply a skin barrier carefully patterned to the stoma and collection appliance.

Institute the following treatment if peristomal skin is broken:

- Change the collection appliance daily.
- Wash the skin.
- Apply compresses of Burow's solution for 30 minutes. Follow with a heat lamp treatment, and apply a protective preparation such as Orabase to broken areas.
- Reapply a skin barrier and appliance.
- Do not use antacids on the skin because they raise the pH and predispose to infection.
- Avoid aluminum paste because it decreases adhesion of the pouch and is hard to remove.

Monitor for signs of yeast infection: irregular patches of deep erythema with papular lesions and the appearance of dry, scaling areas of skin as the process progresses.

NDx: Risk for altered nutrition: less than body requirements related to omission of foods with essential nutrients from the diet because of flatulence, odor, or diarrhea

Planning: Patient outcomes

1. Patient describes components of a nutritionally balanced diet.
2. Patient is able to select a nutritionally balanced diet from foods that are tolerated well.
3. Patient identifies specific foods that are likely causes of flatulence, odor, or diarrhea.

Nursing Interventions

Explain the importance of ingesting 2500 mL of fluid per day.
Instruct in meeting nutritional needs as follows:
- Eat a low-residue diet for 4 to 6 weeks after surgery.

- Progress to a high-carbohydrate, high-protein general diet after this 4- to 6-week period.
- Add new foods one at a time to determine their effects.
- Try each food at least three times before eliminating from diet.
- Consider the effects of specific foods on the gastrointestinal system when selecting the diet:
  - Constipating foods: cheese, nuts, chocolate, corn, raisins
  - Laxative foods: prunes, fresh fruit, broccoli, spinach, green beans, liver, highly spiced foods, beer
  - Gas-forming foods: nuts, cabbage, sauerkraut, corn, cauliflower, broccoli, spinach, peas, beans, apples, avocados, watermelon, cucumbers, carbonated beverages
  - Odor-causing foods: alcohol (particularly beers), onions, beans, cabbage, turnips, asparagus, mushrooms, radishes, cucumbers, eggs, fish, highly spiced foods
  - Deodorizing foods: parsley, beet greens, spinach, buttermilk, yogurt
- Remember that milk and milk products are often not tolerated well and should be limited.

NDx: Risk for body image disturbance related to loss of bowel control, presence of stoma, release of fecal matter onto abdomen, passage of flatus, odor, and need for appliance

Planning: Patient outcomes

1. Patient verbalizes acceptance of self with the colostomy.
2. Patient identifies own strengths.
3. Patient expresses pleasure at visits from relatives and friends.
4. Patient discusses resumption of work, household, and social activities from a positive perspective.

Nursing Interventions

Acknowledge that negative feelings about the colostomy are normal and that it takes time to accept and adjust to this body change.

Avoid any nonverbal behaviors that may convey revulsion, distaste, or pity.

Allow the patient to experience denial while gently fostering acceptance of reality:

- Do not force the patient to look at the stoma or participate in care.
- Do use the terms *colostomy* and *stoma*, describe their appearance, and give brief explanations of the colostomy care being given.
- Touch the stoma to show that it does not hurt, is not easily damaged, and is not revolting.
- Provide an opportunity for the patient to look at or touch the stoma.

Protect the patient from unnecessary embarrassment by ensuring privacy for discussion, teaching, and colostomy care.

Control odor:

- Empty the collection pouch of malodorous flatus or fecal drainage prior to meals and visiting hours.
- Provide good ventilation.
- Do not put pin holes in disposable plastic pouches to allow flatus to escape because this results in unpredictable, uncontrolled odor.

Encourage the patient to be well groomed.

Stress that with some attention to the style of clothing purchased, the ostomy and pouch cannot be noticed.

Foster the patient's sense of control by involving in decision-making.

Encourage the family to treat the patient normally and to engage in a frank discussion of feelings.

NDx: Risk for altered health maintenance related to insufficient knowledge of care of the colostomy, effect on lifestyle, and support services

Planning: Patient outcomes

1. Patient demonstrates correct appliance application.
2. Patient identifies symptoms that should be reported to the health care professional.
3. Patient correctly demonstrates cleaning and deodorizing of the appliance.
4. Patient identifies potential side effects of the colostomy on individual lifestyle without exaggeration or denial.

5. Patient describes available support services, including how to contact the United Ostomy Association.

Nursing Interventions

Teach the patient to care for the colostomy: to identify needed supplies, to empty the pouch, to change the pouch, to control odor, to clean the appliance, and to care for the peristomal skin.

Instruct the patient to:

- Empty the pouch when it is one-third full and at bedtime.
- Set an alarm clock for a few days to awaken in time to empty the pouch.
- Use one hand to support the skin while lifting adhesive with the other when changing the pouch.
- Change the pouch first thing in the morning before eating or drinking because the colostomy is usually not functioning at this time.
- Dispose of pouches in plastic bags, first wrapping them in aluminum foil if it is desired to disguise what is being disposed of.
- Use odor-proof pouch and put deodorant substance such as Nilodor or baking soda in bag PRN.
- Wash reusable appliances with soap and water and expose to fresh air.
- Soak appliances in a commercially available deodorizer if odor persists.
- Resume all activities gradually over 8 weeks.

Refer to ostomy clubs or other support groups.

Additional Interventions

Affirm that sexual intercourse, conception, and pregnancy are all possible following a colostomy.

Recommend emptying appliance before intercourse.

Encourage open discussion of concerns with spouse or significant other.

◆Computed Tomography (CT)

A computed tomography is a noninvasive x-ray used to diagnose pathologic conditions of the head, neck, spine, chest, abdomen, kidneys, and adrenals. An oral or intravenous iodinated contrast dye may be administered prior to the test for better visualization.

PREPROCEDURE CARE

Assessment

- Obtain baseline vital signs.
- Check for allergy to iodinated dye or shellfish.
- Note if an informed consent has been obtained, if required by the institution.
- Check that NPO status has been maintained for 4 hours prior to the procedure.
- Determine the patient's level of understanding about the procedure.
- Observe for signs of increased anxiety such as restlessness or changes in vital signs.

Nursing Diagnoses, Planning, and Nursing Interventions

NDx: Knowledge deficit: Nature of the procedure, potential findings, and follow-up medical management necessary

Planning: Patient outcomes

1. Patient verbalizes the necessity for the procedure.
2. Patient describes the procedure as presented by the physician, radiologist or nurse.

Nursing Interventions

Describe the procedure and the diagnostic equipment using terminology that is easily understandable to the patient.

Explain that feeling somewhat claustrophobic during the testing is quite common.

Tell the patient that some discomfort may be experienced from lying on the hard table for 1/2–1 hour, and some mild nausea may occur from the dye.

Ask the patient to reiterate the information given by the physician and radiologist to check for understanding and to correct misconceptions.

Explain what care will be initiated during the postprocedure time period.

NDx: Anxiety related to fear of the test findings, and the discomfort associated with the testing procedure

Planning: Patient outcomes

1. Patient verbalizes a decrease in anxiety.
2. Patient's vital signs are within normal ranges.
3. Patient rests well prior to the procedure.

Nursing Interventions

Reassure the patient about the necessity for the procedure.

Use comfort measures to promote relaxation.

Allow the patient to verbalize concerns about the potential findings and necessary treatment.

Answer questions honestly, but refrain from giving false reassurance.

Administer a mild sedative (if PRN order available) prior to the testing.

Explain that the discomforts associated with the procedure are usually minimal such as slight stiffness and mild nausea.

Provide an emesis basin at the patient's side.

POSTPROCEDURE CARE

Encourage the patient to drink increased amounts of oral fluids to promote dye excretion and prevent renal complications.

Observe the color, consistency, and amount of urine output.

Check for diarrhea, which may result from oral ingestion of contrast media.

Assess for dyspnea, tachycardia, flushing, rashes, or wheals, which may indicate a reaction to the contrast dye.

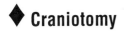

◆ Craniotomy

A craniotomy is an opening in the skull that is created to perform a surgical intervention on the intracranial contents. A bone flap is formed by making several burr holes through which a special saw with a guide wire cuts through the skull from the inside of the skull out, avoiding injury to the brain. The bone flap is replaced at the conclusion of the surgery.

PREOPERATIVE CARE

Provide basic preoperative care as described under that entry.

Assess and document the patient's neurologic status and vital signs to provide a baseline for postoperative comparison.

Assess the patient's and family's understanding of the medical problem and procedure to be performed.

Ascertain whether patient and family expectations in regard to prognosis are realistic.

POSTOPERATIVE CARE

Assessment

- Check vital signs and neurologic signs: temperature, pulse, respirations, blood pressure, pupillary and other reflexes, level of consciousness, arm lifts, hand grips, leg lifts, and ankle plantar flexion and dorsiflexion.
- Observe depth and pattern of respirations.
- Check ABG values.
- Observe for accumulation of oral secretions.
- Assess for abnormal bleeding and clear or yellowish drainage.
- Assess for signs of restlessness and discomfort.
- Observe for seizures.

Nursing Diagnoses, Planning, and Nursing Interventions

NDx: Pain related to surgical trauma of the scalp and cranial tissues

Planning: Patient outcomes

1. Patient rests quietly.
2. Patient reports pain is relieved or manageable.

Nursing Interventions

Administer medications as ordered (narcotics and most barbiturates are contraindicated).

Maintain a quiet, dim environment.

Avoid sudden or jarring movement of the patient.

Apply ice packs to the head as ordered.

Help the patient use alternative pain relief measures such as relaxation techniques.

Report increasingly severe, prolonged, or newly occurring headache to the physician.

NDx: Risk for impaired gas exchange related to post-anesthetic state

Planning: Patient outcomes

1. Patent airway is maintained.
2. Patient maintains regular respiratory pattern of 12 to 24 breaths per minute.

Nursing Interventions

Suction the patient as needed.

Administer O_2 as ordered.

Instruct the conscious patient to breathe deeply but not to cough vigorously.

Turn the patient frequently.

NDx: Risk for altered tissue perfusion: cerebral related to postoperative cerebral edema

Planning: Patient outcomes

1. Patient maintains or improves neurologic status.

Nursing Interventions

Position the patient with the head elevated 30° to 45°.

Position the patient on the back or on the side opposite the incision.

Avoid twisting or flexing of the neck of the unconscious patient.

Never position the patient with the head lowered.

Instruct the patient to avoid coughing, straining, sneezing, and hip flexion.

NDx: Risk for infection related to break in skin integrity

Planning: Patient outcomes

1. Patient is afebrile.
2. Purulent drainage is absent.
3. Incision is clean and approximated.

Nursing Interventions

Monitor temperature and report elevations of 2° or more.

Administer prophylactic antibiotics as ordered.

Use strict aseptic technique when handling the operative site.

Monitor the dressing for blood or cerebrospinal fluid and report to physician.

Instruct the patient to keep the incision clean and dry once the dressing is removed and to avoid scratching it.

Additional Interventions

Offer fluids when the patient is alert and progress to a regular diet as tolerated and ordered.

Apply lightweight ice packs to the eyes to decrease periorbital edema.

Provide total nursing care for the first 48 hours after surgery.

Whenever possible, encourage the patient to participate in care.

◆ Cystoscopy

A cystoscopy is an examination of the urinary bladder and urethra by direct visualization through a fiberoptic scope. Several types of specimens can be obtained during the cystoscopy such as saline washings for cytologic examination and biopsies of suspicious areas. Treatments and surgical excision of tissue or surgical repairs may be completed during the instrumentation. Catheters may be introduced during cystoscopy for drainage, dilation, or splinting of the upper urinary system. Ureteral or bladder stones may be crushed and removed through the cystoscope. Routine cystoscopy is performed under local anesthesia, but regional, spinal, or general anesthesia may be used when the physician prefers it, or when multiple biopsies or other painful procedures are anticipated.

PREOPERATIVE NURSING CARE

Review the history and other completed diagnostic studies.

Assess the patient's anxiety level regarding the cystoscopy, since the nature of cystoscopy provokes great anxiety in some patients, requiring repeated reassurances and explanations.

Evaluate any physical limitations that would prevent the patient from lying in a lithotomy position.

Explain the necessity of the procedure to the patient and the details of what is to be done.

Maintain NPO status after midnight prior to surgery if general anesthesia is to be used.

Teach the patient relaxation methods during the preoperative period for use in the postoperative period.

Complete the routine preoperative care as outlined in Preoperative Nursing Care entry in this text.

POSTOPERATIVE NURSING CARE

After the cystoscopy, monitor I & O carefully.

Encourage increased fluid intake.

Notify the physician if the patient does not void within 8 hours or if excessive bleeding or pain is present.

Note any hematuria or change in the appearance of the urine, although dysuria and frequency are common for 24 to 48 hours.

If an indwelling catheter is present, monitor for patency and measure the output.

Document both the color and amount of urine.

Medicate the patient as necessary for discomfort from bladder spasms.

Give the patient written discharge instructions and review the information verbally in understandable terms.

Explain the home care needed to the family and allow time for questions or concerns.

Refer to the Nursing Care Guide for Patients Undergoing Cystoscopy 30-1 in the textbook.

 Dilation and Curettage

Dilation and curettage (D&C) is a common operative procedure in which the cervix is dilated and the uterine endometrium scraped out. Its uses include diagnosis of uterine malignancies, control of abnormal uterine bleeding, relief of dysmenorrhea, abortion, and emptying of the uterus after an incomplete abortion.

NURSING CARE

Provide basic pre- and postoperative care as described under that entry.

Monitor vaginal bleeding by keeping a pad count and noting degree of saturation. Bleeding is excessive when pads are changed every hour after the first postoperative hour and more than one is saturated in an 8-hour interval.

Monitor for abdominal cramping: assure patient this is expected; give analgesics and/or apply heat to the abdomen as ordered.

Note time and amount of voiding.

Start fluids when alert; progress to normal diet as tolerated.

Instruct the patient in self care as follows:

- Expect bleeding to darken and progressively decrease.
- Consider a few small clots normal.

- Report recurrent bright red bleeding, foul odor, continuous sharp abdominal pain unrelieved by analgesics, fever or chills.
- Avoid strenuous exercise and heavy work. Gradually increase overall activity with return to full routine in 2 weeks.
- Avoid use of tampons for 1 week.
- Avoid sexual intercourse for 2 weeks or until bleeding stops.

◆ Electrocardiography (ECG, EKG)

An ECG is a graphic representation of the electrical impulses of the heart. Electrodes placed on the body surface (limbs and chest) detect the electrical activity of the cardiac cycle in a variety of *lead system* combinations. The 12-lead ECG is composed of three bipolar and nine unipolar leads that record atrial depolarization (*P* wave), ventricular depolarization (*QRS* complex), and ventricular repolarization (*ST* segment and *T* wave). It is used to analyze abnormalities in the electrical conduction system of the heart, which may relate to various disease states. Cardiac disease may be present even if the ECG is normal since some cardiac disorders do not affect the conduction system.

NURSING CARE

Explain the procedure to the patient and allow time for questions.

Tell the patient that food and fluids may be ingested prior to the exam.

Explain that there is no discomfort associated with the test, but it requires the patient to lie still for approximately 5 minutes.

Keep the patient covered as much as possible during the procedure to prevent chilling and unnecessary exposure.

Clean the patient's skin at the sites of electrode placement after the test is completed.

◆ Endoscopy

Endoscopy is the visualization of the inside of a body cavity by means of a tube illuminated by an external light source. Most endoscopic examinations are done with a flexible fiberoptic scope, which can provide an undistorted image of the body cavity even when completely bent. This scope is designed to allow passage of instruments so that pictures can be taken, biopsies obtained, polyps and foreign objects removed, and bleeding areas cauterized. Specific types of endoscopy include bronchoscopy, esophagogastroduo-denoscopy, colonoscopy, retrograde pancreatoscopy, cystoscopy, and arthroscopy. See entries under these headings for further information.

◆ Enteral Nutrition (Tube Feedings)

Enteral feedings are used to maintain weight in patients with severe anorexia, increased metabolic needs, or inability to eat by mouth. They are given by intermittent or continous drip.

ASSESSMENT

- Observe for signs of improved nutritional status: weight gain, increased energy, improved condition of hair, skin, and nails.
- Check for bowel sounds and placement of tube before each intermittent feeding and q 4h during continuous feedings.
- Assess for tolerance of feedings: check for nausea, cramping, abdominal distention, vomiting, diarrhea.
- Check urine for glucose and acetone and check blood glucose daily.
- Check for signs of aspiration (abrupt coughing and gagging with sudden dyspnea; low grade fever and slowly developing cough), hyperglycemia (thirst, polyuria, confusion), dehydration (loss of skin tur-

gor, thirst, change in mentation, rapid weight loss, urinary specific gravity over 1.018).

NURSING DIAGNOSES, PLANNING, AND NURSING INTERVENTIONS

NDx: Altered nutrition: less than body requirements related to inadequate intake or absorption of nutrients

Planning: Patient outcomes

1. Patient maintains weight or shows slow, steady weight gain.
2. Patient is in positive nitrogen balance.
3. Serum levels are within normal range.

Nursing Interventions

Give water in addition to enteral feedings in amount needed to have daily intake exceed output by 500 ml.

Record I & O.

Weigh patient OD at same time and on same scale.

Notify physician of rapid weight gain or loss which can signify overhydration or dehydration, respectively.

If feeding administration rate must be decreased for tolerance, compare calories per day at the new rate with calories per day ordered; record new amount and notify physician if significantly fewer.

NDx: Risk for aspiration related to enteral feeding

Planning: Patient outcomes

1. Abrupt coughing and gagging are absent.
2. Respirations are silent and easy.
3. Lungs are clear on auscultation.

Nursing Interventions

Keep head elevated at least 30° during feeding and for at least one hour after.

Check placement of tube before every intermittent feeding and q 4h during continous feeding; if placement is in question, delay feeding until confirmed.

Check gastric residual before every intermittent feeding and q 2-4h during continuous; discontinue feeding if residual is more than 30 ml; recheck in 30-60 min; if still more than 30 ml, notify physician.

Attempt to reposition tube by rotating it, advancing it a few inches, pulling it back slightly; changing patient's position; or injecting a little air if the plunger cannot be withdrawn or only air is aspirated.

Discontinue feeding and call physician if nausea or vomiting occurs.

NDx: Risk for diarrhea related to intolerance of formula administered

Planning: Patient outcomes

1.   Patient passes formed stool at regular intervals.
2.   Patient denies abdominal cramping.

Nursing Interventions

Build tolerance to feedings by giving slowly over long periods of time initially and gradually increasing rate and time between feedings.

Dilute formula with water PRN; increase to full strength gradually.

Administer feedings at room temperature.

Prevent bacterial contamination of feeding by: using aseptic technique; changing administration set q 12 h; never letting formula hang longer than the recommended time; never storing in the refrigerator longer than 24 hours; and rinsing reusable bags and tubing with warm water before adding new formula.

Additional Interventions

Use a 30 ml syringe to aspirate fluid behind a clog in the feeding tube; if not successful, flush with warm water.

Flush tube with at least 30 ml of water q 3-4h during continuous feedings and at beginning of intermittent feedings to prevent clogging.

Do not flush with fruit juice.

Squeeze or shake container of formula at intervals if thick.

Administer medications by mixing (crush tablets thoroughly) with a small amount of water. Follow each drug with 5 ml of water and give 25 ml of water after last medication. If giving directly into jejunum, dilute with 50-100 ml of water.
Never give bulk forming agents via a feeding tube.

Esophagogastroduodenoscopy

Esophagogastroduodenoscopy is the direct visualization of the esophagus, stomach, and the beginning of the duodenum by means of an endoscope passed through the patient's mouth. It is used in the diagnosis of hiatus hernia, esophageal varices, esophagitis, ulcer disease, polyps, and malignant tumors as well as to identify areas of bleeding and to obtain biopsy specimens. Food and fluids are withheld for 8 hours prior to the procedure or, if an emergency, stomach contents are aspirated. A sedative such as Versed is given IV; the throat is anesthetized; the scope is guided through the mouth to the hypopharynx; the patient is asked to swallow; and the scope is advanced to the area to be examined. It is essential that the patient lie perfectly still during the procedure. Photographs of lesions and brushings for cytologic examination are taken when indicated. The major complication is perforation of the GI tract with excessive bleeding and subsequent infection. Aspiration is a risk if food and fluids have not been withheld prior to the procedure.

NURSING CARE

Following the procedure, check vital signs, level of consciousness, and return of the gag reflex.
Also assess for bleeding and pain.
Report immediately any complaints of sharp, intense pain in the abdomen or chest or a sudden rise in temperature and tachycardia.
Give food and fluids when the gag reflex returns and instruct the patient in the use of gargles or lozenges for a sore throat.

Make certain someone is available to escort the patient home after the sedation has worn off if the procedure was done on an outpatient basis.

◆ Fixation Devices: External and Internal

Treatment of musculoskeletal disorders by simple casting and/or prolonged immobility in traction is not appropriate for all patients or all disorders. In some situations an external or internal fixation device may be used to stabilize the involved bone or joint.

An external fixation device consists of a metal frame with attached metal percutaneous pins that are held rigidly in place by the frame. The percutaneous pins are inserted into or through the bone above and below a fracture or defect in the bone or joint. An external fixation device is used to compress bone fragments and to maintain alignment for bone, joint, or soft tissue healing. Indications for external fixation therapy include: open fractures with nerve and vascular damage, open contaminated fractures with soft tissue damage and infection, severe comminuted fractures, leg lengthening, joints to be removed temporarily, and joint fusions.

Internal fixation devices are surgically inserted directly into or attached onto bone to provide support, to fill in a defect, or to achieve and maintain reduction of fracture fragments. They allow early ambulation of patients with musculoskeletal disorders.

Internal fixation devices include both temporary and permanent pins, rods, nails, screws, plates, and wires. The type of device selected depends on the condition to be treated and the physician preference. Intraoperative fluoroscopy and postoperative radiographic studies are used to ensure proper placement of the device and correct bone alignment.

ASSESSMENT

- For external fixation devices:
  - Assess the pin sites and the neurovascular status of the involved limb.

- Check the stability of the frame and security of the pins at least once every 4 hours until discharge.
- Assess any wounds and soft tissue injuries for odor, drainage, inflammation, or necrotic areas.
- Assess the patient's knowledge about self care after discharge including care of the pin site and fixation device.

• For internal fixation devices:
Preoperatively
- Assess affected body part as a baseline to detect changes in the postoperative period.
- Determine the patient's understanding about the surgery and the postoperative course.
- Ask the patient about feelings of anxiety or other concerns about the surgery.
- Observe for signs of anxiety such as twitching, increased heart rate and respiratory rate, withdrawal, and crying.

Postoperatively
- Monitor vital signs, check that dressings are secure, and observe for excessive drainage.
- Assess the neurovascular status of the affected body part.
- Check the suture site for redness, swelling, purulent drainage, and bleeding.
- Assess the patient for pain and other discomforts.
- Assess knowledge about self care after discharge.

NURSING DIAGNOSES, PLANNING, AND NURSING INTERVENTIONS

NDx: Anxiety related to the application of the device, or surgical intervention, and ability to manage self care and maintain independence with the device in place

Planning: Patient outcomes

1. Patient denies anxiety, fear, or nervousness about self care and management with the device in place.
2. Patient reports feeling relaxed, resting at intervals, and sleeping well.
3. Signs of increased anxiety such as twitching, nervousness, increased respirations and pulse are absent.

Nursing Interventions

Reinforce the physician's explanation about the need for the fixation device and how it will assist the patient to become mobile.

Show a picture of the device to the patient prior to surgery or application to reduce surprise, fear, and anxiety afterwards.

Allow time for questions or verbalization of concerns from the patient or family.

Assist the patient to find strategies that enhance effective coping and increase independence.

Obtain referral for social services, physical therapy, or occupational therapy, if needed, for assistance with adjustment of lifestyle and maintenance of independence.

Seek assistance of clergy or a professional counselor if appropriate.

NDx: Altered health maintenance related to a knowledge deficit about the care for the fixation device and pin-site care (if external), and mobility management (either external or internal)

Planning: Patient outcomes

1. Patient states appropriate information about care and management of the device and when to notify the physician if problems become evident.
2. Patient demonstrates correct pin-site or suture-line care.
3. Patient moves safely with the fixation device intact, using assistive devices if needed.

Nursing Interventions

Teach the patient how to care for the fixation device (if external) and when to notify the physician if problems arise.

Instruct the patient how to assess the neurovascular status of the involved limb.

Demonstrate pin-site or suture-line care to the patient and allow time for the patient to practice it with supervision.

Reinforce the physician's instructions about weight bearing and manipulation of the affected limb.

271

Discuss limitations, if any, and the use of the affected limb.

Encourage the patient to continue with the prescribed exercises to maintain muscle strength and range of motion of joints adjacent to the affected part.

Teach the patient the appropriate use of the assistive device, if applicable, or obtain referral for physical therapy or occupational therapy.

Provide for the patient's safety by assisting with movement until the patient can securely manage alone or with the assistive device.

Help the patient plan modifications of the home environment if needed.

Provide the patient with suggestions on how to modify clothing to fit over the apparatus if external.

Assist with preparations for self care after discharge, discuss how to prepare a safe home environment, and plan modifications if needed.

Allow the patient to practice with self-help aids that may be needed to assist with daily hygiene and grooming tasks or other activities of daily living.

Teach the patient about dosage, frequency of administration, and side effects of any analgesics or other medications prescribed.

NDx: Risk for infection related to the pin sites and other soft tissue injuries or surgical interventions with suture site

Planning: Patient outcomes

1. Patient remains free from infection.
2. Patient's skin shows signs of healing such as new granulation tissue and closure of wounds.
3. Patient verbalizes correct pin-site care.

Nursing Interventions

Teach the patient to watch for signs of localized infection such as redness, swelling, increased pain or drainage at the pin sites, or signs of systemic infection such as fever, increased pulse and respiratory rate, and general malaise.

Teach the patient aseptic pin-site care.

Tell the patient to report any signs of infection to the attending physician.

NDx: Risk for injury related to premature or improper weight bearing and/or failure of the external/internal fixation device

Planning: Patient outcomes

1. Patient denies problems with mobility or use of the affected part.
2. Patient remains free from injury.
3. Patient verbalizes the correct weight-bearing progression regimen.

Nursing Interventions

Reinforce the information about the surgery and the typical postoperative course that the physician presented to the patient.

Explain when weight bearing is appropriate and how to manipulate until that point in time. Teach the patient how to use the assistive device safely.

Obtain an order for a referral for a physical therapist or occupational therapist to work with the patient.

Teach the patient how to readjust in the home environment to maintain safety.

Tell the patient to report any untoward sign to the physician such as sudden severe pain at the site, inability to bear weight at the appropriate time or falls or other blows to the affected area that may occur.

Demonstrate exercises that will help develop strength in preparation for weight bearing.

NDx: Pain related to surgical intervention and muscle spasms from manipulation during placement of the device

Planning: Patient outcomes

1. Patient reports minimal discomfort or pain
2. Patient states methods to decrease pain by using relaxation techniques and the appropriate use of analgesics

Nursing Interventions

Give prescribed analgesics and explain the dosage, frequency, side effects, and expected therapeutic effects of the medication.

Offer analgesics as prescribed just prior to physical therapy and other painful procedures.

Position patient for comfort and reposition frequently.

Encourage the use of relaxation strategies by the patient.

Elevate the extremity for 48 hours postoperatively to reduce swelling unless otherwise ordered.

◆ Gastrectomy

Gastrectomy is the surgical removal of the stomach. In a total gastrectomy, the entire stomach is removed and the esophagus is sutured to either the duodenum or jejunum. In a subtotal gastrectomy, a part of the stomach is removed. Total or subtotal gastrectomy is done to remove benign or malignant tumors of the stomach or to remove a chronic peptic ulcer. It may also be done to stop hemorrhage from a perforated ulcer.

PREOPERATIVE CARE

Provide basic care as described under the Preoperative and Postoperative Care entry in this text.

Assess nutritional and fluid and electrolyte status carefully since the pathology necessitating surgery involves the GI tract.

POSTOPERATIVE CARE

Assessment

- Check vital signs, dressings for drainage, suture line for signs of infection and dehiscence, patency of NG tube, character (normally bloody for 24 hours, then brown-tinged, and finally yellow or clear) and amount (decreases as peristalsis returns, less with total then with subtotal gastrectomy) of drainage.
- Check for fecal odor to gastric aspirate, return of bowel sounds, and passage of flatus.
- Measure abdominal girth to detect abdominal distention.

- Assess tolerance to foods and fluids when oral intake is resumed.
- Record all intake and output and assess overall nutritional status.

Nursing Diagnoses, Planning, and Nursing Interventions

NDx: Risk for ineffective airway clearance related to shallow breathing secondary to diaphragmatic splinting accompanying upper abdominal surgery

Planning: Patient outcomes

1. Patient moves, coughs, and breathes deeply as directed.
2. Lung sounds are clear on auscultation.

Nursing Interventions

Turn, cough, and deep breathe every 2 hours while on bedrest.
Keep head of bed elevated to decrease pull on incision.
Splint incision with pillow when turning, coughing, or deep breathing.
Ambulate as ordered.

NDx: Risk for injury (internal suture line) related to gastric distention, vomiting, or movement of the nasogastric tube

Planning: Patient outcomes

1. Patient is afebrile.
2. Abdomen is soft.
3. Patient states pain is decreasing.

Nursing Interventions

Maintain NG tube suction to prevent gastric distention and vomiting.
Irrigate NG tube gently with NS as ordered to keep it patent.
Reinforce/replace tape anchoring tube to nose PRN.
Notify physician if abdominal girth increases.

NDx: Altered nutrition: less than body requirements related to postoperative dietary restrictions, early satiety, or dumping syndrome

Planning: Patient outcomes

1. Patient ingests a nutritionally well-balanced diet.
2. Patient achieves and maintains recommended weight.

Nursing Interventions

Administer IV fluids as ordered, usually for about 4 days.

When begun on oral intake, start with a clear, warm fluid such as tea since cold liquids tend to cause distress.

Introduce full fluids gradually and progress to a bland diet.

Give six small feedings per day.

Give liquids before or after but not with meals to combat early satiety.

Combat dumping syndrome by instructing the patient to:
- Avoid high carbohydrate foods including fluids like fruit nectar.
- Assume low Fowler's position during meals.
- Lie down for a half hour after eating to delay gastric emptying.
- Avoid fluids with meals.
- Take antispasmodics as ordered to help delay gastric emptying.

Additional Interventions

Administer pain medication as ordered.

Reinforce dressing PRN; if wet with predominantly bloody drainage, change it.

Cleanse and apply water soluble lubricant to naris containing NG tube.

Apply water soluble lubricant to lips to prevent drying and cracking secondary to being NPO and mouth breathing.

Rinse mouth frequently and offer throat lozenges or gum, if allowed, to moisten oral mucous membranes.

Instruct patient to report continuous epigastric distress which increases after eating, or persistent fatigue.

◆ Hysterectomy

Hysterectomy is the surgical excision of the uterus. Vaginal hysterectomy, which is fast and has minimal postoperative discomfort, is done when the uterus is removed because of small fibroid tumors, recurrent bleeding due to endocrine imbalance, and when a vaginal repair is planned simultaneously. Abdominal hysterectomy is done when fibroid tumors are large, when the adnexa are to be removed, and when a women has had previous pelvic surgeries. Risk of postoperative infection and other complications is higher with vaginal hysterectomy, especially in women under 35 or over 60 years of age.

PREOPERATIVE CARE

Provide basic preoperative care as described under the Pre- and Postoperative Care entry.

Assess the patient's understanding of the procedure and its effects (e.g., after hysterectomy, menstruation ceases and pregnancy does not occur; surgical menopause also occurs after hysterectomy with bilateral oophorectomy).

Counsel patients to stop smoking a minimum of 12 to 24 hours prior to surgery.

Administer prophylactic antibiotics as ordered.

Clarify any misconceptions.

POSTOPERATIVE CARE

Assessment

- Make basic assessments of physiologic stabilization as described under the Preoperative and Postoperative care entries.
- Check abdominal dressing and/or perineal pad for bleeding every 15 minutes for 2 hours, every hour for 8 hours, then every 8 hours. Expect a moderate amount of serosanguineous drainage.

- Note time and amount of voiding and check for urinary distention.
- Check for bowel sounds, nausea, vomiting, abdominal distention, belching, gas pain, passage of flatus, and bowel movements.
- Observe for signs of thrombophlebitis: pain, redness, heat, swelling of calf, positive Homans' sign.
- Assess psychological response to the surgery and observe for signs of potential sexual dysfunction.

Nursing Diagnoses, Planning, and Nursing Interventions

NDx: Pain related to tissue trauma secondary to surgical excision of the uterus

Planning: Patient outcomes

1. Patient splints incision when coughing or moving.
2. Nonverbal signs of pain such as grimacing and guarding are absent.
3. Patient reports pain is relieved.
4. Patient gets out of bed, sits, and ambulates without undue discomfort.

Nursing Interventions

Administer prescribed narcotic analgesics at scheduled times for 48 hours.

Promote comfort through positioning, back rubs, etc.

Encourage use of relaxation exercises.

Apply heat to abdomen, ambulate, and insert a rectal tube as ordered to relieve gas pains.

Teach the patient to splint abdominal incision to decrease pain on coughing and moving.

Instruct the patient to pull buttocks together before sitting to decrease vaginal discomfort.

NDx: Risk for altered tissue perfusion related to interruption of venous blood flow

Planning: Patient outcomes

1. Calves are free of heat, redness, and swelling.

2. Homans' sign is negative.
3. Symptoms of pulmonary embolism are absent: respirations are of normal rate and depth, and the patient is free of cyanosis, chest pain, and hemoptysis.

Nursing Interventions

Instruct patient to:
Dorsiflex feet 20 to 25 times each hour while awake and in bed.
Keep legs extended and uncrossed while in bed.
Encourage ambulation as soon as allowed.
Apply antiembolic stockings.

NDx: Risk for altered health maintenance related to insufficient knowledge of discharge instructions

Planning: Patient outcomes

1. Patient describes limitations on activities.
2. Patient lists symptoms to be reported.
3. Patient describes expected emotional reactions.

Nursing Interventions

Instruct the patient to:
Report any bleeding, other than vaginal discharge, or temperature elevation to the health care professional.
Avoid tub baths for 2 to 3 weeks.
Avoid activities that increase pelvic congestion for several months. These include sitting for long periods of time, jogging, fast walking, horseback riding, and douching.
Be prepared for feelings of weakness and fatigue.
Avoid strenuous activities such as heavy lifting and vacuum cleaning for 6 to 8 weeks.
Avoid sexual intercourse for 3 weeks after vaginal hysterectomy and for 6 weeks after an abdominal hysterectomy.
Remember that after an abdominal hysterectomy, abdominal soreness and a feeling that the vagina is narrow and short may occur during intercourse for 3 to 4 weeks.

Recognize that periods of emotional lability and feelings
of depression and sadness are normal.
Return for follow-up appointment.
Provide other basic postoperative care as described under
the Preoperative and Postoperative Care entries.

◆ Ileostomy

An ileostomy is a surgically created opening between
the ileum and the abdominal wall through which malodorous, enzyme rich, caustic, yellow, green, or brown
liquid fecal matter is expelled. Preparation is the same as
for a colostomy. Exactly how much liquid and therefore
what the volume of output is depends on where in the
ileum the ostomy is located. Because the terminal ileum
begins to take over the water absorbing function of the
colon, the closer the ileostomy is to the junction of the
large bowel the less liquid is the output. The three types
of ileostomy are the standard end (Brook's) ileostomy,
ileal pouch-anal canal anastomosis, and continent ileostomy or Kock pouch. A conventional ileostomy expels
flatus and then 1000 to 2000 mL per day of odorless liquid
in 12 to 72 hours. With resumption of oral intake, volume
decreases and effluent turns dark green to yellow to
brown with a distinct odor. In 3 to 6 months it becomes
like fluid paste.

NURSING CARE

Nursing care for a patient having a conventional ileostomy is similar to that for the patient having a
colostomy (See entry). Specific teaching applicable
to the patient who has had a conventional ileostomy
is as follows:
Expect the ileostomy to be noisy initially as a result of
tissue edema but be assured that this will decrease
with time.
Expect undigested foods such as seeds and kernels to pass
through the stoma.
Give meticulous care to the skin surrounding the stoma
because this is more critical with an ileostomy than
with a colostomy owing to the increased danger of
skin excoriation from enzymes in the effluent.

Make ongoing assessments of self for signs of dehydration, hypokalemia, and hyponatremia.

Ingest a mixture of 1 tsp of table salt, 1 tsp baking soda, and 1 quart water as ordered by the physician if diarrhea occurs to correct acidosis secondary to the loss of bicarbonate.

Avoid laxatives.

Maintain accurate fluid intake and output records at all times.

Treat blockage of the ostomy by a mass of undigested high-fiber foods as follows:

- Assume knee-chest position.
- Gently massage area below the stoma.
- Call physician if lumen remains blocked, because a lavage by bulb syringe with 30 to 50 mL of normal saline may be required.
- Adjust pouch, because stoma swells with the blockage.
- Increase fluid intake after removal to compensate for the resultant diarrhea.
- Expect abdominal pain around the stoma for 3 to 5 days.

Intestinal Resection

An intestinal resection is the excision of a part of the small or large intestine. It is used to treat problems such as intestinal malignancy, obstruction, inflammatory bowel disease, perforated diverticulum, and ischemic or traumatic injury. If the two remaining ends of bowel are then surgically joined to reestablish the normal continuity of the bowel, it is an anastomosed resection. If the functioning end of the bowel is brought out onto the abdominal surface, it is a resection with the formation of an ostomy. Preparation for the procedure includes a low-residue diet decreasing to a liquid diet 24 hours before surgery to prevent accumulation of stool; enemas or an oral preparation such as GoLYTELY to empty the bowel; and oral, nonabsorbable antiinfectives to decrease bacteria in the bowel. Fluid and electrolytes are also commonly given to make up for losses. TPN for protein replacement may be needed by some patients.

PREOPERATIVE CARE

Provide basic care as described under Preoperative and
Postoperative Care in this text.

Review normal bowel pattern to establish a baseline for
postoperative assessment of bowel function.

POSTOPERATIVE CARE

Assessment

- Check vital signs, chest excursion, lung sounds,
  color, patency of NG tube, and color, consistency,
  and amount (decreases over 24-48 hr) of drainage.
- Observe for abdominal distention and for drainage
  on the dressing.
- Assess for nausea, pain, dehydration or overhydration, altered electrolyte balance, signs of thrombophlebitis (redness, edema, heat, and pain in the
  calf, positive Homans' sign).
- Measure I & O and daily weight.
- Assess tolerance of oral intake when resumed.
- Assess bowel sounds and question about passage of
  flatus and feces.

NURSING DIAGNOSES, PLANNING, AND NURSING INTERVENTIONS

NDx: Pain related to surgical trauma to the abdomen

Planning: Patient outcomes

1. Patient moves without signs of severe pain such as
   moaning, pallor, and tachycardia.
2. Patient rests quietly without signs of discomfort
   such as clenched hands, groaning, and crying.
3. Patient states pain is relieved.

Nursing Interventions

Give prescribed analgesics as needed.

Position in semi-Fowler's to relieve stress on the suture
line.

Encourage ambulation and use a rectal tube as ordered for
relief of gas pain associated with the return of peristalsis.

NDx: Risk for altered mucous membrane related to NPO status and presence of a nasogastric or nasointestinal tube

Planning: Patient outcomes

1. Oral mucous membrane is moist and free of cracks.
2. Lips are supple, moist, and free of cracks.
3. Patient denies dryness of the mouth.

Nursing Interventions

Assist patient to brush teeth at least three times per day.
Encourage frequent mouth rinses avoiding use of those
    that dry mucous membranes.
Apply water-soluble lubricant to lips.

NDx: Risk for altered nutrition: less than body requirements related to inadequate intake or malabsorption

Planning: Patient outcomes

Patient maintains expected weight.
Patient resumes oral intake of a nutritionally balanced
    diet.
Patient takes nutritional supplements as directed.

Nursing Interventions

Give small amounts of clear fluids when oral intake is
    resumed.
Progress to full fluids and then to a regular diet as toler-
    ated without discomfort such as hiccups, nausea,
    and vomiting.
Give nutritional supplements as ordered.
Alert physician promptly to any weight loss.

NDx: Risk for altered health maintenance related to insufficient knowledge of discharge instructions

Planning: Patient outcomes

1. Patient explains instructions for self care at home.
2. Patient lists symptoms to be reported to the physician.

3.   Patient states time of follow-up appointment.

Nursing Interventions

Instruct patient regarding care of incision, diet, and activities, etc., after discharge, stressing that laxatives must be avoided because of their irritating effects on the bowel.

Instruct patient to report bleeding, abdominal distention, abdominal rigidity, or fever.

Encourage patient to return for follow-up care.

Additional Interventions

Monitor for signs of peritoneal irritation secondary to leaking of the internal suture line.

Instruct in how to splint the wound.

Encourage coughing and deep breathing.

Instruct patient to perform foot and leg exercises ten times each every 2 hours while on bedrest.

Avoid use of knee gatch or pillows under the knees.

Apply antiembolic hose or use sequential compression devices as ordered to promote venous return.

Ambulate patient as ordered.

Instruct patient to avoid crossing legs or sitting for long periods.

 # Joint Replacement

Total joint replacement, or arthroplasty, involves the surgical removal of deformed or diseased joint surfaces and replacement by smooth artificial surfaces made of metal and plastic. The purpose of joint replacement is to relieve pain and to provide increased range of motion and function of the involved joint. Joint prostheses exist for most joints, but replacements for the knee, hip, shoulder, ankle, and wrist, and Silastic implants for the phlanges of the fingers and toes, are the most common. Adverse effects of artificial joints include injury to nerves, producing pain and numbness; infection of the new joint; thromboembolism; loosening of metal or plastic parts; limb length difference; and dislocation of the new joint.

PREOPERATIVE NURSING CARE
Assessment

- Check the neurovascular status of the affected body part as a baseline to detect changes in the postoperative period.
- Determine the patient's understanding of the surgery and the postoperative course.
- Ask the patient about feelings of anxiety or other concerns about the surgery.
- Follow the nursing guidelines in the Preoperative Nursing Care entry in this text.

POSTOPERATIVE NURSING CARE
Assessment

- Monitor vital signs, assessing peripheral pulses and comparing them bilaterally.
- Check that dressings are secure and observe for excessive drainage.
- Check the suture site for redness, swelling, purulent drainage, and bleeding.
- Assess for pain and other discomfort.
- Assess the patient's knowledge about self care after discharge.

Nursing Diagnoses, Planning, and Nursing Interventions

NDx: Anxiety related to placement of a foreign substance in the body and the results of the intervention

Planning: Patient outcomes

1. Patient reports manageable levels of anxiety, fear, or nervousness about the surgery and its potential outcome.
2. Patient reports being relaxed, rests at intervals, and sleeps well.
3. Signs of increased anxiety such as twitching, nervousness, increased respirations and pulse are absent.

Nursing Interventions

Reinforce the physician's explanation about the need for the prosthesis and how it will permit the patient to maintain mobility.

Allow time for questions or verbalization of concerns from the patient or family.

Assist the patient to find strategies that enhance effective coping.

Provide teaching regarding the possible course of rehabilitation.

Seek assistance of clergy or a professional counselor if appropriate.

NDx: Altered health maintenance related to lack of information about self care, potential complications, and ability to complete activities of daily living

Planning: Patient outcomes

1. Patient states appropriate information about self care, avoiding complications, and when to notify the physician if problems become evident.
2. Patient demonstrates correct exercises to maintain strength and range of motion.
3. Patient moves the involved part safely, using assistive devices if needed.

Nursing Interventions

Teach the patient when to notify the physician if problems arise.

Reinforce the physician's instructions about weight bearing and manipulation of the involved part.

Discuss limitations, if any, and the use of the affected limb.

Encourage the patient to continue with the prescribed exercises to maintain muscle strength and range of motion of joints adjacent to the affected part.

Teach the patient the appropriate use of the assistive device, if applicable, or refer the patient to physical therapy or occupational therapy.

Provide for the patient's safety by assisting with movement until the patient can securely manage alone or with the assistive device.

Discuss any obstacles that may interfere with the patient's safe mobility in the home setting.

Help the patient plan modifications of the home environment if needed.

Assist with preparations for rehabilitation or self care after discharge.

Teach the patient about dosage, frequency of administration, and side effects of any analgesics or other medications prescribed.

NDx: Risk for infection related to the wound, surgical intervention, and foreign device

Planning: Patient outcomes

1. Patient remains free from infection.
2. Patient's suture line shows signs of healing such as new granulation tissue and absence of drainage, swelling, or redness.
3. Patient states an understanding of the need to take prophylactic antibiotics prior to some invasive procedures and dental work.

Nursing Interventions

Teach the patient to watch for signs of localized infection such as redness, swelling, increased pain, or drainage at the suture line.

Be certain the patient understands wound care if it is still necessary after discharge.

Tell the patient to report any signs of infection to the attending physician.

Explain about the need to take prophylactic antibiotics prior to undergoing an invasive procedure or dental work.

NDx: Risk for injury related to premature weight bearing and/or failure of the prosthesis

Planning: Patient outcomes

1. Patient denies problems with mobility or use of the affected part.
2. Patient remains free from injury.

Nursing Interventions

Reinforce the information about the surgery and the typical postoperative course that the physician presented to the patient.
Explain when weight bearing is appropriate and how to
  manipulate until that point in time.
Teach the patient how to use the assistive device safely.
Obtain orders for a physical therapist or occupational
  therapist to work with the patient.
Teach the patient how to readjust the home environment
  to maintain safety.
Tell the patient to report to the physician any untoward
  sign such as sudden severe pain at the site, inability to bear weight at the appropriate time, or falls or
  other blows to the affected area that may occur.
Demonstrate exercises that will help develop strength in
  preparation for weight bearing.

NDx: Pain related to surgical intervention and muscle
spasms from manipulation during placement of the device

Planning: Patient outcomes

1. Patient denies discomfort or pain.
2. Patient's affected body part returns to an acceptable
    level of mobility.

Nursing Interventions

Offer analgesics as prescribed, especially prior to physical
  therapy and other painful procedures.
Position the patient for comfort and reposition frequently,
  unless otherwise contraindicated.
Support the affected part and maintain proper alignment
  with pillows or blankets until the patient is able to
  move independently.
Avoid extreme adduction or abduction of the involved
  body part.
Elevate the extremity for 48 hours postoperatively to
  reduce swelling and pressure, unless otherwise ordered.

◆ Laparoscopy

Laparoscopy is a procedure in which the internal organs of the abdomen and pelvis are visualized and examined by means of a laparoscope. The laparoscope is inserted typically under general anesthesia through an incision in the abdominal wall (usually the lower aspect of the umbilicus) after the abdomen has been insufflated with a gas such as carbon dioxide. Laparoscopy is done for diagnostic (evaluation of patients with chronic abdominal or pelvic pain, abdominal neoplasm, metastatic disease) and for therapeutic (bilateral tubal ligation, removal of adhesions, cholecystectomy, ablation of endometrium) purposes. Complications include perforation of the bowel, peritonitis, embolism, and infection.

NURSING CARE

Obtain baseline vital signs prior to the procedure.

Monitor vital signs every 15 minutes until stable following the procedure.

Position the patient supine or in low Fowler's position to decrease pressure of the insufflated gas on diaphragm.

Administer prescribed analgesics for chest and shoulder discomfort.

Give warm saline gargles for relief of sore throat due to intubation.

Allow resumption of activity as tolerated.

Give fluids and light foods as tolerated.

Instruct the patient in self care as follows:

- Apply heat and take analgesics for chest and shoulder discomfort.
- Ambulate to promote resorption of insufflated gas.
- Gargle with warm water and salt to relieve sore throat.
- Avoid lifting for 7 to 10 days.
- Resume full activity over a 3 day period.
- Resume sexual intercourse when comfortable to do so.
- Report oral temperature higher than 100°F (37.7°C), or any redness, swelling, or drainage from the wound.

◆ Lobectomy

A lobectomy is a surgical procedure in which a lobe of a lung is removed. Two chest tubes connected to water-seal drainage systems are placed for postoperative removal of air and fluid from the chest cavity.

PREOPERATIVE CARE

Preoperative care is essentially the same as that prior to a pneumonectomy. (See entry under Pneumonectomy.)

POSTOPERATIVE CARE

Assessment

- Postoperative assessments are essentially the same as those made following a pneumonectomy. In addition, see assessments to be made following the insertion of chest tubes under that entry.

Nursing Diagnoses, Planning, and Nursing Interventions

NDx: Ineffective breathing pattern related to unwillingness to breathe deeply secondary to pain, fear of displacing chest tubes, or depressant effects of anesthesia and analgesics

Planning: Patient outcomes

1. Breath sounds and percussion note over remaining lung tissue are normal.
2. Lung reexpansion is evident on x-ray film.

Nursing Interventions

Position the patient on the back or with the operated side up for the first 48 hours.
Keep the patient elevated in a semi-Fowler's position.
Monitor the respiratory rate every 1 to 2 hours.
Auscultate the lungs every 2 to 3 hours.

Direct the patient in diaphragmatic and pursed lip breathing every 1 to 2 hours.

Coordinate breathing exercises with peak effectiveness of pain medications.

Instruct and assist the patient in splinting the incision anteriorly and posteriorly.

Direct the patient in the use of the incentive spirometer every 2 to 3 hours.

Administer oxygen as ordered.

Monitor ABG values.

Plan frequent rest periods.

See nursing interventions related to care of the chest tubes under that entry.

NDx: Impaired physical mobility related to transection of chest muscles affecting shoulder movement and severe pain in the chest and shoulder secondary to surgery

Planning: Patient outcomes

1. Patient moves affected shoulder through usual active range of motion (ROM).
2. Patient uses affected arm in performing ADL.
3. Patient assumes an erect position.

Nursing Interventions

Perform passive ROM exercises to affected arm at least 2 times every 4 to 6 hours for 24 hours postoperatively.

Instruct and guide the patient in active arm and shoulder exercises 10 to 20 times every 2 hours thereafter.

Encourage the use of the affected arm in self-care activities.

Structure the environment to foster the use of the affected arm.

Encourage the patient to assume a fully erect position.

NDx: Body-image disturbance related to loss of lung tissue and the accompanying change in respiratory function

Planning: Patient outcomes

1. Patient realistically describes changes in physical status resulting from surgery.

2. Patient verbalizes acceptance of the change in respiratory status.

Nursing Interventions

Encourage the patient to verbalize perceptions and feelings about altered respiratory status.

Acknowledge feelings of anger, fear, sadness, and helplessness as real and valid.

Assist the patient in identifying the effect on respiratory status, physical stamina, and function.

Encourage sharing of mutual concerns between patient and significant other.

For additional nursing interventions, and those related to ineffective airway clearance and pain, see the care of the patient with a pneumonectomy.

 # Lumbar Puncture

A lumbar puncture is a procedure in which a sterile needle is inserted into the subarachnoid space at the L-4 to L-5 level in order to determine CSF pressure; obtain samples of CSF; to reduce ICP; or introduce anesthetics and intrathecal medications.

PREPROCEDURE CARE

No special preparation.

POSTPROCEDURE CARE

Nursing Care

Instruct the patient to lie flat for 6 hours following the procedure.

Monitor vital signs and neurological signs.

Assess for headache.

Administer analgesics as ordered.

Maintain IV fluids as ordered.

Encourage oral fluids.

◆ Magnetic Resonance Imaging

MRI uses magnetic fields and radio waves analyzed by computer to produce two- and three-dimensional cross sectional images of the body. It reveals subtle variations in structure such as tumor masses, degenerative changes, areas of necrotic tissue, and blood flow, which often cannot be identified with other types of diagnostic modalities. It does not involve exposure to radiation or to contrast materials.

Patient preparation for an MRI consists of donning a patient gown and removing all metal objects such as hairpins, glasses, jewelry, and dentures. The patient is given ear plugs to protect against the intermittent banging noises that occur during the procedure and is then placed on a nonmagnetic stretcher that slides into a narrow tunnel-like space in the MRI machine. At all times during the 30 to 90 minute procedure, the patient is in verbal communication with the technician.

MRI cannot be done on patients with pacemakers or metallic implants, or on those having an IV infusion.

◆ Mechanical Ventilation

Mechanical ventilation is used to maintain proper levels of oxygen and carbon dioxide in the blood when a patient's own ventilatory ability is inadequate to achieve this goal. Negative pressure ventilators, which exert negative pressure on the chest to expand during inspiration, are used in the care of patients with neuromuscular disorders, such as myasthenia gravis, multiple sclerosis, and muscular dystrophy. Positive pressure ventilators, which exert positive pressure on airways to inflate alveoli during inspiration, are used in the care of patients with chest and lung disorders, such as flail chest, chronic bronchitis, emphysema, and adult respiratory distress syndrome.

Pressure-cycled ventilators, which are set to deliver a preset positive pressure for a specified length of time or until the preset pressure is reached, are generally used for short-term, closely monitored situations, such as in a PACU. Volume-cycled ventilators deliver a constant volume of air with each breath regardless of the positive pressure necessary to attain that volume. Both are positive-pressure ventilators.

ASSESSMENT

- Auscultate lung sounds, assess need for suctioning, and observe for symmetric chest expansion every 2 hours.
- Check vital signs every 2 to 4 hours.
- Assess for signs of hypoxia (restlessness, anxiety, tachycardia, increased respiratory rate, increased work of breathing, cyanosis, confusion), hypercapnia (somnolence, lethargy, tachycardia, confusion, headache), and hypocapnia (muscle spasm, tetany, diaphoresis, light-headedness, tachypnea, cardiac dysrhythmia).
- Assess the patient's synchrony with the ventilator.
- Check ABG values at regular intervals and whenever ventilator settings are changed.
- Observe for signs of decreased cardiac output (weak peripheral pulses, narrowed pulse pressure, slow capillary refill, decreased urinary output, restlessness, decreasing level of consciousness, pallor, fatigue, chest pain) in patients on PEEP.
- Observe for signs of cardiac overload and pulmonary edema if settings for PEEP are decreased.
- Check nasogastric drainage and stool for frank or occult blood and review hematocrit values since stress ulcers are associated with mechanical ventilation.
- Inspect the skin for redness and breakdown.
- Assess joint mobility and nutritional status.
- Assess for anxiety, feelings of powerlessness, and for other emotional responses to the ventilator.
- Assess endotracheal/tracheostomy tube every hour for proper placement and function and at the same time check the ventilator for proper settings and working alarms.

NURSING DIAGNOSES, PLANNING, AND PATIENT OUTCOMES

NDx: Ineffective breathing pattern related to (specify) or inability to sustain spontaneous ventilation related to (specify).

Planning: Patient outcomes

1. ABG values are within patient's normal range.

Nursing Interventions

Maintain ventilator closed-circuit system.

Prevent accidental disconnection of the patient from the ventilator by leaving the alarm on at all times, even during suctioning.

Keep a manual resuscitation bag at the bedside, and manually ventilate the patient if power fails or the ventilator malfunctions.

Respond immediately to any alarm; if the problem cannot be immediately identified and corrected, disconnect the patient and ventilate by hand while problem is further investigated.

Check settings on the ventilator every hour.

Check tubing for condensation and drain collected water to prevent aspiration.

Promote synchronization between patient and ventilator by slowly ventilating by bag for three to six breaths or by verbally coaching the patient as to when to inhale and exhale.

Administer ordered analgesics or sedatives.

NDx: Risk for ineffective airway clearance related to excessive secretions

Planning: Patient outcomes

1. Breath sounds are normal.
2. ABG values are within patient's normal range.

Nursing Interventions

Direct the patient to cough and deep breathe every 2 hours.

Change the patient's position at least every 2 hours.
Position patient on unaffected side or back if only one lung
is affected.
Suction as needed.
Maintain humidification, making certain that the water
level is maintained in the ventilator reservoir.
Perform chest physiotherapy as ordered.
Administer prescribed intravenous or inhaled broncho-
dilators.

NDx: Risk for fluid volume excess related to blocked
insensible water loss

Planning: Patient outcomes

1. Chest sounds are clear.
2. Extremities are free of edema.
3. Vital signs are within patient's baseline range.

Nursing Interventions

Measure I & O.
Weigh patient daily.
Monitor for edema, crackles, hyponatremia, and decreased
hematocrit.

NDx: Impaired physical mobility related to mechanical ventilation

Planning: Patient outcomes

1. Joints have patient's normal range of motion (ROM).
2. Patient moves as directed.

Nursing Interventions

Change patient's position and provide skin care every 2
hours.
Perform active or passive ROM exercises every 8 hours.
Maintain position of function while the patient is on
bedrest to prevent contractures and external hip
rotation.
Use a foot board and have patient wear tie-up shoes or
high-top sneakers to prevent foot drop.

Sit patient in a chair as soon as his or her condition allows.

Walk the patient while ventilating with oxygen via a bag or while pushing the ventilator along when permitted.

NDx: Anxiety related to being on a mechanical ventilator

Planning: Patient outcomes

1. Body posture appears relaxed.
2. Facial expression appears relaxed.

Nursing Interventions

Explain procedures and equipment to patient and family.

Reassure patient and family regarding the dependability of the machine and that close supervision is provided.

Do not leave patient unattended until he or she has anxiety under control and is comfortable with ventilator.

Involve the patient in decision making regarding care to provide a sense of control.

Encourage the use of relaxation exercises, tape recordings, and other stress-reduction techniques.

Provide a diversion suited to the patient's condition and personal preference.

Facilitate discussion of concerns and anxieties with significant others and provide information as needed.

Promote communication between patient and family.

NDx: Risk for altered thought processes related to change in sensory input secondary to limited mobility

Planning: Patient outcomes

1. Patient is oriented to time, place, and person.

Nursing Interventions

Speak frequently to the patient.

Call the patient by name and orient to day, time, date, and place as part of routine care.

Place a calendar and clock within the patient's view.

Dim lighting at bedtime to help distinguish between day and night.

Ask family members to bring in pictures or other personal items that can be placed in the patient's environment.

Provide patient with a window view to allow light and sensory stimulation.

Encourage diversionary activities and visits by significant others.

Plan uninterrupted periods of rest and sleep.

Additional Interventions

Provide oral hygiene every 8h.

Give antacids or other medication ordered to combat stress ulcers.

Administer tube feedings or total parenteral nutrition (TPN) solutions as ordered.

Monitor bowel function.

◆ Modified Radical Mastectomy

Modified radical mastectomy is a treatment for breast cancer that involves the removal of the entire breast, skin, pectoralis minor muscle, and axillary lymph nodes but preserves the major pectoral muscles. Survival rates equal those of patients treated with radical mastectomy, in which the major pectoral muscles are removed.

PREOPERATIVE CARE

Provide basic preoperative care as described under that entry.

Note size and location of any palpable mass, presence of discharge from the nipple, dimpling of the skin, areas of ulceration, and deviation of the direction of the nipple.

Assess the patient's anxiety level, level of coping, and support systems.

Review with the patient information provided by the surgeon regarding the procedure and make certain the patient understands that a wound drainage system and a large pressure dressing will be in place postoperatively, and that the affected arm and hand will be elevated on pillows.

Demonstrate exercises for the affected shoulder and arm and obtain a return demonstration of all exercises.

POSTOPERATIVE CARE

Assessment

Make usual postoperative assessments related to physiologic stabilization.

Check vital signs.

Inspect the dressing and sheets under the patient for bleeding.

Check the wound drainage system and note the color and amount of drainage.

Assess for pain and for mobility of the affected arm.

Inspect the affected arm for signs of infection: redness, warmth and edema.

Assess the level of stress and anxiety the patient and family are experiencing.

NURSING DIAGNOSES, PLANNING, AND NURSING INTERVENTIONS

NDx: Pain related to surgical trauma of the anterior chest

Planning: Patient outcomes

1. Patient takes pain medication as needed.
2. Patient reports reduced pain.

Nursing Interventions

Administer prescribed narcotic analgesics as needed.

Institute comfort measures such as positioning, rubbing the patient's back, and applying heat to the back, shoulder and upper arm as ordered.

Guide the patient in the use of relaxation techniques.

Provide diversionary activities.

Reassure the patient that the pain will decrease to soreness in 48 to 72 hours.

NDx: Risk for infection related to vascular and lymphatic alteration from surgery

Planning: Patient outcomes

1.   Patient explains the need to protect the affected arm from trauma.
2.   Patient lists precautions to be taken to protect the affected arm.
3.   Patient verbalizes understanding of aseptic techniques in caring for dressing, drains, and incision at home.

Nursing Interventions

Explain to the patient that the removal of lymph nodes in the axillary region makes the arm more prone to infection.

Place a sign near the patient's bed and on her Kardex that the affected arm cannot be used for drawing blood, taking blood pressure, or administering IV fluids.

Teach the patient the signs and symptoms of infection and instruct her to report abnormalities to the physician.

Instruct the patient to protect the affected arm and hand from injury as follows:

Avoid:
- Burns while cooking or smoking
- Sunburns
- Injections, vaccinations, blood samples, and blood pressure tests done on the affected arm when possible
- Nicks and scratches
- Cutting cuticles and nails
- Touching hot and cold things
- Elastic cuffs on blouses and sleepwear

Always:
- Carry heavy packages or handbags on the other arm
- Wash cuts promptly with soap and water, apply an antibacterial medication, and monitor for redness, soreness, or other signs of infection
- Wear watches and jewelry loosely on the operated arm
- Wear protective gloves when gardening and when using strong detergents
- Use a thimble when sewing

- Use lotion on cuticles; push cuticles back with a soft cloth and file nails
- Use mitt-type holder when cooking
- Use an electric razor for underarm shaving
- Report signs of swelling, redness, and pain in affected arm

NDx: Risk for impaired physical mobility related to breast surgery

Planning: Patient outcomes

1. Patient states the rationale for exercising the affected arm.
2. Patient demonstrates range of motion exercises.
3. Patient plans progressive exercise regimen 3–5 times daily.
4. Patient lists activities of daily living that enhance arm and shoulder movement.

Nursing Interventions

Start passive range-of-motion exercises of the arm and shoulder on the affected side and provide a soft ball for the patient to squeeze as soon as possible postoperatively.

Encourage the patient to start gradual active range of motion exercises and to begin to use the affected arm and shoulder to care for herself as soon as the suction is removed and permission is obtained from the physician.

Teach the patient appropriate range-of-motion exercises such as those used in the Reach to Recovery Program and discuss how appropriate exercises can be incorporated into daily routines.

NDx: Risk for body image disturbance related to the loss of the breast

Planning: Patient outcomes

1. Patient verbalizes feelings, concerns and questions about change in body image.
2. Patient views incision, if able, prior to discharge.
3. Patient is receptive to information about prostheses.
4. Patient expresses positive feelings about self.

Nursing Interventions

Encourage the patient to talk about her feelings.

Acknowledge and accept feelings of loss, grief, fear of rejection.

Encourage the patient to look at the incision.

Provide the patient with information about obtaining both a temporary and permanent breast prosthesis.

Provide the patient with information about breast reconstruction.

Additional Interventions

Explain to the patient that mild to severe lymphedema can occur in the affected arm at any time after surgery.

Instruct the patient not to overdo arm exercises and to facilitate venous return by elevating the arm.

Encourage discussion about sexual activities and handle it in a sensitive and open manner.

Nasogastric Intubation

Nasogastric intubation refers to the insertion of a tube through the nose into the stomach. It may be done to remove toxic substances by suction, to instill irrigating solutions or medications, to control bleeding, or to administer external feedings. It is also done to remove gastric contents when the GI tract is unable to propel or absorb its secretions or until a suture line in the GI tract is healed.

ASSESSMENT

- Assess function of tube inserted to remove gastric contents q 4h by checking for drainage and that the patient is free of feelings of fullness or nausea. Irrigate with NS to check patency PRN.
- Check amount, color (normal is yellow-green), and consistency of drainage.
- Observe for passage of flatus, bowel movement, signs of fluid and electrolyte imbalance, and irritation of naris from the tube.

- Measure I & O, including amounts of irrigating fluid instilled and returned.

NURSING DIAGNOSES, PLANNING, AND NURSING INTERVENTIONS

NDx: Risk for altered oral mucous membrane related to mouth breathing and limitation on oral intake

Planning: Patient outcomes

1. Oral mucous membrane is pink and moist.
2. Lips are supple, moist, and free of cracks.
3. Patient denies soreness or dryness of mouth and lips.

Nursing Interventions

Assist patient to brush teeth and rinse mouth every 4 hours while awake.

Use a soft toothbrush.

Avoid lemon and glycerin swabs as well as commercial mouthwashes because they are drying.

Clean the mouth of the unconscious patient with saline or hydrogen peroxide-moistened swabs four to six times each day.

Apply a water-soluble lubricant to the lips to keep them supple and prevent cracking.

Allow patient to "mist" the mouth with a spray bottle of water or offer gum, small amounts of Gatorade, warm saline gargles, or anesthetic throat lozenges to help wet mucous membranes of the mouth and soothe irritated pharynx if permitted.

Do not allow the patient to swallow sips of water or suck on ice chips unless specifically ordered.

NDx: Risk for fluid volume deficit related to drainage rather than reabsorption of gastrointestinal secretions

Planning: Patient outcomes

1. Skin turgor is firm.
2. Mucous membranes are moist.
3. Urinary output is at least 50 ml/hr.
4. Urinary specific gravity is between 1.003 and 1.035.

5. Serum electrolyte levels and acid-base parameters are within normal range.

Nursing Interventions

Monitor laboratory data and skin turgor for signs of dehydration.

Administer replacement fluids and electrolytes as ordered.

Obtain daily weights.

Monitor central venous pressure or other hemodynamic parameters to ensure adequate but not over-replacement of fluid.

NDx: Risk for impaired tissue integrity related to mechanical irritation from the NG tube

Planning: Patient outcomes

1. Skin and mucous membranes of the nares are free of erythema.
2. Skin and mucous membranes of the nares are intact.
3. Bleeding from the nares is absent.

Nursing Interventions

Cleanse the area around the nares gently using warm water or saline.

Remove any crusts.

Apply a protective water-soluble lubricant.

Prevent pull on the tube by looping an elastic band around it, then looping the tube above the elastic around the patient's ear, and using a safety pin inserted through the elastic band to pin the tube to the patient's gown or pajamas.

Reinsert the tube through the opposite naris or change position of tube over the ear if irritation occurs.

Remove the tape anchoring the tube in place daily. Wash the area thoroughly, wipe with an alcohol swab, shave male patients, and apply a new tape.

Use a transparent, moisture- and vapor-permeable dressing such as Op-Site, which can remain in place for as long as seven days, if skin irritation is a problem.

Additional Interventions

Mark the tube at the end of the naris right after insertion
so a change in the tube's position can be identified.

Irrigate tube as ordered to maintain patency:

Use type and amount of solution specified by the physician.

Follow strict sterile technique if the tube is in place to
protect a suture line.

Instill irrigating fluid manually, then reattach to suction.

If the patient is discharged with the tube in place to the
home setting, make a referral to a home health
agency for nursing assistance and education about
tube maintenance and feedings.

Pneumonectomy

A pneumonectomy is the surgical removal of an entire
lung. It is done to treat bronchogenic carcinoma, lung
abscess, bronchiectasis, or unilateral tuberculosis when
the problem is so extensive that all involved tissue cannot
be removed by lobectomy. A chest tube is generally not
inserted during a pneumonectomy; rather, the space is left
to fill with serosanguineous fluid, which eventually solidifies.

PREOPERATIVE CARE

Provide basic preoperative care as described under that
entry.

Perform a complete respiratory assessment. Include history of smoking and exposure to other respiratory
irritants and the amount of exertion required to
induce dyspnea.

Observe the patient for signs of anxiety.

Assess the patient's understanding of the planned surgery
and expected outcomes.

Provide the patient with basic information about the
perioperative experience.

Teach the patient how to perform breathing exercises,
coughing, splinting, and arm and shoulder exercises.

POSTOPERATIVE CARE

Assessment

- Check respiratory rate, heart rate, temperature, blood pressure, CVP readings, and urinary output.
- Observe for signs of respiratory dysfunction: slow, rapid, shallow, or irregular respirations; use of accessory muscles; orthopnea; duskiness or cyanosis; restlessness; irritability; confusion; and somnolence.
- Auscultate the chest for adventitious breath sounds and for diminished or absent breath sounds.
- Check ABG values and chest x-ray results.
- Assess fluid and electrolyte status.
- Check the dressing for the amount and color of drainage.
- Inspect the incision for signs of infection: redness, heat, induration, swelling, lack of approximation, and drainage.
- Monitor for dysrhythmias.
- Observe for signs and symptoms of pulmonary edema: severe dyspnea, tachycardia, dull percussion over unoperated areas, adventitious breath sounds, persistent cough with frothy or blood-tinged sputum, cyanosis, and apprehension.
- Observe for signs and symptoms of mediastinal shift: severe dyspnea, restlessness, agitation, rapid or irregular pulse, cyanosis, displacement of the trachea from the midline, and a change in the point of apical impulse.

Nursing Diagnoses, Planning, and Nursing Interventions

NDx: Ineffective breathing pattern related to unwillingness to breathe deeply secondary to pain and the depressant effects of anesthesia and analgesics

Planning: Patient Outcomes

1. Breath sounds and percussion note over the remaining lung are normal.
2. ABG values are within normal range.

Nursing Interventions

Position the patient on the back or with the unoperated
  side up to promote maximum ventilation of the
  remaining lung and to help keep the fluid that
  accumulates in the pleural space below the level of
  the bronchial stump.
Direct the patient in diaphragmatic and pursed lip breathing and the use of the incentive spirometer every 1-2
  hours.
Assist the patient to splint the incision during breathing
  exercises.
Coordinate breathing exercises and coughing with peak
  effectiveness of pain medication.
Administer oxygen as ordered.
Monitor ABG values and oxygen saturation via pulse
  oximetry.
Provide frequent rest periods.

NDx: Ineffective airway clearance related to increased
secretions secondary to respiratory tract irritation and
poor cough effort secondary to pain and the depressant
effects of anesthesia and analgesics

Planning: Patient Outcomes

1.   Respirations are easy and quiet at a rate of 12 to 20
     per minute.
2.   Breath sounds and percussion note over remaining
     lung are normal.
3.   ABG values are within normal range.

Nursing Interventions

Assist the patient to cough, deep breathe, and turn every
  1-2 hours.
Assist the patient into a sitting position when coughing.
Assist the patient to splint the incision when coughing.
Coordinate breathing exercises and coughing with the
  peak effectiveness of pain medications.
Monitor breath sounds before and after deep breathing
  and coughing exercises.
Monitor the amount, color, and viscosity of expectorate.
Monitor ABG values.

Guide the patient in diapraghmatic breathing exercises, and perform percussion, vibration or postural drainage if ordered.

Do not percuss or vibrate over the operative area.

Administer humidification and minibulizer therapy as ordered.

Suction as necessary.

NDx: Pain (chest and shoulder) related to surgical trauma to muscles, nerves, and other tissues

Planning: Patient outcomes

1. Patient states pain is relieved.
2. Patient moves easily.
3. Patient coughs effectively.

Nursing Interventions

Administer prescribed narcotic analgesics as needed around the clock for the first 24 hours after surgery.

Administer analgesics before the pain becomes severe or 30-40 minutes before painful exercises.

Avoid medicating the patient to the point of inability to cough effectively or respiratory depression.

Administer oral analgesics as ordered after the first 48-72 hours.

Assist the patient to splint the incision.

Support the affected arm and shoulder with pillows or a sling.

Promote comfort and the use of relaxation exercises or guided imagery.

Maintain a calm, quiet environment.

Additional Interventions

Give oral fluids as soon as the patient is alert, and progress to regular prescribed diet as tolerated.

Weigh the patient daily.

Report temperature of 102°F or higher or lower than 98°F.

Monitor for signs of complications such as pulmonary edema, cardiac dysrhythmias, and mediastinal shift.

Notify physician immediately if sputum is excessive or if it contains bright red blood.

Instruct the patient as follows:

- Perform breathing exercises as taught for the first 3 weeks at home.
- Perform arm and shoulder exercises five times a day.
- Practice standing fully erect in front of the mirror until normal posture is restored.
- Expect soreness in the chest and shoulder for several weeks.
- Use hot soaks or a heating pad to relieve chest or shoulder pain.
- Take prescribed or recommended over-the-counter analgesics if additional relief is needed.
- Expect altered sensation around the incision for several weeks.
- Expect feelings of weakness and fatigue for the first 3 weeks after surgery.
- Space activities to allow for frequent rest periods.
- Avoid heavy lifting (more than 20 lb) until muscles of the chest wall have healed completely in 3 to 6 months.
- Build up tolerance to walking by using a moderate pace and by gradually increasing distance and duration.
- Stop any activity that causes chest pain, shortness of breath, or excessive fatigue.
- Stop or decrease smoking if a smoker.
- Avoid exposure to smoke, fumes, aerosol sprays, and other respiratory tract irritants.
- Avoid exposure to colds and other respiratory infections.
- Obtain annual influenza vaccine and pneumonia vaccine as recommended by physician.
- Report signs of respiratory infection: persistent fever, increased sputum production, shortness of breath, or increased discomfort or decreased mobility in affected arm and shoulder.
- Return for follow-up evaluation of wound healing and respiratory function on (specify date and time).

For additional interventions related to impaired physical mobility and body image disturbance, see the care of the patient with a lobectomy.

◆ Preoperative Nursing Care

The preoperative period begins when it is determined that surgery is the best course of treatment and concludes when the patient enters the operative suite. Diagnostic studies are completed, preoperative teaching is initiated, body system disorders are stabilized, and consent for surgery is obtained.

A common surgical risk evaluation is completed during the preoperative period. Common components of the evaluation include:

1. Thorough history and physical examination
2. Psychosocial assessment, including coping mechanisms and support systems
3. Economic status
4. Nutritional status
5. Fluid and electrolyte balance
6. Immune status
7. Cardiovascular status
8. Respiratory status
9. Renal function
10. Hepatic function
11. Endocrine function
12. Hematologic status
13. Pregnancy
14. Therapeutic drug use
15. Drug, alcohol, and nicotine use

Specific diagnostic exams provide information about the need for surgical intervention and its extensiveness. Additional preoperative activities for which the nurse may assume full or partial responsibility include:

- surgical consent
- food and fluid restriction
- elimination
- skin/site preparation
- preanesthesia evaluation
- preanesthesia medication
- checklist of preoperative information

ASSESSMENT

- Obtain history of hospitalization and surgical experiences.

- Determine the patient's knowledge base about the planned surgery.
- Check vital signs.
- Observe for nonverbal signs of anxiety such as nervousness, withdrawal, and increasing pulse rate.
- Ask about significant others, coping mechanisms, and other support systems.

NURSING DIAGNOSES, PLANNING, AND NURSING INTERVENTIONS

NDx: Anxiety related to hospitalization, surgery, surgical outcome, and impact on lifestyle

Planning: Patient outcomes

1. Patient asks questions and verbalizes concerns.
2. Patient verbalizes reduced apprehension about the impending surgical procedure.
3. Patient's vital signs are within normal ranges.

Nursing Interventions

Provide opportunities for the patient and significant others to ask questions and express concerns.

Provide information without giving false or inappropriate hope.

Reinforce explanations from the physician.

Refer questions and concerns that cannot be answered to other members of the health care team.

Utilize the assistance of clergy or other support personnel to counsel the patient.

NDx: Knowledge deficit: Diagnosis, diagnostic procedures, planned surgery, expected outcomes, admission procedures, preoperative and postoperative routines, and expectations

Planning: Patient outcomes

1. Patient verbalizes understanding of diagnosis, diagnostic procedures, planned surgery, expected outcomes, and admission procedures.
2. Patient cooperates with the testing and admission procedures.

3. Patient verbalizes an understanding of the preoperative and postoperative routines and expectations.
4. Patient demonstrates postoperative health maintenance exercises.

Nursing Interventions

Explain all tests and nursing interventions.
Reinforce the physician's explanations.
Review hospital policies that affect the patient and significant others.
Instruct the patient about preoperative and postoperative health maintenance exercises that he or she will be expected to perform such as breathing deeply, coughing, and use of the incentive spirometer.
Reinforce instructions and allow the patient to ask questions to correct misunderstandings.
Supervise the patient's demonstration of the pulmonary exercises, correct any errors, and reinforce correct technique.

Postoperative Nursing Care

The postoperative care period begins when the patient is transferred from the PACU to the postsurgical unit. Nursing care is determined by the differences in individuals (age, previous medical history, sex, etc.), the type of surgery and location of incision(s), and the anesthesia administered. The goals of nursing care during this time period are to promote physical comfort and wound healing, to prevent injury and complications, and to prepare the patient for discharge. As the patient progresses through the postoperative period, care progresses from acute observation and intervention to self care and health teaching.

ASSESSMENT

- Monitor vital signs on arrival to the unit and compare the results with the preoperative and intraoperative data.

- Continue to monitor vital signs until stable or as prescribed by the physician or institutional policy.
- Complete a head-to-toe assessment.
- Examine dressings for placement, adherence, and drainage.
- Check beneath the patient for drainage or bleeding.
- Determine the placement of tubes, drains, or other such equipment; connect to the appropriate receptacles and ensure proper functioning.
- Note the amount and characteristics of all drainage.
- Check the parenteral infusion to ensure the accuracy of the type and rate, and the infusion site for signs of infiltration, or other complications of intravenous therapy.
- Assess for pain, noting the type, duration, location, intensity, and need for analgesics.
- Check the patient's respiratory function, administer oxygen as needed, and observe for signs of respiratory difficulty.

NURSING DIAGNOSES, PLANNING, AND NURSING INTERVENTIONS

NDx: Risk for ineffective breathing pattern related to tracheobronchial obstruction by secretions or hypoventilation secondary to the effects of general anesthesia, postoperative analgesics, pain, and positioning

Planning: Patient outcomes

1. Patient maintains patent airway as evidenced by normal breath sounds.
2. Patient maintains spontaneous unlabored respirations of more than 10/minute and less than 30/minute.
3. Patient remains free of dyspnea and cyanosis.

Nursing Interventions

Reposition the patient side-to-side every hour until fully conscious.

Arouse the patient frequently.

Have the patient take deep breaths and cough every 15 to 30 minutes, splinting the abdomen as needed.

Encourage the use of incentive spirometry when the patient is fully awake.

Auscultate the thorax for adventitious breath sounds.
Offer pain medication at prescribed intervals.

NDx: Pain related to surgical incision and manipulation of internal structures during surgery

Planning: Patient outcomes

1. Patient verbalizes relief of pain or decreased pain to a tolerable level.
2. Patient rests well at intervals after administration of prescribed analgesic.

Nursing Interventions

Determine the location, duration, and intensity of the pain.

Position the patient for maximum comfort.

Encourage the patient to request medication for pain as needed, and offer or administer the prescribed analgesic at regular intervals during the first 48 hours postoperatively.

Utilize guided imagery and distraction to keep the patient from focusing on the pain.

Evaluate the effectiveness of the pain medication to provide relief.

NDx: Risk for infection related to surgical incision, wound drain, and/or bedrest

Planning: Patient outcomes

1. Patient remains free of manifestation of wound infection as evidenced by the absence of fever, wound redness, purulent or malodorous drainage, or edema.
2. Patient demonstrates proper wound care technique and states the signs of wound infection.
3. Patient remains free of manifestations of a respiratory infection as evidenced by the absence of dyspnea, tachypnea, or adventitious breath sounds.

Nursing Interventions

Use universal precautions and aseptic technique during dressing changes.

Instruct the patient on appropriate handwashing and
dressing changes.

Examine the wound for early signs of infection and report
them immediately.

Culture any suspicious drainage.

Change moist dressings promptly.

Encourage a high-protein, high-vitamin diet to aid in
wound healing.

Encourage the patient to cough and breathe deeply frequently, and to use the incentive spirometer to
prevent respiratory infections.

Have the patient move frequently in bed and encourage
early ambulation as allowed to prevent the complications of prolonged bedrest.

◆ Prostatectomy

A prostatectomy, the removal of the prostate gland,
may be simple (only the enlarged portion of the gland is
removed), total (the entire gland and its capsule are excised), or radical (the entire prostate, its capsule, seminal
vesicles, a cuff of the bladder neck, and sometimes pelvic
lymph nodes are removed). The most common surgical
approach is the transurethral prostatectomy (TURP). Other
surgical approaches include the suprapubic (abdominal
and bladder incision), retropubic (low abdominal incision)
and perineal (perineal incision) prostatectomies.

TURP is used to treat symptomatic benign prostatic
hypertrophy when the prostate is only moderately enlarged and occasionally for prostate cancer when the
patient is a poor surgical risk. A cystoscope and resecto-
scope are inserted into the urethra to scrape out the
enlarged portion of the gland. A three-way Foley catheter
is inserted upon completion of the procedure and an
irrigating solution (saline or glycine) is continuously run
in and out of the bladder to keep the operative area clear
and prevent blockage of the catheter. There is no external
surgical incision.

PREOPERATIVE CARE

Provide basic preoperative care as described under that
entry.

Administer a Fleet or soapsuds enema as ordered.

Instruct the patient not to take aspirin or non-steroidal antiinflammatory drugs for one week prior to surgery, because of increased risk of bleeding.

POSTOPERATIVE CARE
Assessment

- Make usual postoperative assessments related to physiologic stabilization.
- Check abdominal or perineal dressings every 15 minutes for 2 hours, then every hour for 8 hours, or more frequently as indicated.
- Check vital signs, central venous pressure, laboratory data, and true urinary output.
- Assess for signs of urethral catheter obstruction: increase in bladder spasms or pain, absence of urine and normal saline irrigant outflow from the indwelling urinary catheter, and distention of the lower abdomen on palpation.
- Observe the color of urinary output from the urethral catheter and for the presence of bloody drainage at penile meatus.
- Observe for signs of TURP syndrome (hypervolemic dilutional hyponatremia): restlessness, muscle twitching, visual disturbances, confusion, disorientation, nausea, vomiting, elevated blood pressure, and bradycardia followed by hypotension and cardiovascular collapse.

Nursing Diagnoses, Planning, and Nursing Interventions

NDx: Risk for urinary retention related to obstruction of urinary drainage tubes and/or surgical trauma to the bladder neck and prostatic urethra

Planning: Patient outcomes

1. Urinary drainage tubes are patent and draining.
2. Bladder distention is absent.
3. Depending on the type and extent of prostatectomy, patient voids continently in amounts of more than 90-120 mL per voiding within 8 hours of catheter removal or has a post-voiding residual urine volume of less than 50 mL.

Nursing Interventions

Maintain the flow of normal saline irrigant at the prescribed rate to keep the urine pink-tinged to clear.

Empty the urinary drainage bag frequently.

Instruct the patient not to lie on the drainage tube.

Check the position of the catheter and drainage tube frequently for kinking.

Keep the tube in a straight line from the bed to the collection bag clip or pin the tube to the bed sheet to prevent looping or coiling and undue pressure on the catheter.

Position the drainage bag on the same side to which the patient is turned while in bed to ensure proper gravity drainage.

Irrigate the catheter by hand as ordered if bladder spasms occur and continuous irrigation is absent.

Do not speed up the irrigant in an attempt to dislodge the obstruction if there is no urinary outflow.

Remove catheter (when ordered) early in the day, preferably before breakfast.

Give the patient a urinal and tell him to use it at the first urge to void.

Record time and amount of voiding for the first 8 to 10 hours after catheter removal.

NDx: Risk for fluid volume excess related to dilutional hyponatremia secondary to absorption of irrigating fluid during TURP

Planning: Patient outcomes

1. Patient is free of agitation and confusion.
2. Blood pressure and pulse are stable and within patient's normal range.
3. Serum sodium and potassium levels and serum osmolarity are within normal limits.
4. Pulse oximetry is within normal limits for the age and condition of the patient.

Nursing Interventions

Monitor the patient for signs of hyponatremia (see **Assessments**).

Monitor vital signs and report a drop in pulse rate and/or an elevation in blood pressure.

Monitor serum electrolytes and report abnormal results.

Assist the patient into a sitting position if dyspnea and pulmonary congestion develop.

Slow the IV rate to KVO if dyspnea and pulmonary congestion develop.

Anticipate the physician's order and secure IV hypertonic saline solution if dyspnea and congestion develop.

Record intake, output, and daily weight after administration of diuretics and hypertonic solutions.

NDx: Pain related to surgical tissue trauma and bladder spasms

Planning: Patient outcomes

1. Patient states that discomfort is lessened or relieved.

Nursing Interventions

Administer analgesics and antispasmodics as ordered.
Keep the catheter patent and draining to relieve bladder spasms.
Provide physical and psychological comfort measures.
Maintain a quiet, restful environment.
Encourage relaxation techniques.

NDx: Risk for altered health maintenance related to insufficient knowledge of self care after prostatectomy

Planning: Patient outcomes

1. Patient lists signs and symptoms to be reported.
2. Patient describes limitations on activity and sexual intercourse and states date of return to work.
3. Patient describes measures to prevent constipation and straining during bowel movements.
4. Patient states reason for use and directions for each discharge medication.
5. Patient states the date of his follow-up visit.

Nursing Interventions

Teach the patient as follows:

- Bloody urine is common immediately after surgery. Small pieces of tissue or blood clots can be passed during urination for up to 2 weeks after surgery.
- Strenuous exercise and sports activities such as tennis, golf, swimming, and lifting objects heavier than 20 lb must be avoided for 6 weeks. These activities can stimulate bleeding.
- Abstinence from sexual intercourse is recommended for a minimum of 3 weeks. Check with the physician before resuming this activity.
- Showering rather than bathing in a tub is recommended. Use of hot tubs should also be discouraged to limit dilation of pelvic blood vessels.
- Driving an automobile and sitting for long periods of time in an automobile are restricted for a minimum of 3 weeks. Check with physician before attempting either activity.
- Return to work usually occurs at 4 to 6 weeks depending on the type and extent of prostatectomy performed and the nature of the work.
- Report promptly abrupt episodes of frank bleeding to the physician.
- Report increases in bloody urine not cleared by drinking fluids (up to 32 oz in 30 minutes) that last for a few hours or one or two voidings.
- Notify physician if urinary stream decreases or if urinating becomes difficult.
- Take medications, especially antibiotics if prescribed, on time as ordered.
- Avoid straining at bowel movement because this can initiate bleeding.
- Maintain a high intake of nonalcoholic fluids (2 to 2.5 L/day) to ensure soft, regular bowel movements, to limit clot formation, and to prevent infection.
- Include fresh vegetables, fruits, whole-grain products (Shredded Wheat), and bran in a well-balanced diet.
- Report signs of constipation early to the physician, who usually orders a stool softener. Avoid use of enemas and suppositories, which can stimulate bleeding; a mild laxative may be used.

- Report signs of urinary tract infection: fever (higher than 37.6°C [99.8°F]), chills, painful urination, back or side pain (flank area), and general malaise.

Additional Interventions

Maintain the sterility of the irrigating solution and equipment; label solution with date and time and discard any older than 24 hours.

Use strict sterile technique when irrigating the urethral catheter and changing wound dressings.

Keep penile meatus and catheter junction clean and free of bloody drainage.

Cleanse the skin around the suprapubic catheter (if present) with an antibacterial agent and cover with a dry sterile dressing if ordered.

Encourage oral fluids to 2500 mL per day unless contraindicated.

Monitor for signs of urinary tract infection (elevated temperature, chills, dysuria, pyuria).

Place the call light near the patient and encourage him to use it to call for help.

Encourage the patient to eat a high-fiber diet.

Tape the urethral catheter to the patient's thigh to prevent inadvertent tension on it and resultant trauma to the bladder.

Instruct the patient to move slowly and carefully in bed to avoid displacement of the catheter.

Assist the patient OOB and carefully place urinary drainage bags and normal saline irrigant in front of him.

Encourage the patient to ambulate early and consistently.

Give sitz baths for cleanliness and comfort as ordered following perineal prostatectomy.

Discuss sexuality and temporary retrograde ejaculation with the patient. Include significant other in discussion if appropriate.

Avoid all rectal treatments (with the exception of B & O suppositories) for 48-72 hours postoperatively.

Note: Nursing Interventions for patients undergoing procedures requiring external surgical incisions include special attention to the wound, additional drains and catheters, and skin care. Patients with abdominal incisions may have an NG tube to low suction in place for 3-4 days postoperatively.

Pulmonary Function Studies

Pulmonary function studies measure the functional ability of the lungs by comparing the patient's lung volumes and capacities with those of other people of the same age, sex, height and race. They are used to assess risk of respiratory complications in surgical patients; diagnose and monitor the course of specific pulmonary disorders; evaluate the effect of medications; and determine need for mechanical ventilation.

NURSING IMPLICATIONS

Provide the patient with information and instructions as follows:
- Equipment is complex but the test is simple—lips are sealed around a mouthpiece; a nose clip is placed over the nostrils; and directions are given to perform various inhalation and exhalation maneuvers.
- Fatigue is not unusual after testing.
- Omit medications which may affect respiratory function (e.g., sedatives, narcotics, bronchodilators) for 4 hours before testing.
- Do not eat a meal immediately before the test.
- Wear loose clothing for the test.

Pulse Oximetry

Pulse oximetry is a noninvasive procedure for monitoring arterial blood oxygen saturation levels (SaO_2). It is frequently used in the perioperative periods and in intensive care for patients on mechanical ventilation. It is also used while transporting critical patients within the hospital. It may also be used during stress testing and in testing drug effects for patients with respiratory disorders. A light beam passes through the tissues as the sensor measures the amount of light absorbed. The oxygen saturation is reported as a percentage, with 95% or higher considered normal.

NURSING CARE

Explain the equipment and rationale for testing oxygen
saturation to the patient.

Slightly rub the patient's fingertip (or upper earlobe) to
increase the blood flow and attach the monitor.

Record the data (as specified by the institution).

Radiation Therapy

Radiation therapy utilizes the effects of ionization to
damage and kill cancer cells. Since normal cells as well as
malignant cells can be damaged by radiation, the goal of
therapy is to deliver a lethal dose of radiation to malignant
cells while minimizing the amount of radiation to which
normal cells are subjected.

Depending on the characteristics of the tumor, radiation therapy may be used for either cure or palliation. It
may be used alone or in conjunction with surgery and/or
chemotherapy.

Radiation may be given by external beam (teletherapy)
or internally by implanting radioactive material directly
adjacent to or within the tumor (brachytherapy) (see Cervical Cancer in Section 1 for discussion of internal radiation therapy).

ASSESSMENT

- Assess patient's understanding of radiation therapy,
  its goals, and its potential side effects.
- Observe for skin changes at radiation site: redness,
  tanning, dry or moist desquamation, itching, pain.
- Observe for side effects related specifically to the
  area of the body being irradiated:

Head and Neck

- Inflammation, ulceration, or infection of the oral
  mucous membrane, condition of teeth, oral pain,
  ability to eat, take fluids, swallow, amount and
  consistency of saliva, changes in taste (decreased,
  absent, unpleasant or metallic) nausea and vomiting, alopecia.

Chest or Back

- Sore throat, dysphagia, upper chest pain secondary to esophagitis, dyspnea, dry cough, hemoptysis and fever secondary to pneumonitis.

Upper Abdomen

- Nausea and vomiting.

Lower Abdomen

- Cramping and diarrhea.

Pelvis

- Diarrhea, cystitis, vaginal dryness, stenosis, premature menopause, loss of libido, and sterility.

Hematopoietic System

- Anemia, leukopenia, and thrombocytopenia.

NURSING DIAGNOSES, PLANNING, AND NURSING INTERVENTIONS

NDx: Risk for altered health maintenance related to insufficient knowledge of treatment, side effects, self-care measures, and required follow-up

Planning: Patient outcomes

1. Patient describes expected effects of radiation.
2. Patient states the symptoms of side effects most likely to occur.
3. Patient describes the relationship of symptoms to the radiation therapy, noting that specific symptoms will disappear when the radiation therapy is completed.
4. Patient describes or demonstrates appropriate interventions to control specific side effects.
5. Patient states symptoms that should be reported to the health care professional.

Nursing Interventions

Reinforce explanations of the purpose of the radiation, treatment procedure, and possible side effects.

Instruct patients receiving external radiation therapy in self-care and comfort measures as follows:

- Wear loosely fitting clothing.
- Gently wash the affected area with a mild soap and pat dry.
- Avoid the use of lotion, perfume, and deodorants.
- Avoid pressure on the irritated area.
- Avoid exposure to sun.
- Avoid swimming in saltwater or chlorinated water.
- Avoid applications of heat or cold to irritated areas.
- Use a water-soluble lubricant for dry desquamation.
- Use either the open or partially open treatment for moist desquamation.
  - Open treatment: Keep area clean, dry, uncovered, and exposed to the air.
  - Partially open treatment: Keep area clean and covered with a nonadhering dressing. Change dressing frequently to keep wound surface clean and dry.
- Use cool, moist compresses or water-soluble lubricants for itching.
- Take antihistamines and use topical antipruritic lotions as ordered by the physician.
- Perform good oral hygiene after eating and at bedtime using a soft toothbrush, nonabrasive toothpaste, and dental floss.
- Increase fluids to at least 2500 mL/day unless otherwise restricted.
- Decrease smoking.
- Do a daily self-examination of the mouth and report any changes.
- Rinse the mouth frequently with mouthwash for xerostomia. Use a mouthwash that does not contain a drying agent such as alcohol.
- Breathe through the nose to avoid the drying effect of mouth breathing.
- Suck sour, hard candies to help stimulate saliva and create a pleasant taste.
- Remove thick oral secretions with a swab, and use an oral gavage bag to irrigate the mouth.
- Eat a liquid or blenderized high-protein diet at room temperature if dysphagia or esophagitis is a problem.

- Wash hands properly.
- Keep the fingernails clean and short.
- Identify and immediately report any sign of infection, such as fever, severe fatigue, or purulent skin drainage.

Thoracentesis

Thoracentesis is the aspiration of fluid or air from the pleural space by means of a specialized needle inserted through the chest wall at a site selected based on x-ray and percussion. As a diagnostic procedure it is done to obtain a specimen of fluid from the pleural space and as a therapeutic procedure to relieve respiratory distress or instill medication. During the procedure the patient is in a sitting position; following the procedure the patient is on bedrest and a chest film is taken to check for pneumothorax.

NURSING CARE

Assess the patient's ability to assume the required position and comply with directions.

Obtain baseline vital signs before the procedure.

Monitor pulse and respirations during the procedure.

Direct patient to sit still and avoid talking, coughing, or deep breathing during the procedure.

Suggest panting if an urge to cough is experienced.

Record total amount of fluid withdrawn, noting its color and viscosity.

Check for signs of hemorrhage and pneumothorax: tachycardia, dyspnea, hypotension, swelling at needle insertion site, faintness, vertigo, tightness in the chest, uncontrollable cough, and blood-tinged, frothy sputum.

Thyroidectomy

A thyroidectomy is the surgical removal of all or part of the thyroid gland as a treatment for hyperthyroidism or cancer of the thyroid gland. The surgical excision may incorporate the use of lasers with fiberoptic scopes.

PREOPERATIVE NURSING CARE

Assessment

- Determine the patient's level of understanding about the disorder and emotional status, especially if the diagnosis is cancer of the gland.
- Complete the preoperative assessment as detailed in the Preoperative Nursing Care entry in this text.

POSTOPERATIVE NURSING CARE

Assessment

- Check vital signs frequently.
- Identify signs and symptoms of hemorrhage and respiratory obstruction such as vital sign changes, frequent swallowing, dyspnea, or gasping.
- Observe for signs of parathyroid damage and laryngeal nerve damage such as tetany, convulsions, hoarseness, and respiratory difficulty.
- Look for early signs of thyroid crisis (thyrotoxicosis) such as fever, restlessness, tachycardia, sweating, and pulmonary edema.
- Auscultate lung sounds and heart sounds.
- Assess for pain, noting intensity, duration, and relief methods.

Nursing Diagnoses, Planning, and Nursing Interventions

NDx: Risk for inefficient airway clearance related to tracheolaryngeal obstruction secondary to complications of subtotal thyroidectomy: hemorrhage, edema, laryngeal nerve damage, parathyroid damage

Planning: Patient outcomes

1. Patient maintains a clear airway as evidenced by stable vital signs, regular respirations, and unlabored breathing pattern.
2. Patient is able to speak and swallow without difficulty.

Nursing Interventions

Instruct the patient to support the head when moving in the bed.

Apply an ice collar and place the patient in semi-Fowler's position.

Monitor vital signs, looking for subtle changes reflecting complications.

Have the patient speak every 2 hours to determine voice quality.

Administer humidified oxygen.

Check the dressing every 1 to 2 hours for the first 24 hours.

Evaluate the patient frequently for restlessness, irritability, numbness, tingling of the fingers, toes, ears, and circumoral area, muscle twitching, or a positive Chvostek's sign or Trousseau's sign.

Keep equipment for emergency tracheostomy and calcium gluconate, succinate, or chloride parenteral administrations at the bedside.

NDx: Pain related to surgical incision and edema

Planning: Patient outcomes

1. Patient reports decrease or absence in pain.
2. Patient is able to move neck, as allowed, without excessive discomfort.

Nursing Interventions

Administer analgesics as prescribed.

Instruct patient about relaxation exercises to promote pain relief.

◆ Total Parenteral Nutrition (Hyperalimentation)

Total parenteral nutrition (TPN), also called intravenous hyperalimentation (IVH) or simply hyperalimentation, is the IV administration of nutrients in amounts needed to produce a state of anabolism. It is used when nutritional needs cannot be met via the GI tract. It may therefore be used in cases of inflammatory bowel disease, pancreatitis, trauma, extensive burns, acute renal failure, or following extensive bowel surgery. Because the solutions are highly concentrated and hypertonic, administration into a wide diameter vessel with rapid blood flow is necessary.

ASSESSMENT

Assess baseline condition at start of therapy: observe for signs of nutritional deficiency, fluid and electrolyte imbalance, and note weight.

Check for sharp chest pain, decreased breath sounds, rapidly expanding hematoma, tracheal compression, and respiratory distress immediately following catheter insertion.

Check temperature every 4 hours and check insertion site for erythema, skin ulceration, or drainage.

Observe for signs of vitamin and trace element deficiency or toxicity.

Check serum glucose every 4 to 6 hours using bedside glucose monitoring; observe for signs of hyperglycemia (diuresis, dry skin, thirst) or hypoglycemia (weakness, diaphoresis, pallor).

Assess for therapeutic responses to TPN therapy: weigh the patient daily; review laboratory data; and observe for signs of improved healing.

NURSING DIAGNOSES, PLANNING, AND NURSING INTERVENTIONS

NDx: Altered nutrition: less than body requirements related to inability to take in needed amounts of nutrients via the GI tract

Planning: Patient outcomes

1. Patient is in positive nitrogen balance.
2. Patient gains specified amount of weight per week.

Nursing Interventions

Use a controller or pump to administer prescribed solutions at a constant rate around the clock (60–80 mL

328

per hour is usual initial rate, which is increased by 25 mL/hr/day according to tolerance).

Check rate every 30 minutes and reset as necessary.

Never adjust rate to compensate for past increase or decrease.

Mark container in hourly amounts to aid in assessing accuracy of flow rate.

Measure I & O.

Weigh patient qd at same time, on same scale, in same clothing.

NDx: Risk for infection related to in-line contamination or migration of organisms along the catheter from the insertion site

Planning: Patient outcomes

1. Patient is afebrile.
2. Insertion site is free of erythema, edema, and drainage.
3. Skin around insertion site is intact.

Nursing Interventions

Guard against in-line contamination:
- Keep all prepared solutions refrigerated until used.
- Examine new containers carefully for cracks or small punctures.
- Inspect solutions against a bright light for turbidity or particulate matter.
- Change IV tubing and filters every 24 hours at same time as solution container is changed.
- Use TPN line only for TPN.

Guard against infection originating at the site of insertion:
- Cleanse the site according to agency protocol using strict aseptic technique and apply an occlusive dressing.
- Seal all edges of dressing with tape.
- Place a slit piece of tape under the catheter for occlusion.
- Change the dressing every 48 hours or 3 times per week and whenever wet, contaminated, or if the airtight seal is broken.
- Tape all tubing junctions.

- Anchor filter to dressing to eliminate pull on insertion site.
- Use a plastic drape or thin, transparent waterproof dressing such as OpSite PRN to keep dressing dry.
- Take temperature every 6 hours; report elevations to the physician.
- If temperature spikes, culture and change the IV tubing and hang new solution immediately.

Additional Interventions

Maintain patient in flat position when changing tubing. Instruct him or her to perform a Valsalva maneuver when catheter is open to air.

◆ Tracheostomy

A tracheostomy is an artificial opening into the trachea created to establish an airway. Tracheostomies are done to bypass complete upper airway obstruction as from pharyngeal tumors or laryngeal edema, to allow for long-term mechanical ventilation, and to decrease the work of breathing in paralyzed, weak, or critically ill patients. They may be temporary or permanent.

ASSESSMENT

- Following a tracheostomy, observe respiratory rate, rhythm, depth, chest excursion, cough, amount and appearance of tracheal secretions, and frequency of need for suctioning.
- Review ABG values if available.
- Check placement of tracheostomy tube and pressure in the cuff every 8 hours. Check the pressure by attaching a manometer to the cuff port and note if the minimal occlusive volume is increased or decreased.
- Check seal created by the cuff every 2 to 4 hours. Signs of a leak are a harsh, gurgling sound during expiration heard with a stethoscope over the trachea; warm air exiting the patient's mouth during

expiration; and the patient being able to make sounds.
- Check that dressing and tapes are dry and intact.
- Check for signs of infection: fever; redness, swelling, or purulent drainage from wound; leukocytosis.
- Assess for complications: pneumothorax (cough, sharp chest pain, tachycardia), pneumomediastinum (dyspnea, crepitus, face and neck edema), and cardiac tamponade (increased CVP, narrowed pulse pressure, paradoxical pulse, hypotension, dyspnea, decreased level of consciousness).

NURSING DIAGNOSES, PLANNING, AND NURSING INTERVENTIONS

NDx: Anxiety related to the tracheostomy procedure and its effects on body functions

Planning: Patient outcomes

1. Facial expression and body posture are relaxed.
2. Patient is able to rest quietly.
3. Patient attends to explanations and directions.

Nursing Interventions

Clarify information regarding the tracheostomy with patient and family, e.g., speaking will not be possible with the basic tracheostomy tube in place; suctioning will be needed to clear secretions.

Recognize that anxiety over accidental suffocation is common; counteract it by reassuring patient about the effectiveness of breathing through a tracheostomy, the close observation that will be provided, the availability of the call bell, and the large number of people functioning on a daily basis with a tracheostomy.

NDx: Risk for ineffective breathing pattern related to tracheal obstruction

Planning: Patient outcomes

1. Respiratory rate is 14 to 20 per minute.
2. Chest movement is smooth, symmetric, and of normal depth.

3. Breath sounds are clear.
4. Cyanosis is absent.

Nursing Interventions

Keep a replacement tracheostomy tube and obturator at the bedside in case of accidental dislodgement of the tube placed at time of surgery.

Do not change tapes or deflate cuff for 24 hours.

Do not change tube for at least 1 week.

Suction PRN to maintain patency (q 5-10 minutes immediately postop, later q 2-3 hours).

Avoid unnecessary suctioning.

Suction patients sensitive to decreased oxygen levels more often but for a shorter time.

Document time of suction, characteristics of secretions, respiratory status, and patient's response.

Keep a manual resuscitation bag and adapter mask and scissors to snip neck tape in an emergency at the bedside.

NDx: Risk for infection related to bacterial contamination of the tracheal wound

Planning: Patient outcomes

1. Tracheostomy site is intact and free of redness, edema, or drainage.
2. Purulent tracheal secretions are absent.
3. Patient is afebrile.

Nursing Interventions

Use strict sterile technique when caring for the tracheostomy.

Cleanse the tracheostomy and surrounding area:
- Remove the inner cannula and soak it in half-strength hydrogen peroxide solution.
- Suction outer cannula; follow with deep breathing either by the patient or via a manual resuscitation bag.
- Remove soiled dressing and use gauze and peroxide solution to remove secretions and crust from around the tube.

- Use peroxide-soaked swabs to cleanse under the neck plate and openings in its sides.
- Cleanse the inner cannula with a brush and pipe cleaners; rinse in sterile saline or water.
- Dry thoroughly and replace in the outer cannula.
- Change tracheostomy tapes.

Prepare clean tapes before removing the soiled ones. Cut the tape with about two-thirds left on one side and one-third on the other, then make a make a horizontal slit 1 inch from each end.

Insert the slit end of the tie through the side opening of the outer cannula.

Pull the opposite end through the slit and draw securely on opposite side.

Hold the tube while this is being done.

Tie the tapes on the side of the neck.

Slip a 3 x 3-inch gauze pad folded into a V shape or factory-made split sponge between the neck and the tracheostomy tube to provide padding and to absorb secretions.

Never cut a gauze pad for this use because frayed threads can be aspirated.

Additional Interventions

Select an alternative method of communication with the patient before the procedure if possible.

Use the selected method consistently.

Orient significant others to selected communication method.

◆ Traction

Traction is a pulling force applied to a body part while countertraction pulls in the opposite direction. Traction can be applied to the body by manual, skin, or skeletal means. Manual traction is used to reduce a fracture or dislocated joint but is only effective while the pull is maintained by the individual applying the traction. For long-term application of traction, skin or skeletal traction is instituted. Skin traction is used only for temporary traction in adults because the skin cannot tolerate the weight for long periods of time. Traction is used as a therapeutic intervention for reducing a fracture, to lessen muscle spasms and prevent contractions, to maintain alignment and reduction while a bone heals, to prevent or correct a deformity, to lessen the chance of necrosis due to pressure on the articular surfaces of an injured joint, and to rest the joint after a fracture or dislocation.

ASSESSMENT

- Assess the patient's neurovascular status frequently by checking pulses proximal and distal to the site of the traction attachment.
- Note the color, texture, and temperature of the skin.
- Look for swelling, which may indicate constriction of the extremity.
- Ask the patient about pain, numbness, or tingling in the affected part.
- Assess the traction equipment for proper alignment, attachment, weight, and countertraction.
- Note if the ropes and weight hang freely.
- Assess the equipment in light of the principles of traction.
- Check if the patient is positioned properly in the bed for the type of traction being maintained.
- Observe for signs of pressure complications on areas such as the elbows, back of the head, back, buttocks, heels, and under slings or wraps.
- Assess for signs of the hazards of immobility.
- Note the amount of movement the patient is able to accomplish.
- Ask if the patient is completing range-of-motion exercises at regular intervals.
- Check the positioning of the foot and watch for evidence of foot drop.

NURSING DIAGNOSES, PLANNING, AND NURSING INTERVENTIONS

NDx: Anxiety related to fear of the equipment and unknown recovery potential, and discomfort

Planning: Patient outcomes

1. Patient denies anxiety, fear, or nervousness about the traction therapy and potential outcome of the therapy.

2. Patient appears relaxed and is able to rest at intervals and to sleep well.
3. Signs of increased anxiety such as twitching, nervousness, increased respirations and pulse, or withdrawal from participation in care are absent.

Nursing Interventions

Explain the purpose of all the traction equipment to the patient.

Teach the patient how to use the trapeze for readjustment of position in the bed.

Explain the necessity of maintenance of body and traction alignment.

Explain the steps of the procedure and the reason for it prior to performing any procedure on the patient.

Allow the patient time to ask questions and relay concerns.

Check vital signs and watch for changes indicating increased anxiety.

Teach the patient relaxation methods and strategies to cope with the fears of hospitalization.

Encourage the patient to complete range-of-motion exercises to help relieve discomfort from the static position and to maintain muscle tone and joint motion.

Provide diversional activity for the patient to relieve the boredom and anxiety bedrest.

NDx: Pain related to inability to move well or change position easily in bed due to the traction therapy, pressure from the pulling force or method of attachment of the apparatus, and/or discomfort at site of injury

Planning: Patient outcomes

1. Patient denies pressure, pain, or discomfort.
2. Patient is able to exercise and move somewhat within the confines of the traction equipment.

Nursing Interventions

Reposition the patient, as allowed, for comfort and relief of pressure.

Teach the patient how to move in the bed with the use of the overhead trapeze.

Explain how much movement is allowed.

Give prescribed pain or sedation medications as needed.

Give the medication for pain prior to performing procedures with the patient that cause increased discomfort.

Be certain the traction equipment is in proper alignment with the appropriate weight.

Incorrect use of the equipment may aggravate the patient's discomfort as well as cause harm to the patient.

Additional Interventions

Perform pin-site care as described in Table 19-7 in the textbook to prevent infection at the site of the insertion of pins, wires, or tongs.

◆ Treadmill (Exercise Stress Testing)

A treadmill is a noninvasive test used to determine cardiac functioning during physical activity. The patient's electrocardiogram (ECG), heart rate, and blood pressure are monitored while the patient walks on the treadmill. The incline and speed are increased until the target heart rate (80-90% of the maximum heart rate for sex and age) is achieved, or until the patient presents symptoms such as chest pain, extreme fatigue, or changes on the ECG.

PREPROCEDURE CARE

Assessment

- Check and record the baseline vital signs.
- Determine the patient's level of understanding about the procedure.
- Check if NPO status has been maintained for 4 hours prior to the procedure.
- Assess for appropriate clothing and shoes to complete the testing.
- Determine if the patient has anxiety about the testing procedure.

NURSING DIAGNOSES, PLANNING, AND NURSING INTERVENTIONS

NDx: Knowledge deficit: Nature of the exercise procedure, potential findings, and follow-up medical management necessary

Planning: Patient outcomes

1. Patient verbalizes the necessity for the procedure.
2. Patient describes the procedure as presented by the physician, radiologist, or nurse.

Nursing Interventions

Describe the procedure and the diagnostic equipment using terminology that is easily understandable to the patient.

Tell the patient to alert the nurse (technician) if any pain or extreme fatigue is experienced.

Explain that the test will be discontinued when symptoms are apparent.

Ask the patient to reiterate the information given by the physician to check for understanding and to correct misconceptions.

Explain what care will be initiated during the postprocedure time period.

NDx: Anxiety related to fear of the stress of the exercise associated with the test and the test findings

Planning: Patient outcomes

1. Patient verbalizes a decrease in anxiety.
2. Patient's vital signs are within normal ranges prior to the testing.
3. Patient states feeling comfortable about initiating the procedure.

Nursing Interventions

Reassure the patient about the necessity for the procedure.
Tell the patient that the test will be discontinued if untoward symptoms appear.

Reassure the patient that the exercise will not be continued beyond his or her capacity.

Allow the patient to verbalize concerns about the potential findings and necessary treatment.

Answer questions honestly, but refrain from giving false reassurance.

POSTPROCEDURE CARE

Monitor vital signs and ECG for 30 minutes to 1 hour after stress testing.

Allow the patient to rest in a quiet atmosphere during this post-test period.

Clean the electrode sites on the patient's skin prior to discharge.

Ultrasonography

Ultrasonography is a noninvasive procedure that uses high frequency, inaudible sound waves to form images of internal structures. Sound waves are directed at the area to be studied by a transducer that is rubbed slowly on the lubricated skin surface or is in contact with the eye. As the sound waves hit internal structures, they are reflected back and converted to an image on a screen. Photographs of these images can be taken as desired. This procedure is used to visualize soft tissues and does not expose the patient to radiation. It is used to determine the size, shape, location, and/or movement of structures such as the spleen, pelvic organs, heart, liver, gallbladder, pancreas, kidney, and the internal eye. It allows masses to be located and their internal consistency (solid vs cystic) to be determined.

NURSING CARE

Ultrasonography is a painless procedure which requires no specific preparation except in the case of abdominal studies. For these, patients are instructed to avoid carbonated beverages and large amounts of carbohydrates for 48 hours to decrease internal gas. In some other cases the patient may be NPO for 8 hours or have an enema or carthartic ordered. Ultrasonography should always be scheduled before tests using barium. When ultra-sonography is done to visualize organs of the female reproductive system, the patient must have a full bladder to serve as a reference point for structures to be studied. Thus patients are instructed to drink a quart of water an hour before the test and not to urinate after drinking the water until the test is over.

◆ Wounds/Grafts

Closure of wounds may occur or be initiated in several ways:

Granulation — healing from the edges inward.

Side-to-side approximation — suturing of the edges of the wound.

Skin flaps — a flap of tissue raised from one area of the body and transferred to another.

Skin grafts — transplanted skin to cover the wound area: an autograft is from the self; a homograft is from one person to another; a heterograft is from an animal to a human.

Closure depends on the location, size, and type of wound, as well as the patient's general condition, age, previous history of disease, and nutritional status. Wound care is based on the same factors and the physician's preferences.

ASSESSMENT

- Check that all dressings are intact.
- Observe for purulent drainage, foul odor, bleeding, and redness.
- Evaluate circulation peripheral to the wound.
- Assess grafts for adherence, epithelialization, vascularization, and granulation.
- Assess the donor site if an autograft.
- Observe for systemic signs and symptoms of infection.

NURSING DIAGNOSES, PLANNING, AND NURSING INTERVENTIONS

NDx: Risk for infection related to possible invasion of microorganisms secondary to breaks in skin

Planning: Patient outcomes

1. Patient remains free of infection as evidenced by absence of fever, daily increase in wound granulation and healing, and lack of signs of infection in the wound.
2. Patient demonstrates correct wound care prior to discharge.

Nursing Interventions

Maintain strict asepsis when handling patient or performing wound care.

Cleanse wound as ordered, and assess and record untoward findings.

Teach the patient appropriate wound care and observe the patient's technique prior to discharge.

Section III

Pharmacologic Agents

◆◆ ◆◆ ◆◆ ◆◆

Generic Name
Acetaminophen/Codeine

Trade Name
Tylenol with Codeine, Phenaphen with Codeine

Class
Narcotic and opioid analgesic, Schedule III

Action
Acetaminophen blocks the generation of pain impulses while the codeine binds with opiate receptors at many sites in the central nervous system, resulting in an alteration of both perception of and emotional response to pain through an unknown mechanism.

Uses
Mild to moderately severe pain.

Dosage
1–2 tabs q 4 h prn.

Side Effects
Dizziness, sedation, nausea, vomiting, constipation, urinary retention, rash, respiratory depression.

Interactions
Potentiation with alcohol, central nervous system depressants, monoamine oxidase inhibitors, anticholinergics, tricyclic antidepressants.

Nursing Implications
Administer the medication before pain reaches its peak in order to maximize the effectiveness of the drug.
Monitor vital signs to detect respiratory changes.
Check bowel sounds for decreased peristalsis.
Instruct patient not to perform any hazardous activities (such as driving) after taking the medication.

Geriatric Considerations
Check the older adult for side effects from the codeine. Dosage may need to be decreased.
Institute safety measures to prevent injury since risk of side effects is increased.

Generic Name
Albuterol (Salbutamol)

Trade Name
Proventil, Ventolin, Salbutamol

Class
Bronchodilator agent, beta-adrenergic agonist

Action
Acts on beta 2-adrenergic receptor sites to relax the bronchial smooth muscle and promote dilation.

Uses
Prevention and treatment of bronchospasm and exercise-induced asthma.

Dosage
1 to 2 inhalations every 4–6 h or 2 inhalations 15 min. before the start of exercise. 2–4 mg po tid or qid, not to exceed a maximum dose of 8 mg qid. 4–8 mg PO every 12 h when taking the extended release tablets. Maximum dose is 16 mg bid.

Side Effects
Nervousness, tremor, palpitations, tachycardia, nausea, vomiting, muscle cramps.

Interactions
Action of albuterol enhanced by CNS stimulants. Digitalis and levodopa increase the risk for dysrhythmias. MAO inhibitors and TCAs increase the risk of cardiovascular symptoms and should not be given. Beta blockers, including propranolol, have a mutual antagonistic effect. Effectiveness of antihypertensives, antipsychotic, and beta-blocking agents is decreased.

Nursing Implications
Use inhalation and tablets together if necessary.
Instruct the patient to:
    Perform inhalation correctly.
    Wait 2 minutes between puffs.
    Use the bronchodilator inhaler first, then wait 5 minutes
        to use the steroid inhaler.

Discontinue the drug if bronchospasms occur.

Store medication in a light-resistant container.

Administer with caution in hyperthyroidism, diabetes, cardiovascular disorders, hypertension, and patients with unusual responses to adrenergics.

Geriatric Considerations

Lower dose required. Older adults are likely to have a chronic cardiovascular disorder in which symptoms may be aggravated by using this drug. Watch for enhanced CNS stimulation effects such as restlessness, nervousness, insomnia, and anxiety.

Generic Name

Alprazolam

Trade Name

Xanax

Class

Antianxiety agent, Schedule IV

Action

Depresses the CNS at the limbic and subcortical levels of the brain. Enhances the activity of gamma-aminobutyric acid (GABA).

Uses

Treatment of anxiety disorders and tension. Used as adjunctive therapy in the management of anxiety associated with depression and panic disorders. Not used for everyday stress or for longer than 4 months.

Dosage

0.25 mg–0.5 mg PO tid. Maximum total dose is 4 mg in divided doses.

Side Effects

Drowsiness, headache, confusion, lightheadedness, dry mouth, nausea, constipation, vomiting, transient hypotension, tachycardia, hostility.

Alcohol and other CNS depressants cause additional CNS depression. Cimetidine increases sedative effects. Serum levels of tricyclic antidepressants are increased.

Nursing Implications

Instruct the patient to:

> Avoid activities that require alertness and psychomotor coordination until CNS effects are known.
>
> Continue drug unless discontinued by physician as withdrawal symptoms can occur if drug is abruptly stopped.

Do not administer to patients with acute narrow-angle glaucoma, psychoses, or anxiety-free psychiatric disorders.

Geriatric Considerations

Reduce daily dosage because of susceptibility to CNS effects. Starting dose is 0.25 mg bid or tid; increase gradually if necessary.

Generic Name

Aminophylline

Trade Name

Theophylline
Immediate release: Aerolate, Slo-Phyllin, Theolair
Extended release: Slo-Bid, Theo-Dur, Theo-24, Uniphyl

Class

Bronchodilator

Action

Directly relaxes smooth muscle of bronchial airways and pulmonary blood vessels, producing relief of bronchospasm. Stimulates cardiac muscle and the central nervous system. Produces diuresis through a combined action of increased renal perfusion and increased sodium and chloride ion excretion. Also stimulates skeletal muscle and increases gastric acid secretion.

Uses

Used for prevention and relief of symptoms of bronchial asthma and to manage reversible bronchospasm due to chronic bronchitis and emphysema.

Dosage

Initial dosage calculated on basis of lean body weight. Dosage is subsequently adjusted based on peak serum theophylline concentrations, clinical condition and presence of toxicity.

Chronic bronchospasm: PO: Adults: Initially, 16 mg/kg or 400 mg/day (whichever is less) in 2–4 divided doses (6–12 h intervals). May increase by 25% every 2–3 d up to maximum of 13 mg/kg/d (>16 yr). Doses above maximum based on serum theophylline concentrations, clinical condition, and presence of toxicity.

Acute bronchospasm in patients not currently on theophylline: 6 mg/kg PO/loading dose.

Adults: Initially, 5 mg/kg (theophylline), then begin maintenance theophylline dosage based on patient group. Young adult smokers 3 mg/kg q 6 h. Healthy, nonsmoking adults 3 mg/kg q 8 h. Older patients, patients with cor pulmonale 2 mg/kg q 8 h. Patients with CHF, liver disease 1–2 mg/kg q 12 h.

Acute bronchospasm in patients currently on theophylline: IV/PO: Adults: Obtain serum theophylline level. If not possible and patient in respiratory distress, not experiencing toxicity, may give 2.5 mg/kg dose. Maintenance: Dosage based on peak serum theophylline concentration, clinical condition, presence of toxicity.

Side Effects

Frequent: Momentary change in sense of smell during IV administration; shakiness, nervousness, restlessness, increased heart rate, mild diuresis, nausea, and vomiting.

Interactions

Smoking, charcoal-broiled food, high-protein, low-carbohydrate diet may decrease theophylline level. Level also decreased by barbiturates, carbamazepine, phenytoin and rifampin. Aminophylline decreases therapeutic effectiveness and levels of lithium. Altered lab values:

May produce false-positive elevation of uric acid serum level. Levels increased by allopurinol, beta blockers, calcium blockers, cimetidine, erythromycin, quinolones.

Nursing Implications

Give with food to avoid GI distress.

Instruct patient to increase fluid intake to decrease viscosity of secretions.

Offer emotional support since there is a high incidence of anxiety due to difficulty in breathing and the sympathomimetic response to the drug.

Monitor respiratory rate, depth, rhythm, and character as well as quality and rate of pulse.

Assess lung sounds for wheezes.

Monitor arterial blood gases.

Observe lips and fingernails for blue or dusky color in light skinned patients; gray in dark skinned patients.

Observe for clavicular retractions and hand tremor.

Evaluate for clinical improvement (quieter, slower respirations, cessation of clavicular retractions).

Monitor theophylline blood serum levels (therapeutic serum level range: 10–20 mg/mL).

Test for peak serum concentration 1 h after IV, 1–2 h following immediate release dose, 3–8 h following extended release. Obtain level just before next dose.

Geriatric Considerations

The maintenance dose in the elderly must be decreased to 0.3–0.6 mg/kg/h.

Generic Name

Amoxicillin trihydrate

Trade Name

Amoxil, Trimox, Polymox, Biomox, Sumox, Wymox

Class

Antiinfective (Broad-spectrum penicillin)

Action

Inhibits cell wall synthesis during active multiplication.

Uses

Amoxicillin-sensitive infections including ear, respiratory or genitourinary tract, skin, soft tissue, and acute uncomplicated gonorrhea.

Dosage

750 mg to 1.5 g PO daily in divided doses given q 8 h.
Gonorrhea: 3 g once.
Endocarditis prophylaxis: 3 g 1 h before procedure, then 1.5 q 6 h after initial dose.

Side Effects

Frequent: Nausea, diarrhea.
Less frequent: Urticaria, superinfection, blood dyscrasias, hyperactivity, anaphylaxis.

Interactions

May produce false-positive Clinitest. Potentiated by probenecid.

Nursing Implications

Use cautiously in patients with other drug allergies.
Obtain specimen for culture and sensitivity tests prior to first dose.
Instruct patient to:
Take with food to minimize gastrointestinal distress.
Notify physician if rash, fever, or chills develop.
Take medication exactly as prescribed and complete course of treatment, even after feeling better.
Tell patient that amoxicillin may cause the tongue to discolor or darken during therapy, but this is not significant.

Geriatric Considerations

Elderly patients are at an increased risk for developing bacterial and fungal superinfections with large doses and/or prolonged therapy, so observe for any signs and symptoms of infection.

Generic Name
Ampicillin

Trade Name
Ampicin, Omnipen, Principen, Penbritin, Polycillin, Supen, Totacillin

Class
Penicillins (Antimicrobial and antiparasitic agents)

Action
Inhibits cell wall synthesis during active multiplication (bactericidal).

Uses
Systemic infections, acute and chronic urinary tract infections caused by susceptible strains of gram-positive and gram-negative organisms, meningitis, and uncomplicated gonorrhea.

Dosage
Systemic infections, urinary tract infection: 250–500 mg PO qid; 2–12 IM or IV daily, divided into doses given q 4–6 h.
Meningitis: 8–14 g IV daily in divided doses q 3–4 h.
Uncomplicated gonorrhea: 3.5 g PO with 1 g probenecid given as a single dose.

Side Effects
Frequent: Nausea, diarrhea.
Less frequent: Blood dyscrasias, vomiting, glossitis, stomatitis, hypersensitivity (erythematous maculo-papular rash, urticaria, anaphylaxis).
Local: Pain at injection site, vein irritation, thrombophlebitis

Interactions
May cause a false-positive Clinitest.
Increased blood levels with probenecid.
Increased incidence of skin rash with allopurinol.
May potentiate the effect of warfarin.

Nursing Implications
Obtain specimen for culture and sensitivity tests prior to first dose.

Ask patient prior to giving first dose if he or she has had any allergic reactions to this drug.

Instruct patient to take medication exactly as prescribed and to finish full course of treatment, even if feeling better.

Tell patient to call the physician if any rash, fever, or chills develop.

Administer medication 1–2 h before meals or 2–3 h after meals to avoid food interfering with absorption.

Mix with dextrose 5% in water or saline solution for IV administration. Don't mix with other drugs or solutions as they may be incompatible.

Give IV intermittently to prevent vein irritation.

Give ampicillin at least 1 h before bacteriostatic antibiotics.

Tell patient not to use any leftover penicillin for a new illness or share it with family and friends.

Geriatric Considerations

Decreased renal elimination in the elderly increases the half-life of the drug so the dosage may need to be decreased for these patients.

Assess for signs and symptoms of superinfection such as continued fever, poor wound healing, and signs of sepsis.

Generic Name
Atenolol

Trade Name
Tenormin

Class
Antihypertensive, beta-adrenergic blocker

Action
Blocks response to beta stimulation in the heart and depresses renin secretion.

Uses
Hypertension, reduce risk of reinfarction in patients with acute myocardial infarction, decrease incidence of supraventricular tachycardia during coronary artery bypass.

Dosage

Hypertension: 50–100 mg PO daily. (Dosage adjustment necessary if patient's creatinine clearance is below 35 mL/mm.)

Acute MI: 5 mg IV over 5 min., followed by another 5 mg IV 10 min. later. After additional 10 min., administer 50 mg PO; follow with 50 mg PO in 12 h. Thereafter, 100 mg PO daily for at least 7 days.

Coronary artery bypass: 50 mg PO daily starting 3 days before surgery.

Side Effects

Frequent: Bradycardia, hypotension.

Less frequent: Heart failure, bronchospasm, myocardial infarction, heart block, dizziness, fatigue, GI upset, depression, cold extremities.

Interactions

Additive effect with catecholamine-depleting drugs, prazosin, digoxin, verapamil, general anesthesia. Increased rebound hypertension with clonidine withdrawal. May block epinephrine. Concurrent use with thyroid may decrease effectiveness.

Nursing Implications

Explain that the full antihypertensive effect may not appear for 1–2 weeks after initiating therapy.

Check patient's apical pulse before giving the medication; hold if less than 60/min. and notify physician.

Monitor blood pressure frequently.

Instruct patient:

To take the drug at a regular time each day. Instruct patient about the disease and the importance of taking the medication exactly as prescribed.

To check with the physician or pharmacist before taking any over-the-counter drugs.

Assess for shock and hypoglycemia since the drug masks common signs of these conditions.

Geriatric Considerations

Reduction of dosage may be necessary since older patients are more sensitive to the hypotensive effects of antihypertensive drugs.

Observe closely for orthostatic hypotension, which would lead to increased risk of falling.

Atropine sulfate

Trade Name
Atropine Sulfate

Class
Cholinergic-blocking agent (Anticholinergic agent)

Action
Immobilizes acetylcholine at the parasympathetic neuroeffector junction, which blocks all or some of the receptor sites.

Uses
Control of symptomatic bradycardia, adjunctive treatment of peptic ulcer, irritable bowel syndrome, antidote for anticholinesterase insecticide poisoning, and as a preoperative medication to reduce secretions and inhibit cardiac vagal response.

Dosage
0.5–1 mg IV push, repeat every 5 min. to a maximum of 2 mg for dysrhythmias, 0.4–0.6 IM 45–60 min. before anesthesia, 0.4 mg–1.6 mg PO q 4–6 h for GI disorders.

Side Effects
Side effects vary with dose. Dry mouth is most common. Other side effects include: drowsiness, headache, restlessness, ataxia, disorientation, tachycardia, palpitations, mydriasis, photophobia, blurred vision, thirst, constipation, nausea, vomiting, urinary retention, dizziness, insomnia, excitement, hallucinations.

Interactions
Antihistamines, amantadine, glutethimide, meperidine, antiarrhythmics, antiparkinsonian agents, tricyclic antidepressants, and phenothiazines cause an increase in anticholinergic action. Cholinergic drugs, ketoconazole, levodopa, and antacids decrease absorption of atropine sulfate. Digoxin levels may be increased if slowly dissolving digoxin tablets are administered. Methotrimeprazine produces extrapyramidal effects. Potassium chloride tablets increase the risk of mucosal lesions.

Monitor I & O.

Have patient with prostate hypertrophy void before administering since urinary retention can occur.

Monitor for tachycardia, which can lead to ventricular fibrillation in the cardiac patient.

Administer IV push directly into a large vein or over 1–2 min. Be aware that paradoxical bradycardia will appear initially then disappear within 2 min.

Have physostigmine salicylate nearby to treat atropine overdose.

Instruct patient to:

Wear dark glasses in sunlight.

Carry out good dental hygiene due to dry mouth.

Do not administer to patients with narrow-angle glaucoma, obstructive uropathy, GU and GI obstruction, myasthenia gravis, paralytic ileus, intestinal any, unstable cardiovascular status, acute hemorrhage, and toxic megacolon.

Administer with caution to patients with Down's syndrome because of sensitivity to the drug.

Geriatric Considerations

Increased incidence of excitability, agitation, confusion, constipation, and urinary retention because of slow drug metabolism.

Generic Name

Azithromycin

Trade Name

Zithromax

Class

Antiinfective, macrolide antibiotic

Action

Inhibits protein synthesis causing cell death; bacteriostatic.

Uses

Lower respiratory infections, acute bacterial exacerbations of COPD, uncomplicated skin infections, nongonococcal urethritis, and cervicitis caused by *Chlamydia trachomatis*.

Dosage
Respiratory and skin infections: PO 500 mg on the first day then 250 mg/d for 4 more days.
Nongonococcal urethritis and cervicitis: PO single 1 g dose.
Children: not established.

Side Effects
Headache, diarrhea, nausea, abdominal discomfort.

Interactions
Decreased effectiveness if taken with aluminum- and magnesium-containing antacids. May decrease effects of theophylline. May increase anticoagulant effects of warfarin.

Nursing Implications
Assess patient for infection at the beginning and throughout the course of therapy.
Obtain specimens for culture and sensitivity tests prior to beginning therapy.
Instruct the patient to take on an empty stomach.
Instruct patient regarding the importance of completing the full course of therapy as prescribed, even if the signs and symptoms of the infection subside.
Advise patient to report signs of superinfection (black, furry tongue growth, vaginal itching or discharge, loose or foul-smelling stools).
Counsel patients being treated for sexually transmitted diseases about appropriate precautions.

Geriatric Considerations
Generally safe.

Generic Name
Buspirone

Trade Name
BuSpar

Class
Antianxiety

Action
Binds to serotonin and dopamine receptors in the brain. Also increases norepinephrine metabolism in the brain.

Uses
Management of anxiety.

Dosage
PO 15 mg/d in 3 divided doses. May increase by 5 mg/d (not to exceed 60 mg/d). Usual dose is 20–30 mg/d.

Side Effects
Dizziness, insomnia, lightheadedness, headache, drowsiness, excitement, tinnitus, sore throat, chest pain, paresthesia, sweating.

Interactions
Concurrent use with MAO inhibitors may cause hypertension. CNS depressants may increase sedative effect.

Nursing Implications
Instruct patient to take with food to reduce gastric irritation.
Explain to the patient that an antianxiety effect is not expected for 1–2 weeks.
Advise patient to avoid alcohol or other antidepressant medications.
Monitor the effectiveness of therapy through follow-up examinations and documentation of increased well-being with a decrease in subjective feelings of anxiety.
Maintain safety precautions with ambulation due to the potential of dizziness and lightheadedness.
Do not discontinue abruptly.

Geriatric Considerations
Initial dose should be smaller and increments should be gradual.

Generic Name
Captopril

Trade Name
Capoten

Class
Antihypertensive, angiotensin converting enzyme (ACE) inhibitor

Action
Reduces blood pressure primarily through suppression of the renin-angiotensin-aldosterone system by inhibiting ACE in the plasma thereby resulting in systemic vasodilation; in hypertension, reduces peripheral arterial resistance. In HF increases cardiac output and decreases peripheral vascular resistance, pulmonary capillary wedge pressure, heart size.

Uses
Used in treatment of hypertension alone or in combination with other antihypertensives and as adjunctive therapy for HF in combination with cardiac glycosides and diuretics.

Dosage
PO Adults: Initially, 12.5–25 mg bid to tid. After 1–2 weeks, may increase to 50 mg bid to tid, diuretic therapy may be added if no response in additional 1–2 weeks. If taken in combination with diuretic, may increase to 100–150 mg, 2–3 times/d after 1–2 weeks. Maintenance: 25–150 mg 2–3 times/d. Maximum: 450 mg/d.

Side Effects
More frequent: Dry cough, hypotension.
Less frequent: Headache, dizziness and fatigue, rash, diarrhea, nausea, weakness, loss of taste perception (usually returns in several months, even if therapy continues), proteinuria.

Interactions
Alcohol and diuretics given with captopril may cause a severe hypotensive episode. Captopril may increase lithium concentration and toxicity. Hyperkalemia may

occur with potassium-sparing diuretics and potassium supplements. NSAIDs and aspirin may decrease hypotensive effect.

Nursing Implications

Schedule renal function tests before beginning therapy.

Take BP at regular intervals and before each dose; observe for fluctuations.

Assist with ambulation if dizziness occurs.

Place patient in supine position if marked hypotension occurs.

Assess for anorexia due to decreased taste.

Monitor CBC, electrolytes, BUN, creatinine, and urinalysis results.

Schedule a CBC and differential prior to start of drugs, every 2 weeks for 3 months, and periodically thereafter for patients with renal impairment, autoimmune disease, or for those taking drugs that affect leukocytes or the immune response.

Instruct patient to:

Take drug 1 h before meals.

Continue taking drug until physician states otherwise.

Refrain from driving or operating heavy machinery until drug effects are established.

Change position gradually.

Avoid alcohol, hot showers, and baths.

Consult a physician or nurse before taking OTC drugs.

Monitor weight.

Eat a low-sodium diet.

Take BP at the same time every day, record in diary, and report changes to physician.

Geriatric Considerations

Antihypertensive drugs should be started with smaller than usual doses and increased by smaller increments at less frequent intervals since the elderly are more susceptible to volume depletion and sympathetic inhibition.

Use caution in ambulation and take precautions to prevent falls as the elderly are also more susceptible to hypotension due to impaired cardiovascular reflexes.

Generic Name
Cefaclor

Trade Name
Ceclor

Class
Second-generation cephalosporin (Antiinfective, antibiotic)

Action
Inhibits cell wall synthesis, promoting osmotic instability. Usually bactericidal.

Uses
Treatment of specific, serious infections caused by gram negative bacteria. These include otitis media, respiratory, urologic, and gynecologic infections, septacemia, as well as infections of the skin, skin structures, bones, and joints.

Dosage
250–500 mg PO q 8 h.

Side Effects
Frequent: Nausea, diarrhea, cramping, maculopapular rash.
Less frequent: Blood dyscrasias, dizziness, headache, somnolence, vomiting, anorexia, pseudomembranous colitis, vaginitis, vaginal moniliasis, dermatitis, fever, cholestatic jaundice, and hypersensitivity.

Interactions
Used with probenecid, may inhibit excretion and increase blood levels of cefaclor.

Nursing Implications
Obtain specimen for culture and sensitivity tests prior to administering first dose.
Instruct patient to take the drug exactly as prescribed and complete the full course of treatment, even though feeling better.
Instruct patient to notify the prescribing health care provider if a skin rash develops.
Monitor for superinfection if a large dose or prolonged therapy is ordered.

Store reconstituted suspension in the refrigerator and shake well before using.

Instruct patient to take with meals.

Consider that urine glucose determinations may be false-positive with Clinitest.

Geriatric Considerations

Decreased renal elimination in the elderly increases the half-life of the drug so the dosage may need to be decreased for these patients.

Assess for signs and symptoms of superinfection such as continued fever, poor wound healing, and signs of sepsis.

Generic Name
Cefadroxil monohydrate

Trade Name
Duricef, Ultracef

Class
Cephalosporin (Antiinfective, antibiotic)

Action
Inhibits cell wall synthesis, promoting osmotic instability. Usually bactericidal.

Uses
Treatment of susceptible urinary tract, skin, skin structure, bone, and joint infections, pharyngitis, tonsillitis, septicemia.

Dosage
500 mg to 2 g PO daily, depending on the infection being treated. Usually given qid or bid.

Side Effects

Frequent: Nausea, vomiting, diarrhea, maculopapular and erythematous rashes.

Less frequent: Blood dyscrasias, dizziness, headache, malaise, paresthesias, pseudomembranous colitis, anorexia, vomiting, glossitis, abdominal cramps, anal pruritus, tenesmus, oral candidiasis, genital pruritus, moniliasis, dyspnea, and hypersensitivity.

Interactions
Increased blood levels possible with probenecid.

Nursing Implications
Obtain specimen for culture and sensitivity tests prior to giving first dose. Increase dosage interval if creatinine clearance is less than 50 mL/min. so that drug doesn't accumulate.
Instruct patient to:
Take medication exactly as prescribed and for complete course of treatment even if feeling better.
Notify prescribing health care provider if skin rash develops.
Take medication with food or milk to decrease gastrointestinal discomfort. Monitor patient for superinfection when giving large doses or prolonged therapy. Tell patient that urine glucose determinations may be false-positive with Clinitest.

Geriatric Considerations
Decreased renal elimination in the elderly increases the half-life of the drug so the dosage may need to be decreased for these patients.
Assess for signs and symptoms of superinfection such as continued fever, poor wound healing, and signs of sepsis.

Generic Name
Cefuroxime sodium

Trade Name
Kefurox, Zinacef, Ceflin

Class
Cephalosporin (Antiinfective and antiparasitic agents)

Action
Inhibits cell wall synthesis, promoting osmotic instability. Usually bactericidal.

Uses
Treatment of susceptible bacterial septicemia, lower respiratory or urinary tract infections, skin and skin structure

infections, meningitis, bone and joint infections, gonorrhea. Surgical prophylaxis.

Dosage

Usual dose: 750 mg to 1.5 g q 8 h for 5–10 d.
Life-threatening infections: 1.5 g IM or IV q 6 h.
Bacterial meningitis: Up to 3 g IV qh.
Uncomplicated urinary tract infection: 125–250 mg PO q 12 h.

Side Effects

Frequent: Diarrhea, nausea, vomiting, maculopapular and erythematous rashes, urticaria.

Less frequent: Headache, malaise, paresthesia, dizziness, pesudomembranous colitis, anorexia, glossitis, dyspepsia, abdominal cramps, genital pruritus, and moniliasis.

At injection sites: Pain, induration, sterile abscesses, temperature elevation, tissue sloughing.

IV: Phlebitis and thrombophlebitis.

Interactions

Avoid concomitant furosemide, ethacrynic acid, other nephrotoxic drugs.

Concomitant aminoglycosides may potentiate nephrotoxicity.

May cause false-positive Clinitest.

Potentiated by probenecid.

Nursing Implications

Contraindicated by hypersensitivity to other cephalosporins.

Use cautiously in patients with impaired renal function; dosage should be reduced.

Absorption is enhanced by food.

Obtain specimen for culture and sensitivity tests prior to administering first dose.

Monitor for superinfections if given in large doses or for prolonged therapy, particularly when given to high-risk patients.

Administer reconstituted IV cefuroxime over 15–30 min.

Geriatric Considerations

Since elderly patients may have significantly lower renal function than younger adults, renal function should be monitored by checking the BUN and serum creatinine levels. The dosage may need to be lowered in order to adjust for decreased renal function.

Generic Name
Cephalexin

Trade Name
Keflex, Keflet, Keftab, Cefanex

Class
Cephalosporin (Antimicrobial and antiparasitic agents)

Action
Inhibits cell wall synthesis, causing osmotic instability. Usually bactericidal.

Uses
Treatment of susceptible infections including otitis media and those involving skin and skin structure, bone and respiratory or genitourinary tract.

Dosage
250–500 mg PO q 6 h.

Side Effects
Frequent: Nausea, anorexia, diarrhea, maculopapular and erythematous rashes, urticaria.
Less frequent: Blood dyscrasias, dizziness, headache, malaise, paresthesia, pseudomembranous colitis, vomiting, glossitis, dyspepsia, abdominal cramps, genital pruritus and moniliasis, vaginitis, dyspnea, and hypersensitivity.

Interactions
May cause false-positive Clinitest. Potentiated by probenecid.

Nursing Implications
Use cautiously in those with impaired renal function or with history of sensitivity to penicillin.

Obtain specimen for culture and sensitivity tests before
administering first dose.

Instruct patient to:

Take medication exactly as prescribed, even after feeling better.

Take with food or milk to lessen gastrointestinal discomfort.

Monitor for superinfection with large doses, prolonged
therapy, or high-risk patients.

Geriatric Considerations

Since elderly patients may have significantly lower renal
function than younger adults, monitor renal function in
these patients by checking their BUN and serum creatinine levels. The dosage may need to be adjusted for
decreased renal function.

Generic Name

Cimetidine hydrochloride

Trade Name

Tagamet, Duractin

Class

Antiulcer agent, histamine H_2 antagonist

Action

Decreases gastric acid secretion by inhibiting the action of
histamine at the H_2 receptor sites on the parietal cells in
the stomach.

Uses

Short-term treatment of duodenal ulcer, benign gastric
ulcers, gastroesophageal reflex, and hypersecretory conditions. Prophylaxis against GI bleeding in critically ill
patients.

Dosage

300–800 mg PO daily or qid with meals and hs for up to 8
weeks. 400 mg hs for maintenance therapy; IV dose 300 mg
diluted with 20 mL of 0.9% normal saline solution, dex-

trose 5% and 10% in water, lactated Ringer's solution, or 5% sodium bicarbonate injection. IV push over 1–2 min. q 6 h or 300 mg diluted in 50 mL of dextrose 5% solution infused over 15–30 minutes q 6 h 300 mg IM q 6 h. IV continuous dose is 900 mg per day diluted in 100–1000 mL of compatible diluent. Use infusion pump giving a total volume of 250 mL per 24 h. Do not use sterile water for injection.

Side Effects

Confusion, dizziness, headache, bradycardia, jaundice, acne-like rash, diarrhea, constipation, fatigue, muscle aches.

Interactions

Antacids decrease absorption. Warfarin, lidocaine, propranolol, phenytoin, theophylline, and some benzodiazepines may have a decreased effect.

Nursing Implications

Instruct the patient taking the drug PO to:
    Take at least 1 h before or after antacids.
    Take the drug PO with meals to increase therapeutic effect.
    Take at bedtime if medication is ordered to be taken as a single dose.
    Avoid smoking, which increases gastric acid secretion.
Schedule cimetidine to be given after hemodialysis for consistent blood levels.
Prepare patient for expected discomfort if given IM.
Monitor serum drug levels frequently.

Geriatric Considerations

Increased susceptibility to cimetidine-induced mental confusion, disorientation, and agitation.

Generic Name
Ciprofloxacin

Trade Name
Cipro, Ciloxan

Class
Quinolones (Antimicrobial and antiparasitic agents)

Action
Interferes with the enzyme DNA gyrase, which is needed for the synthesis of bacterial DNA (bactericidal).

Uses
Susceptible infections, including lower respiratory tract, skin and skin structures, bone, joint; infectious diarrhea.

Dosage
Mild to moderate urinary tract infections: 250 mg PO or 200 mg IV q 12 h.

Severe or complicated urinary tract infections, mild to moderate bone and joint infections, respiratory tract infections, skin and skin structure infections, infectious diarrhea: 500 mg PO or 400 mg IV q 12 h.

Severe or complicated bone or joint infections, respiratory tract infections, skin and skin structure infections: 750 mg PO q 12 h.

Side Effects
Common: Nausea, diarrhea, rash, restlessness.

Less common: Vomiting, abdominal pain, headaches, dizziness, photosensitivity, crystalluria.

IV: Thrombophlebitis, burning pruritus, paresthesia, erythema, swelling.

Interactions
May elevate theophylline plasma levels.

Potentiated by probenecid.

Avoid concomitant antacids, iron, zinc, sucralfate (oral form).

Monitor oral anticoagulants, phenytoin.

Nursing Implications
If the patient takes theophylline or consumes large quantities of caffeine, observe closely as this drug inhibits the metabolism of these substances and may contribute to some of the central nervous system side effects.

Assess for history of allergy before administering drug.

Obtain specimen for culture and sensitivity tests prior to initial dose.

Administer 2 hours after a meal or 2 hours before or after
antacids, sucralfate, or products that contain iron.

Dilute vials (injection concentrate) before use.

If patient has central nervous system disorders or is at an
increased risk for seizures, monitor closely as seizures and psychosis have been reported in patients
with these conditions.

Tell patient to discontinue breastfeeding during treatment since the drug is excreted in breast milk.

Tell patient to avoid hazardous tasks since the drug may
cause dizziness or lightheadedness.

Advise patient to drink plenty of fluids to decrease chance
of crystalluria.

Monitor CBC and differential, platelet count, BUN level,
serum creatinine level, and liver function tests.

Geriatric Considerations

Reduced renal function in the elderly may require the
dosage to be lowered for these patients.

Instruct patients to maintain adequate hydration as allowed by any other disorders that they may have.

Assess for central nervous system side effects that may
cause safety risks (e.g., dizziness, shakiness, changes
in vision).

Review patient's other medications and counsel as necessary. If questions about drug incompatibilities arise,
consult physician or pharmacist.

Instruct patient to keep health-care providers informed of
all drugs being taken (including over-the-counter
drugs).

Generic Name
Clarithromycin

Trade Name
Biaxin, Biaxin Filmtabs

Class
Antiinfective, macrolide antibiotic

Action
Inhibits protein synthesis, causing cell death; bacteriostatic.

Uses
Upper and lower respiratory tract infections, uncomplicated skin and soft tissue infections.

Dosage
Adult: 250–500 mg PO q 12 h for 7–14 d.
Children: Not established.

Side Effects
Headache, diarrhea, nausea, abdominal discomfort, distorted taste, dyspepsia.

Interactions
May increase theophylline and cCarbamazepine levels.
May increase the effect of oral anticoagulants.

Nursing Implications
Instruct patient to take with food if GI effects occur.
Administer (instruct patient to take) around the clock.
Instruct patient regarding the importance of completing the full course of therapy as prescribed, even if the signs and symptoms of the infection subside.
Assess patient for infection at the beginning and throughout the course of therapy.
Obtain specimens for culture and sensitivity tests prior to beginning therapy.
Advise patient to report signs of superinfection (black, furry tongue growth, vaginal itching or discharge, loose or foul-smelling stools).

Geriatric Considerations
Generally safe.

Generic Name
Co-trimoxazole, Sulfamethoxazole-Trimethoprim

Trade Name
Apo-Sulfatrim, Bactrim, Cotrim, Bactrim DS, Cotrim D.S.,
Septra, Septra DS, Septrin, Sufamethoprim, Uroplus S,
Sulfametho-prim DS, Sulfamethoprim, Sulmeprim, Sulfa

Class
Sulfonamide, antiinfective

Action
Inhibits the production of folic acid, which stops the
multiplication of new bacteria.

Uses
Treatment and prevention of urinary tract infections, chronic
bronchitis, shigellosis, traveler's diarrhea, otitis media.

Dosage
One double strength tablet PO q 12 h for 10–14 days or
longer; as a single dose 1–3 double strength tablets; IV
dose is 8–10 mg/kg/day bid or qid. Dosages called "DS"
or "DF" indicate double strength.

Side Effects
Headache, seizures, nausea, diarrhea, vomiting, anorexia,
abdominal pain, hematuria, oliguria, jaundice, photosensitivity, pruritus, urticaria, skin rash, fever, crystalluria,
hemolytic anemia, phlebitis at IV site. Side effects occur
more frequently in AIDS patients.

Interactions
Ammonium chloride and ascorbic acid increase risk of
crystalluria. Effect of oral anticoagulants is enhanced.
Effect of oral contraceptives is decreased. The hypoglycemic effect of oral hypoglycemic agents is decreased. Sodium bicarbonate, salicylates, NSAIDs, methotrexate,
phenytoin increase blood levels of sulfonamides.

Nursing Implications
Collect culture and sensitivity tests before starting initial
    dose.

Instruct patients taking the drug PO to:
  Take with meals.
  Drink 3 quarts of fluid per day to prevent crystal formation.
  Take full prescription.
  Report side effects to health care provider.
Never administer IM or bolus injection.
Dilute IV infusions in D5W; administer separately over 60–90 minutes within 2 hours of reconstitution
Monitor for superinfection.
Report early signs of blood dyscrasia — skin rash, sore throat, mouth sores, and fever.
Administer with caution in patients with renal or liver disease, severe allergies or asthma, and blood dyscrasias.
Do not administer to patients with porphyria, megaloblastic anemia, pregnancy, renal dysfunction, or those taking thiazide diuretics or antidiabetic sulfonylureas.

Geriatric Considerations

Cause renal dysfunction in kidneys already impaired due to crystal formation. Common reactions that occur include: Skin reactions and bone marrow depression.

Generic Name
Diazepam

Trade Name

Apo-Diazepam, E-Pam, Meval, Diazepam Intensol, Navodipam, Rival, Valium, Q-Pam, Valrelease, Vasepam, Zetran, Vivol

Class

Antianxiety agent, benzodiazepine

Action

Action not fully understood. Depresses the limbic and subcortical levels of the brain by inhibiting the ability of excitatory neurotransmitters to stimulate seizure activity.

Uses

Treatment of seizure disorders, tension, skeletal muscular spasms, and anxiety as well as for preoperative sedation and hypnotic effects.

Dosage

Adults: 2–10 mg PO, bid, tid, qid, or extended release capsules 15–30 mg/d, 5–20 mg IV, IM. As an initial dose push 2–5 mg/min. May repeat every 5–10 min. for a maximum dose of 60 mg for seizures or repeat dose every 3–4 h if necessary.

Elderly: 2–5 PO daily or bid; increase as needed.

Side Effects

Lethargy, drowsiness, ataxia, slurred speech, dizziness, hangover, fainting, tremors, hypotension, blurred vision, diplopia, nausea, abdominal distention, vomiting, bradycardia, urticaria, rash, respiratory depression, pain, and phlebitis at injection site.

Interactions

Alcohol and other CNS depressants enhance the CNS depressive effect. Cimetidine, disulfiram, and isoniazid can increase sedation. Phenobarbital potentiates the effect of both drugs. CNS stimulants decrease the antianxiety effect.

Nursing Implications

Avoid mixing the injectable form with other drugs due to incompatibility.

Do not store diazepam in a plastic syringe.

Do not give IM, may be painful.

Administer direct IV or IV push in large veins at a rate not exceeding 5 mg/min.

Monitor for signs of extravasation.

Check respirations every 5–15 minutes during IV administration and before each repeated IV dose.

Recognize that seizures may recur in 20–30 minutes after IV administration due to redistribution of drug.

Instruct patients to:

Avoid activities that require alertness until the CNS effects are known.

Avoid drinking alcohol and taking other drugs.

Never give medication to others.

Monitor for the possibility of abuse and addiction.

Administer with caution in patients with blood dyscrasias, depression, renal or liver damage, and open-angle glaucoma.

Do not administer to patients with acute alcohol intoxication, acute glaucoma, psychosis, myasthenia gravis, or those in shock or coma.

Geriatric Considerations

Reduce dosage due to increased susceptibility to side effects and toxicity due to slow metabolism.

Generic Name
Diclofenac sodium

Trade Name
Voltaren, Voltaren SR

Class
Nonsteroidal anti-inflammatory agent

Action
Inhibits prostaglandin synthesis thereby producing analgesic, anti-inflammatory, and antipyretic effects.

Uses
Ankylosing spondylitis, rheumatoid arthritis, and osteoarthritis.

Dosage
100–200 mg PO, bid or tid.

Side Effects
Headache, tinnitus, abdominal pain, dyspepsia, diarrhea, GI bleeding, constipation, nausea, indigestion, fluid retention, rash, dermatitis, appetite changes, drowsiness, petechiae.

Interactions
Alcohol, anticoagulants, and steroids increase the risk of bleeding. Cyclosporine, lithium, digoxin, and methotrexate may have decreased renal clearance leading to toxic-

ity. Diuretics may have reduced effectiveness. Change in daily dosage of oral hypoglycemics and insulin may be necessary. Potassium-sparing diuretics may have enhanced potassium retention leading to hyperkalemia.

Nursing Implications

Administer with food or after meals to prevent GI irritation.

Avoid crushing, chewing, or breaking the tablets as they are enteric-coated.

Teach the patient the signs and symptoms of GI bleeding (pain in epigastrium, weight loss, blood in stools, blood in emesis) and hepatotoxicity (abdominal pain or tenderness, pruritus, anorexia) as well as the importance of reporting them immediately to the physician.

Monitor liver function studies periodically for elevations.

Do not administer to patients with hypersensitivity to NSAIDs, aspirin, diclofenac, history of urticaria, asthma, or any other allergic reaction.

Geriatric Considerations

Give small dosages with gradual increments. Give with food to decrease the GI effects.

Generic Name
Digoxin

Trade Name
Lanoxin, Lanoxicaps

Class
Cardiac glycoside, isotropic, antiarrhythmic

Action
Increases force of myocardial contraction and cardiac output. Decreases rate of conduction while increasing refractory period of AV node. Increases influx of calcium ions from extracellular to intracellular cytoplasm.

Uses

Improves blood supply to vital organs including the kidneys and produces a diuretic effect. Prophylactic management and treatment of HF; controls ventricular rate in atrial fibrillation and atrial flutter. Treatment and prevention of recurrent paroxysmal atrial tachycardia. Also used as rapid digitalization in these disorders.

Dosage

IV: Adults: 0.4–0.6 mg initially then 0.1–0.3 mg q 4–8 h as needed. Maintenance 0.125–0.5 mg daily as a single dose or in divided doses.

Tablet: Adults: Rapid digitalization: 0.75–1.25 mg divided into 2 or more doses, each administered at 6-hour intervals. Slow: 0.125–0.5 mg once a day for 7 d. Maintenance: 0.125–0.5 mg once a day.

Side Effects

Dysrhythmias, bradycardia, fatigue. There is a cumulative effect with a very narrow margin of safety between a therapeutic and toxic effect. The most common early manifestations of toxicity in adults are GI disturbances (anorexia, nausea, vomiting, abdominal pain, diarrhea) and neurologic abnormalities (headache, fatigue, drowsiness, apathy, disorientation, insomnia, depression, nightmares, and confusion). Other symptoms of toxicity include blurred vision or visual disturbances such as seeing a yellow, green, or white halo around objects or lights and dysrhythmias.

Interactions

Adrenocorticoids (corticosteroids), mineralocorticoids, amphotericin B (parenteral), ACTH, and potassium-depleting diuretics increase risk of inducing hypokalemia and digitalis toxicity. Antacids, especially aluminum and magnesium types, may decrease absorption 25–35%.

Nursing Implications

Assess apical pulse for 60 sec before each dose.

Withhold drug and contact prescribing health care provider if pulse is 60/bpm or below.

Monitor pulse for bradycardia, which may be the first clinical sign of toxicity and ECG for dysrhythmias for 1–2 h after IV administration of digoxin.

Assess for GI and neurologic signs of toxicity q 2–4 h
during digitalization and daily during maintenance.
Monitor serum potassium, magnesium levels.
Schedule and monitor for therapeutic plasma Digoxin
level (0.5–2.0 schedule/mL).

Geriatric Considerations
The elderly are more susceptible to this drug and the side
effects of increased weakness, dizziness, fainting episodes, and falls. Advise elderly to avoid milk, cheeses,
yogurt, and ice cream for at least 2 hours before and after
taking Digoxin because these foods reduce absorption.

Generic Name
Diltiazem hydrochloride

Trade Name
Cardizem, Cardizem SR, Cardizem CD, Dilacor XR

Class
Calcium channel blocker, antianginal, coronary vasodilator

Action
Prevents the influx of calcium ions through the slow
channels of the membrane of myocardial muscle and
vascular smooth muscle during membrane depolarization. The slowed calcium ion influx reduces vascular
tone and mildly decreases the force of myocardial contraction. Dilation of coronary arteries and arterioles is
achieved, thereby improving oxygen supply to myocardial tissue and ultimately inhibiting coronary artery
spasm. Further dilation of peripheral arterioles reduces
cardiac afterload (peripheral resistance), a hemodynamic
function that also lessens oxygen requirements of the
myocardial tissue. SA nodal function, and AV nodal
conduction are also decreased because of the inhibited
influx of calcium ions to the SA and AV nodes.

Uses
Treatment of coronary artery spasm (Prinzmetal's or variant angina, chronic stable angina or effort-associ-

ated angina). Increases exercise tolerance. Suppresses atrial tachydysrhythmias.
Extended Release: Treatment of essential hypertension.

Dosage

Prinzmetal's variant angina, chronic unstable angina: Initially, 30 mg PO tid or qid daily. Increase gradually up to 180–360 mg/d in 3–4 divided doses.
IV: 0.25 mg/kg over 2 min.; may repeat in 15 min. with 0.35 mg/kg; continuous infusion at 10 mg/h.

Side Effects

Occasional: Dizziness, headache, nausea, skin flushing, rash, bradycardia.
Less frequent: Edema of extremities, allergic skin reaction, shortness of breath, wheezing, severe hypotension, tachycardia.

Interactions

Alcohol, antihypertensives and beta-adrenergic-blocking agents, including ophthalmic preparations, may enhance hypotensive effects. Nicotine may reduce effectiveness. Metabolism of carbamazepine, cyclosporine, digitalis, and theophylline may be impaired by calcium channel blockers, leading to increased serum levels and possible toxicity.

Nursing Implications

Give before meals.
Check BP for hypotension.
Assess pulse for strength/weakness, irregular rate.
Monitor ECG for cardiac changes, particularly for prolongation of P–R interval.
Notify prescribing health care provider of any significant interval changes.
Monitor patient closely for other side effects.

Geriatric Considerations

The elderly are more susceptible to this drug and the side effects of increased weakness, dizziness, fainting episodes, and falls. Maximum daily dosage is 180 mg.

Generic Name
Doxepin hydrochloride

Trade Name
Adapin, Sinequan, Zonalon

Class
Tricyclic antidepressant, antianxiety

Action
Increases the amount of norepinephrine or serotonin, or both, in the central nervous system by blocking their reuptake by the presynaptic neurons.

Uses
Treatment of depression and anxiety.

Dosage
Initially, 25–150 mg PO daily as single or divided doses, up to a maximum of 300 mg daily. Entire dose may be given at bedtime.

Side Effects
Frequent: Drowsiness, dizziness, orthostatic hypotension, tachycardia, ECG changes, blurred vision, dry mouth, constipation, urine retention, sweating.
Less frequent: Excitation, tremors, weakness, confusion, headache, nervousness, hypertension, tinnitus, glossitis, mydriasis, nausea, vomiting, anorexia, paralytic ileus, rash, urticaria.
After abrupt withdrawal of long-term therapy: Nausea, headache, malaise.

Interactions
Decreased tricyclic antidepressant levels with barbiturates.
Increased levels with cimetidine.
Increased hypertensive effect if used with epinephrine or norepinephrine.
Severe excitation, hyperpyrexia, or seizures may occur if taken with monoamine oxidase inhibitors.
Increased tricyclic antidepressant levels with methylphenidate.

Reduce dosage if increased signs of psychosis occur.

Record changes in mood.

Monitor for suicidal tendencies.

Instruct patient to:

> Avoid activities requiring alertness and good psycho-motor coordination until central nervous system effects are determined.

> Remember that the effect of the medication may not be seen for 2 weeks or more; full effect may take up to 4 weeks.

> Relieve dry mouth with sugarless hard candy or gum.

> Avoid using alcohol or other depressants while on this drug.

> Avoid over-the--counter medications without first consulting the physician.

> Change position from lying to sitting or sitting to standing slowly because of the possibility of orthostatic hypotension.

Increase fluids and, if needed, suggest a stool softener.

Dilute oral concentrate with 120 mL of water, juice, or milk (incompatible with carbonated beverages)

Check for urine retention and constipation.

Geriatric Considerations

Drug dosage in the elderly should be low, initially, and gradually increased while monitoring the patient's response to the drug.

Instruct patient about possible orthostatic hypotension and provide a safe environment to decrease risk of injury due to side effects of the medication.

Assess for urinary retention.

Generic Name
Doxycycline hyclate

Trade Name

Doryx, Doxy Caps, Doxy 100, Doxy 200, Doxychel Hyclate, Doxy Tabs, Vibramycin, Vibra-Tabs.

Class

Tetracycline, antiinfective agent

Action

Inhibits protein synthesis by binding with the 30S ribosomal subunit of microorganisms to produce a bacteriostatic effect.

Uses

Treatment of infections caused by gram-negative and gram-positive organisms such as: chlamydia, gonorrhea, syphilis in patients allergic to penicillin, trachoma, Lyme disease, and infections due to rickettsiae and mycoplasma.

Dosage

100–300 mg initially PO q 12 h or in divided doses, followed by 100 mg daily or bid for as long as prescribed. 200 mg IV as initial dose daily or bid, then 100–200 mg IV daily or bid.

Side Effects

Epigastric distress, diarrhea, nausea, sore mouth, photosensitivity, maculopapular and erythematous rashes, urticaria, increased pigmentation, anorexia, vomiting, and thrombophlebitis at IV site.

Interactions

Laxatives and antacids that contain calcium, aluminum, and magnesium decrease the absorption rate of the antibiotic. Effectiveness of oral contraceptives is decreased. Ferrous sulfate, sodium bicarbonate, alcohol, carbamazepine, and phenobarbital decrease the effectiveness of the antibiotic. Tetracyclines may enhance the effect of oral anticoagulants.

Nursing Implications

Obtain culture and sensitivity tests before administering initial dose.

Administer the antibiotic 1 hour before or 2 hours after a laxative, antacid, or ferrous sulfate.

Monitor for superinfection.

Reconstitute a 100-mg vial with 10 cc of sterile water for injection when administering IV and use within 72 hours.

Recognize that using the Clinitest method for urine testing will produce false-positive results when doxycycline is administered parenterally.

379

Avoid giving antibiotic within 1 hour of bedtime as this
may cause dysphagia.
Instruct patient to:
Take full prescription even when symptoms subside.
Carry out good oral hygiene.
Take with milk or foods when GI irritation occurs.
Avoid exposure to sunlight.

Geriatric Considerations
Reduced drug dosage is necessary with renal dysfunction.

Generic Name
Enalapril maleate

Trade Name
Vasotec

Class
Antihypertensive, angiotensin converting enzyme (ACE)
inhibitor

Action
Depresses the functioning of the renin–angiotensin–
aldosterone mechanism by inhibiting angiotensin converting enzyme (ACE) in the plasma; in hypertension,
reduces peripheral arterial resistance; in HF increases cardiac output and decreases peripheral vascular resistance,
BP, pulmonary capillary wedge pressure, and heart size.

Uses
Used alone, or in combination with other antihypertensives, for initial therapy of essential hypertension in patients with normal renal function and as adjunctive therapy
for HF in combination with cardiac glycosides and diuretics.

Dosage
PO for hypertension: Initially, 5 mg/d and increased
based on response. Maintenance: 10–40 mg/d as a single
dose or in two divided doses. In patients who are sodium
and fluid depleted (because of diuretics or renal failure)
the initial dose is reduced to 2.5 mg/d. Titrate up to

maximum of 40 mg/d. In treatment of HF, oral dose initially is 2.5 mg once or twice daily. Increased according to patient response. Maintenance dose is 5–20 mg PO, in a single or twice daily dosage. For injection as an adult antihypertensive, administer 1.25 mg over 5 min. every 5 h. Reduce to 0.625 mg initially in patients who are fluid and sodium depleted.

Side Effects

More frequent: Dry cough, headache, dizziness, and fatigue.

Less frequent: Rash, diarrhea, nausea, weakness, loss of taste perception (usually returns in several months, even if therapy continues).

Interactions

Alcohol and diuretics given with Vasotec may cause a severe hypotensive episode. Vasotec may increase lithium concentration and toxicity. Hyperkalemia may occur with potassium-sparing diuretics and potassium supplements. NSAIDs and aspirin may decrease hypotensive effect. Rifampin decreases effects of Vasotec.

Nursing Implications

Schedule renal function tests before beginning therapy.

Take BP at regular intervals and before each dose; observe for fluctuations.

Assist with ambulation if dizziness occurs.

Place patient in supine position if marked hypotension occurs.

Assess for anorexia due to decreased taste.

Monitor CBC, electrolytes, BUN, creatinine, and urinalysis results.

Schedule a CBC and differential prior to start of drugs, every 2 weeks for 3 months, and periodically thereafter for patients with renal impairment, autoimmune disease, or who are taking drugs that affect leukocytes or the immune response.

Instruct patients to:

Take drugs 1 hour before meals.

Never discontinue or skip doses.

Refrain from driving or operating heavy machinery until drug effects are established.

Change position gradually.

Avoid alcohol, hot showers, and baths.

Never take OTC drugs without consulting the prescribing health care provider.

Monitor weight.

Eat a low-sodium diet.

Take BP at the same time every day, record in diary, and report changes to physician.

Geriatric Considerations

Antihypertensive drugs should be started with smaller than usual doses and increased by smaller dosages at less frequent intervals since the elderly are sensitive to volume depletion and sympathetic inhibition. Use caution in ambulation and take precautions to prevent falls as they are also more susceptible to hypotension due to impaired cardiovascular reflexes.

Generic Name
Erythromycin

Trade Name

Apo-Erythro base, E-Mycin, ERYC, Eryc Sprinkle, Ery-Tab, Erythromid, Robimycin Robitabs, Novorythro, PCE Dispertabs, Ilotycin

Class

Antiinfective, bacteriostatic agent

Action

Inhibits bacterial protein synthesis by binding to the 50S ribosome.

Uses

Acute pelvic inflammatory disease; mild to moderately severe respiratory tract, skin, and soft tissue infections; otitis media; legionnaires' disease; urethral, endocervical, and rectal infections; chlamydial infection, pertussis, diptheria, rheumatic fever.

Dosage

250– 500 mg PO q 6–12 h for 7 d. 500 mg–1 g IV q 6 h for at least 7 d.

Nausea, diarrhea, vomiting, abdominal cramping, abdominal pain, fever, jaundice, urticaria, rashes, anaphylaxis.

Interactions

Carbamazepine blood levels are increased, therefore increasing the risk of toxicity. Clindamycin and lincomycin antagonize the effects of erythromycin so they are not used together. Oral anticoagulant blood levels are increased; prothrombin time must be monitored. Theophylline decreases the effect of erythromycin and increases the chance for theophylline toxicity.

Nursing Implications

Obtain culture and sensitivity tests before first dose.
Administer erythromycin IV over 60 minutes after reconstituting according to manufacturer's directions.
Note concentration before administering suspensions.
Monitor for signs and symptoms of superinfection.
Instruct patient in self-administration of oral erythromycin as follows:
  Take with a full glass of water (no juices) 1 hour before or 2 hours after meals for effective absorption (enteric-coated tablets may be taken with meals).
  Chew chewable tablets, do not swallow whole.
  Take drug for as long as prescribed.
  Report severe diarrhea, nausea, vomiting, hives or skin rash to the prescribing health care provider.

Geriatric Considerations

Increased risk of side effects.

Generic Name
Etodolac (Ultradol)

Trade Name
Lodine

Class
Nonsteroidal anti-inflammatory agent

Action

Inhibition of prostaglandin biosynthesis.

Uses

Acute and chronic management of osteoarthritis and pain.

Dosage

Acute pain: 200–400 mg PO q 6–8 h prn not to exceed 1200 mg daily. For patients who weigh 132 lb (60 kg) or under, total daily dose should not be greater than 20 mg/kg.

Side Effects

Malaise, depression, nervousness, dizziness, anemia, palpitations, flushing, blurred vision, tinnitus, photophobia, dyspepsia, abdominal pain, diarrhea, vomiting, constipation, nausea, gastritis, melena, peptic ulcer with or without bleeding or perforation, ulcerative stomatitis, pruritus, rash, hypertension, edema, flatulence, anorexia. Lab tests may reveal a false positive for urinary bilirubin, decreased serum uric acid levels, and borderline or elevated liver function tests.

Interactions

Antacids may decrease peak serum levels of the drug. Cyclosporine impairs elimination of etodolac and increases risk of nephrotoxicity. Elimination of digoxin, lithium, and methotrexate is impaired, resulting in increased blood levels and increased risk of toxicity. Warfarin has a decreased protein-binding effect without altering its clearance. No dosage adjustment is necessary, although prothrombin times need to be monitored.

Nursing Implications

Instruct patient to:
    Take with milk or meals to decrease GI distress.
    Report signs of GI bleeding to prescribing health care provider immediately.
Administer with caution in patients who have a history of GI bleeding, ulceration, and perforation, and renal and hepatic impairment.
Do not administer to patients with hypersensitivity to the drug, or with a history of NSAID-induced asthma, rhinitis, urticaria, or other allergic reactions.

May be increased risk of side effects due to decreased renal and liver function.

Generic Name
Famotidine

Trade Name
Pepcid, Pepcidine

Class
Antiulcer agent, histamine H_2 receptor antagonist

Action
Inhibits the release of histamine (H_2) at the receptor site located on the parietal cells in the stomach, thereby reducing acid secretion.

Uses
Treatment of duodenal ulcer, Zollinger-Ellison syndrome, intractable ulcers, hypersecretory conditions, and GERD (gastroesophageal reflux disease).

Dosage
20 mg, PO IV q 6–12 h (daily and at bedtime)

Side Effects
Headache, dizziness, diarrhea, nausea, constipation, dryness, flatulence, rash, muscle aches, irritation at IV site.

Interactions
None identified.

Nursing Implications
Instruct the patient to:
   Take with food or antacid.
   Take no longer than 8 weeks unless specifically ordered.
   Avoid cigarette smoking to further decrease gastric acid secretion.
Store suspension form at 86°F (30°C) and once opened discard in 30 days.

Administer IV injection by straight IV push after diluting
with 2 cc of sterile water for injection, 0.9% sodium
chloride injection, 5% or 10% dextrose injection, or
5% bicarbonate injection, or lactated Ringer's injection.
Administer IV infusion over 15–30 minutes with 20 mg of
famotidine in 100 cc of a compatible diluent.
Refrigerate IV injection at 35.6–46.4°F (2– 8°C).

Geriatric Considerations
Reduced dosage is recommended due to decreased renal
function in the older adult. Risks of side effects such as
disorientation, agitation, and confusion are increased.

Generic Name
Ferrous sulfate

Trade Name
Feosol, Slow Fe, Ferralyn, Fer-Iron

Class
Antianemic, iron supplement

Action
Provides elemental iron.

Uses
Treatment of iron deficiency.

Dosage
300–325 mg PO tid or qid or may give 1 delayed release
capsule (160–525 mg) PO bid.

Side Effects
Frequent: Nausea, constipation, black stools, epigastric
pain.
Less frequent: Vomiting, elixir may stain teeth.

Interactions
Decreased absorption with antacids, levodopa, penicil-
lamine, quinolones, tetracyclines, and vitamin E.
Response may be delayed if used concomitantly with
chloramphenicol.

Increased absorption is possible with vitamin C.

Nursing Implications
Instruct patient to:
  Take 1 hour before or 2 hours after meals for maximum effectiveness.
  Take with orange juice to promote absorption.
  Dilute liquid preparations in juice or water but not in milk or antacids.
  Take elixir preparations through a straw to avoid staining the teeth.
  Avoid crushing or chewing sustained release preparations.
  Avoid taking the medication with yogurt, cheese, eggs, milk, whole grain breads, cereals, coffee, and tea as these may impair the absorption of oral iron medication
  Continue regular dosing schedule if a dose is missed.
  Never double dose.
  Note color and amount of stool.
Instruct parents to be aware of potential for iron poisoning in children.
Explain measures to prevent constipation.
Monitor hemoglobin and hematocrit during therapy.

Geriatric Considerations
Assess for constipation.
Instruct patient to prevent constipation by:
  Increasing fluid intake, fruit and fruit juices, fiber (whole grains, vegetables, edible seeds, fruits), and level of exercise.
  Taking with foods (although absorption may be decreased) if necessary to decrease gastrointestinal upset.

Generic Name
Fluoxetine hydrochloride

Trade Name
Prozac

Class
Antidepressant

Action
Selectively inhibits the reuptake of serotonin in the CNS.

Uses
Trade: Treatment of depression.
Unlabeled uses: treatment of obesity, bulimia, obsessive-compulsive disorders.

Dosage
Initially, 20 mg PO qd in the morning. After several weeks may increase by 20 mg/d. If more than 20 mg/d, administer bid. Maximum dose is 80 mg/d.

Side Effects
Headache, dizziness, agitation, sweating, insomnia, nausea, diarrhea.

Interactions
MAO inhibitors may increase Prozac levels. Prozac may elevate plasma levels of tricyclic antidepressants, lithium, digitoxin, or oral anticoagulants. Concurrent use with alcohol is not recommended.

Nursing Implications
Inform patient that the therapeutic effects may take 1–4 weeks to be evident.
Emphasize the importance of follow-up examination.
Monitor suicidal patients closely at the beginning of therapy.

Geriatric Considerations
May require a lower dose or less frequent dose. Start with a low dose, gradually increase over several weeks if necessary.

Generic Name
Furosemide

Trade Name
Lasix, Myrosemide

Class
Loop diuretic

Action
Decreases reabsorption of electrolytes, increases potassium excretion, renal blood flow, peripheral venous capacitance. Decreases calcium, magnesium levels, peripheral resistance.

Uses
Treatment of pulmonary edema, and edema of HF, liver disease, ascites, nephrotic syndrome, and hypertension.

Dosage
PO: 20–80 mg/d given as single dose in morning. May increase in 20–40 mg increments q 6–8 h. Maximum: 600 mg.

IM/IV: 20–40 mg given as single injection. May increase in 20-mg increments no sooner than 2 h after previous dose.

Acute Pulmonary Edema: IV: 40 mg IV given over 1–2 min. If satisfactory response is not reached in 1 h, may increase to 80 mg IV, given over 1–2 min.

Hypertension: PO: Initially, 40 mg bid then based on patient response.

Interactions
Additive hypotension with antihypertensives or nitrates. Additive hypokalemia with other diuretics, mezlocillin, piperacillin, amphotericin B, and glucocorticoids. Hypokalemia may increase risk of cardiac glycoside toxicity. Decreases lithium excretion, may cause toxicity. Increased risk of ototoxicity with aminoglycosides. May increase the effectiveness of oral anticoagulants.

Side Effects
Frequent: Increase in urinary frequency and volume. Nausea; gastric upset with cramping, diarrhea, or constipation; electrolyte disturbances; dehydration.

Occasional: Dizziness, lightheadedness, headache, blurred vision, paresthesia, photosensitivity, rash, weakness, urinary frequency/bladder spasm, restlessness, diaphoresis, orthostatic hypotension.

Rare: Flank pain, Stevens-Johnson syndrome, thrombocytopenia, agranulocytosis, leukopenia, neutropenia, anemia, ECG changes, chest pain.

Nursing Implications

Check vital signs, especially BP for hypotension, before administration.

Assess baseline electrolytes, particularly check for low potassium levels.

Assess for edema, skin turgor, change in mental status, cardiac dysrhythmias. Hyponatremia may result in confusion, thirst, cold/clammy skin. Instruct patient to expect increased frequency and volume of urination. Instruct patient to report irregular heartbeat, signs of electrolyte imbalances (noted above), hearing abnormalities (such as sense of fullness in ears, ringing/roaring in ears)

Instruct patient to:

Eat foods high in potassium such as whole grains (cereals), legumes, meat, bananas, apricots, orange juice, potatoes (white, sweet), raisins.

Avoid sun and sunlamps.

Geriatric Considerations

Dosage may need to be lowered in the elderly since they are often more sensitive to the effects of loop diuretics than other adult patients.

Monitor blood pressure carefully and observe closely for orthostatic hypotension, which could lead to increased risk of falling

Monitor electrolyte balance carefully.

Counsel regarding dietary needs as necessary to maintain appropriate potassium balance.

Generic Name
Gemfibrozil

Trade Name
Lopid

Class
Antilipemic

Action
Inhibits peripheral lipolysis and reduces triglyceride synthesis in the liver.

Uses
Treatment of hypertriglyceridemia and severe hypercholesterolemia unresponsive to diet and other drugs. Also used to reduce the risk of coronary heart disease in patients intolerant of or refractory to treatment with bile acid sequestrants or niacin.

Dosage
1.2 g daily in 2 divided doses 30 min. before morning and evening meals.

Side Effects
Frequent: Abdominal and epigastric pain, diarrhea, nausea.

Less frequent: Anemia, leukopenia, blurred vision, headache, dizziness, vomiting, flatulence, bile duct obstruction, elevated enzymes, rash, dermatitis, pruritus, painful extremities.

Interactions
Enhanced clinical effects of oral anticoagulants may occur.

Nursing Implications
Instruct patient to:

Take the medication one-half hour before breakfast and dinner.

Avoid driving or performing other hazardous activities until the central nervous system effects of the drug are known.

Learn about proper dietary management, weight control, and exercise.

Observe bowel movement for evidence of steatorrhea or other signs of bile duct obstruction.

Monitor CBC and liver function tests periodically during the first 12 months of therapy.

Monitor blood glucose levels in diabetic patients. Contraindicated for patients with gallstones.

Refer patients to dietitian as appropriate to assist them in developing a diet that will enhance their ability to lower their serum triglyceride level.

Tell patient to monitor blood glucose levels closely.

Instruct patient to report the development of any unexpected sign or symptom, such as increased hypoglycemia, bleeding, pain associated with gallstones.

Generic Name
Glipizide

Trade Name
Glucotrol, Minidiab

Class
Antidiabetic agent, oral hypoglycemic agent

Action
Lowers the blood sugar by stimulating the production of insulin from the beta cells of the pancreas, reducing glucose production by the liver, and increasing the number of insulin receptor sites.

Uses
Used in non–insulin-dependent diabetes mellitus (Type 2).

Dosage
Initially, 5 mg PO daily before breakfast. Patients with liver disease may be started on 2.5 mg. Usual maintenance dose is 10–15 mg. Maximum dose is 40 mg. For replacement of insulin therapy: If insulin dose is more than 20 units daily, patient may be started on usual dose of oral drug plus 50% of insulin. If dosage of insulin is less than 20 units, then insulin may be discontinued.

Side Effects
Hypoglycemia, dizziness, vomiting, nausea, constipation, rash, pruritus, facial flushing, cholestatic jaundice, photosensitivity.

Interactions

Anabolic steroids, chloramphenicol, clofibrate, guanethidine, MAO inhibitors, phenylbutazone, probenecid, salicylates, and sulfonamides increase hypoglycemic activity. Beta blockers and clonidine prolong hypoglycemic effect and mask the symptoms of hypoglycemia. Corticosteroids, glucagon, rifampin, and thiazide diuretics decrease the hypoglycemic response. Hydantoins increase blood levels of Glucotrol. Oral anticoagulants increase the hypoglycemic effect and increase the anticoagulant effect.

Nursing Implications

When transferring from insulin to glipizide therapy instruct the patient to:

Monitor serum glucose before meals.

Take 30 minutes before meal.

Adhere to specific diet, weight reduction, exercise, and personal hygiene programs. Take measures to avoid infections, e.g., avoid crowds and persons with upper respiratory infections.

Report symptoms of hyperglycemia and hypoglycemia to the prescribing health care provider.

Recognize that insulin therapy may be needed during periods of high stress; e.g., fever, infections, and surgery.

Do not administer to patients with diabetic ketoacidosis with or without coma.

Administer with caution in patients with kidney and liver disease, hypersensitivity to sulfonamides, and who are pregnant.

Geriatric Considerations

Initial dosage begins at 2.5 mg daily and is then titrated to serum glucose levels. May have an increased risk of side effects due to multi-drug therapy.

Generic Name
Glyburide

Trade Name
Diabeta, Micronase, Glynase PresTabs

Class
Antidiabetic agent (Oral hypoglycemic)

Action
Stimulates the release of insulin from the pancreatic beta cells and reduces glucose output by the liver.

Uses
Indicated as an adjunct to diet to lower blood glucose in patients with non–insulin-dependent diabetes mellitus (Type 2).

Dosage
Elderly or debilitated: Initially, 1.25 mg daily.
Others: Initially, 2.5–5 mg daily with breakfast. Increased 2.5 mg at weekly intervals if needed based on blood glucose.
Maintenance: 1.25–20 mg daily in single or divided doses (if over 10 mg daily).

Side Effects
Hypoglycemia, nausea, heartburn, epigastric fullness, cholestatic jaundice, rash, pruritus, facial flushing, photosensitivity.

Interactions
Increased hypoglycemic activity with anabolic steroids, chloramphenicol, clofibrate, guanethidine, monoamine oxidase inhibitors, phenylbutazone, salicylates, and sulfonamides.
Prolonged hypoglycemic effect and symptoms of hypoglycemia masked with beta blockers and clonidine.
Decreased hypoglycemic response with corticosteroids, glucagon, rifampin, and thiazide diuretics.
Interaction with hydantoins may cause an increase in the blood levels of hydantoins.
Increased hypoglycemic activity or an enhanced anticoagulant effect with oral anticoagulants.

Nursing Implications
Instruct patient:
  Regarding the disease: The importance of following the therapeutic regimen, adhering to specific diet, weight

reduction, exercise, and personal hygiene programs, and avoiding infection.

How and when to perform self-monitoring of blood glucose levels.

How to recognize hypoglycemia and hyperglycemia.

That during periods of stress, such as infection, fever, surgery, or trauma, insulin may be required.

To take this medication about 30 minutes before eating since its absorption is delayed by food.

Monitor for hyperglycemia if patient is receiving insulin therapy.

Geriatric Considerations

Enhanced sensitivity to the side effects of this drug may occur with elderly patients so encourage patients to take appropriate safety measures (watch for symptoms of hypoglycemia and act appropriately to alleviate this).

Instruct patient to be consistent in timing of meals and medication administration since food delays the absorption of this drug.

Generic Name
Heparin

Trade Name
Calciparine, Calcilean (heparin calcium)
Liquaemin Sodium, Hep-Lock (heparin sodium)

Class
Anticoagulant

Action
Inhibits blood coagulation by preventing conversion of fibrinogen to fibrin, and prothrombin to thrombin by enhancing inhibitory effects of antithrombin III.

Uses
Prophylaxis and treatment of various thromboembolic disorders: Deep vein thrombosis, pulmonary emboli, atrial fibrillation with embolization. Treatment for acute and chronic consumptive coagulopathies and peripheral arte-

rial thromboembolism. Prophylaxis for open heart surgery, myocardial infarction, disseminated intravascular coagulation, and as an anticoagulant in transfusion and dialysis procedures. Also used in very low doses to maintain patency of IV catheters (heparin flush).

Dosage

Deep vein thrombosis/MI: IV push 5000–10,000 U q 4 h then titrated to APTT or ACT level. Follow-up IV infusion 1000 U/h titrated to APTT or ACT level.

Pulmonary embolism: IV push 7500–10,000 U q 4 h then titrated to APTT or ACT level. Follow-up IV infusion.

Open heart surgery: IV infusion 150–300 U/kg.

Therapeutic anticoagulation of all disorders depends on results of APTT.

Side Effects

Frequent: Bleeding, diarrhea, nausea, vomiting, anorexia, stomatitis, abdominal cramps, rash, ecchymosis, and fever.

Less frequent: Hepatitis, hematuria.

Rare: Hemorrhage and thrombocytopenia.

Interactions

Antagonizes the effect of corticosteroids; decreased effect of heparin with digitalis, tetracyclines, and antihistamines; increased effect of heparin with aspirin, dextran, and oral anticoagulants.

Nursing Implications

Assess the patient to determine that heparin is not contraindicated by preexisting conditions such as: Blood dyscrasias, liver disease (with hypoprothrombinemia), kidney disease, peptic ulcer, chronic ulcerative colitis, and active bleeding; individuals undergoing eye, spinal cord, or brain surgery since even minor bleeding may cause serious consequences; individuals with continuous drainage of the stomach or small intestine, threatened abortion, subacute endocarditis, severe hypertension, or hypersensitivity to the drug.

Assess blood studies: HCT, platelets, occult blood in stools q 3 mo. and APTT and ACT qd at the same time.

Check blood pressure and watch for increasing signs of
    hypertension.
Administer IV undiluted.
Antidote is protamine sulfate.

Geriatric Considerations
Elderly patients should usually start at lower doses due to
the increase in bleeding complications and mortality associated with anticoagulant use in this age group.

Generic Name
Human Insulin

Trade Name
Human, Novolin

Class
Antidiabetic agent

Action
Increases glucose transport across muscle and fat cell
membranes to reduce blood glucose level. Promotes conversion of glucose to glycogen.

Uses
Treatment of Type I diabetes mellitus (insulin dependent), ketosis-prone diabetics, diabetes mellitus inad-
equately controlled by diet and oral hypoglycemics, and
diabetic ketoacidosis (use regular insulin only).

Dosage
Adjusted according to patient's blood and urine glucose
concentrations.

Side Effects
Frequent: Lipoatrophy, lipohypertrophy
Less frequent: Hypoglycemia, hyperglycemia (rebound,
    or Somogyi effect), urticaria, itching, swelling, red-
    ness, stinging, warmth at injection site, anaphy-
    laxis.

Interactions

Prolonged hypoglycemic effect with alcohol, beta blockers, clofibrate, fenfluramine, guanethidine, monoamine oxidase inhibitors, salicylates, and tetracycline.

Diminished insulin response with corticosteroids, epinephrine, dextrothyroxine, and thiazide diuretics.

Nursing Implications

Instruct patient:

Regarding the importance of accuracy in measuring amount of insulin to be injected.

To use, as necessary, aids such as magnifying sleeve, dose magnifier, etc. to improve accuracy.

Not to alter the order of mixing insulins or change the model or brand of syringe or needle.

To store insulin in a cool area, although it does not have to be refrigerated.

That whenever NPH or Lente is mixed with regular insulin in the same syringe, administer it immediately to avoid binding.

Not to use insulin that has changed color or has become clumped or granular in appearance.

To check expiration date on vial before using contents.

Regarding proper use of equipment for performing self-monitoring of blood glucose.

Regarding choosing an appropriate site for injection as well as the process for preparing and injecting the insulin.

About the nature of the disease: The importance of following the therapeutic regimen, adhering to the specific diet, weight reduction, exercise, personal hygiene, and avoiding infection; timing of injection and eating.

To recognize hypoglycemic symptoms.

To wear Medic Alert at all times; to carry ample insulin and syringes on trips; to have carbohydrate (sugar or hard candy) on hand for emergency; to take note of time zone changes for dose schedule when traveling.

Not to smoke within 30 minutes after insulin injection.

Geriatric Considerations

Observe patient preparing and administering insulin to ensure that no visual, physical, or mental impairment interferes with ability to correctly perform this activity.

Instruct family member, neighbor, etc. how to correctly prepare and administer insulin in case the patient is unable to do this.

Provide ample time for teaching and return demonstrations by patient.

Provide information concerning diabetes in literature that is at the appropriate reading level for the patient.

Utilize pamphlets, books, etc. with illustrations.

Generic Name
Hydrochlorothiazide

Trade Name
Esidrix, HydroDIURIL, Mictrin, Oretic, Thiuretic, Urozide, Natrimax, Novohydrazide, Apo-Hydro, Dichlotride, Diuchlor, HCTZ

Class
Thiazide diuretic, antihypertensive

Action
Increases urinary excretion of sodium and water by inhibiting reabsorption of sodium in the ascending limb of the loop of Henle.

Uses
Treatment of HF and hypertension.

Dosage
25–100 mg PO daily or intermittently. Dose is increased or decreased based on blood pressure. Maximum dose 200 mg/d.

Side Effects
Volume depletion, dehydration, orthostatic hypotension, anorexia, nausea, fluid and electrolyte imbalances including hypokalemia, dilutional hyponatremia, hypochloremia, hyperuricemia, photosensitivity, rash, hypersensitivity reactions, confusion, ECG changes, muscle weakness, poor skin turgor, tachycardia, hyperglycemia.

Interactions

Cholestyramine and colestipol cause decreased intestinal absorption. Diazoxide increases hyperglycemic, hyperuricemic and antihypertensive effects. Hypoglycemic agents may need dosage readjustments based an blood glucose levels. Corticosteroids enhance the hypokalemic effect. NSAIDs and oral contraceptives decrease the diuretic effect. Antihypertensives and vasopressors enhance the hypotensive effects.

Nursing Implications

Administer hydrochlorothiazide as far apart as possible from cholestyramine or colestipol.

Administer in AM for prevention of nocturia.

Check for edema.

Monitor intake and output, weight, BP, serum electrolytes including serum potassium, BUN, and creatinine.

Monitor serum uric acid if the patient has gout.

Instruct the patient to:

Use a sunscreen when exposed to sunlight.

Avoid sudden changes of position in relationship to gravity to prevent orthostatic hypotension.

Report signs of hypokalemia (muscle weakness, abdominal cramps).

Eat high-potassium foods such as citrus fruits, tomatoes, bananas, dates, and apricots.

Be alert for signs of digitalis toxicity if patient is also taking this drug.

Discontinue thiazide before parathyroid function tests are performed.

Administer with caution in severe renal disease, impaired hepatic function, and chronic hepatitis.

Do not administer to patients with anuria and hypersensitivity to thiazides and sulfonamide derivatives.

Geriatric Considerations

Susceptible to excessive diuresis, hypotension, and electrolyte imbalances. Use smallest effective dose to prevent hypovolemia.

Generic Name
Hydrocodone Bitartrate

Trade Name
Hycodan, Hycomine, Hydrocet, Lorcet, Lortab, Triaminic Expectorant DH, Tussionex, Vicodin, Zydone

Class
Narcotic analgesic; antitussive, Schedule III

Action
Acts mostly an the central nervous system, altering both the perception of and emotional response to pain. Also suppresses the cough center in the medulla.

Uses
Relief of moderate to moderately severe pain. May also be used to relieve cough.

Dosage
Analgesic: 5–10 mg q 4–6 h as needed.
Cough: 5 mg q 4–6 h as needed.
Maximum: 15 mg per dose.

Side Effects
Potential for abuse, central nervous system and respiratory depression, lightheadedness, nausea, vomiting, constipation, urinary retention, rash, hepatotoxicity (overdose).

Interactions
Potentiation with monoamine oxidase inhibitors, tricyclic antidepressants, alcohol, central nervous system depressants, anticholinergics.

Nursing Implications
Instruct patients to:
  Avoid activities requiring alertness until central nervous system effects are determined.
  Never exceed the recommended dosage.
  Limit alcohol intake with this drug.
  Use with aspirin or acetaminophen to increase analgesia.

Since urinary retention may be more pronounced in elderly patients, question them about voiding, pain in the bladder area, or sensations of inadequate bladder emptying; palpate for bladder distention.

Instruct patients to void before each dose.

Monitor blood pressure frequently since hypotension is more common in the elderly.

Observe safety precautions to prevent injury.

Generic Name
Hydrocortisone

Trade Name
Cortef, Cortenema, Hycort, Hydrocortone, Hytone

Class
Corticosteroid agent

Action
Stabilizes leukocyte lysosomal membrane to decrease the signs and symptoms of inflammation. Other actions include suppression of the immune response, stimulation of the bone marrow, and metabolization of fats, proteins, and carbohydrates.

Uses
Treatment of adrenal insufficiency, severe inflammation, ulcerative colitis, proctitis, and shock.

Dosage
In chronic states: 5–40 mg PO in daily divided doses (maximum 80 mg qid may be given), 100–500 mg IM or IV then 50–100 mg; repeat as necessary. Acute life-threatening diseases PO 60–240 mg daily individual doses or 1 enema per day (100 mg) for 21 days hs. Soft tissue and intra-articular infections 5–75 mg, depending on size of joint. Daily dose is titrated to lowest effective dose. Increased dosage may be necessary with fever, trauma, emotional problems, and surgery. Dosage is tapered slowly with long-term use.

Side Effects

Euphoria, hypertension, insomnia, cataracts, edema, glaucoma, increased appetite, nausea and vomiting, GI irritation, hyperglycemia, osteoporosis, muscle weakness, fatigue, delayed wound healing, mental irregularities, potential hypokalemia, acne, hirsutism, increased susceptibility to infection, insomnia, nervousness, hyperglycemia, personality changes, HF.

Interactions

Antihistamines, barbiturates, chloral hydrate, glutethimide, phenytoin, rifampin decrease the effect of hydrocortisone. Phenylbutazone, indomethacin, and aspirin increase the risk of bleeding and GI irritation. Adrenergics, anticholinergics, TCAs, and meperidine increase risk of increased intraocular pressure. Effectiveness of oral anticoagulants is altered. A decline in antibody response and an increased risk of neurologic complications occur following administration of live attenuated virus vaccines. Potassium-depleting diuretics enhance the potassium-wasting effect.

Nursing Implications

Administer the daily dose in the morning for better results and decreased toxicity.

Administer PO drug with foods to prevent GI irritation.

Administer IM deeply and rotate sites.

Do not give subcutaneously.

Dilute medication according to manufacturer's directions for IV push and give over 30 seconds to several minutes.

Change IV solution every 24 hours.

Monitor blood pressure, weight, serum electrolytes, and serum glucose levels for steroid-induced hyperglycemia.

Inspect skin for petechiae.

Assess for depression or psychotic periods when taking high-dose therapy.

Instruct the patient to:

Never discontinue the drug suddenly without physician or prescribing health care provider approval.

Carry an identification card in case supplemental steroids are needed.

Recognize symptoms of adrenal insufficiency and Cushingoid symptoms.

Practice safety measures to avoid falls and soft tissue
trauma.

Avoid exposure to persons with contagious diseases.

Give a diet low in sodium and high in potassium and
protein if ordered.

Administer with caution to patients with GI alteration,
renal disease, hypertension, osteoporosis, vaccinia,
varicella, diabetes, exanthema, Cushing's syndrome,
thromboembolic disorders, myasthenia gravis, seizures, cancer, HF, ocular herpes simplex, tuberculosis, emotional instabilities, psychotic tendencies,
hypoalbuminemia.

Do not administer to patients with hypersensitivity, systemic fungal infections, and sulfites (in the injectable form), which can cause an allergic reaction.

Geriatric Considerations

Need to weigh the risk/benefit ratio of steroid therapy
since diseases that can be aggravated by steroids are
common among the elderly.

Generic Name
Ibuprofen

Trade Name
Advil, Medipren, Motrin, Nuprin, Rufen, Trendar

Class
Nonsteroidal anti-inflammatory drug

Action
Produces anti-inflammatory, analgesic, and antipyretic
effects, possibly through inhibition of prostaglandin synthesis.

Uses
Mild to moderate pain, arthritis, primary dysmenorrhea,
gout, and postextraction dental pain.

Dosage
200–800 mg PO tid or qid not to exceed 3.2 g/d.

Side Effects

Frequent: Headache, drowsiness, dizziness, peripheral edema, epigastric distress, nausea, occult blood loss, peptic ulceration, tinnitus.

Less frequent: Prolonged bleeding time, aseptic meningitis, visual disturbances, reversible renal failure, elevated enzymes, pruritus, rash, urticaria, edema, bronchospasm.

Interactions

Decreased effectiveness of diuretics is possible.

Increased plasma levels or pharmacologic effects of oral anticoagulants and lithium is possible.

Nursing Implications

Instruct patient:

That full therapeutic effect for arthritis may be delayed for 2–4 weeks.

Regarding signs and symptoms of gastrointestinal bleeding and instruct them to report these to the physician immediately.

To take the medication with meals or milk to reduce gastrointestinal adverse reactions.

That using ibuprofen while taking aspirin, alcohol, or steroids may increase the risk of gastrointestinal adverse reactions.

Not to exceed 1.2 g/d when using over-the-counter brands.

Not to self-medicate for extended periods without consulting a health care provider.

Do not administer to asthmatic patients with nasal polyps.

Monitor renal and hepatic function periodically during long-term therapy.

Geriatric Considerations

Monitor renal function. Decreased renal function in the elderly may require that the dosage be lowered.

Instruct patient to inform physician of all medications being taken.

Generic Name
Imipramine

Trade Name
Tofranil, Tripramine, Janimine

Class
Tricyclic antidepressant

Action
Increases the amount of norepinephrine or serotonin, or both, in the central nervous system by blocking their reuptake by the presynaptic neurons.

Uses
Treatment of depression.

Dosage
75–100 mg PO or IM daily in divided doses with 25–50 mg increments up to 200 mg maximum daily dosage.
Elderly and adolescents: Initial dose of 30–40 mg daily, with a maximum of 100 mg.

Side Effects
Frequent: Drowsiness, dizziness, orthostatic hypertension, tachycardia, ECG changes, blurred vision, dry mouth, constipation, urine retention, sweating.
Less frequent: Excitation, tremors, weakness, confusion, headache, nervousness, hypertension, tinnitus, mydriasis, nausea, vomiting, anorexia, paralytic ileus, rash, urticaria.
After abrupt withdrawal of long-term therapy: Nausea, headache, malaise.

Interactions
Decreased tricyclic antidepressant levels with barbiturates.
Increased serum levels with cimetidine.
Increased hypertensive effect if used with epinephrine or norepinephrine.
Severe excitation, hyperpyrexia, or seizures may occur if taken with monoamine oxidase inhibitors.
Increased tricyclic antidepressant blood levels with methylphenidate.

Instruct patient:

That full therapeutic effect for arthritis may be delayed for 2–4 weeks.

To avoid activities requiring alertness and good psychomotor coordination until central nervous system effects are determined.

That there will be a delay of 2 weeks or more before a noticeable effect is seen and that the full effect may take up to 4 weeks.

To relieve dry mouth with sugarless hard candy or gum.

To avoid over-the-counter medications without first consulting the prescribing health care provider.

About possible orthostatic hypotension.

Not to suddenly stop taking the medication.

Reduce dosage if signs of psychosis increase.

Record changes in mood.

Monitor for suicidal tendencies.

Geriatric Considerations

Initial dosage in the elderly should be small with a gradual increase while the patient is monitored for appropriate response and untoward side effects.

Use of a nighttime dose may alleviate daytime side effects.

Instruct patient to be aware of safety risks associated with decreased alertness and psychomotor skills as well as orthostatic hypotension.

Monitor for urine retention and constipation.

Increase fluid intake and suggest a stool softener if necessary.

Tell patient to inform prescribing health care provider of all medications (prescription and over the counter) currently being taken.

Generic Name
Indapamide

Trade Name:
Lozol

Class
Thiazide diuretic

Action

Inhibits sodium reabsorption in the cortical diluting site of the nephron. Also has a direct vasodilating effect that may be a result of calcium channel-blocking action.

Uses

Treatment of edema and hypertension.

Dosage

2.5–5.0 mg PO qd.

Side Effects

Electrolyte disorders (particularly hypokalemia and hyponatremia), hyperglycemia, hyperuricemia, gout, dysrhythmias, headache, nervousness, blurred vision, muscle cramps, dizziness, fatigue, orthostatic hypotension, GI disturbances.

Interactions

Increased antihypertensive, hyperglycemic, hyperuricemic effects with diazoxide. Decreased diuretic effectiveness with nonsteroidal anti-inflammatory drugs.

Nursing Implications

If patient has severe renal disease, impaired hepatic function, and progressive hepatic disease, monitor side effects very carefully.

Monitor I & O, weight, BP, and serum electrolytes regularly.

Instruct patient to:

Eat a diet that is high in potassium and to watch for signs and symptoms of hypokalemia.

Take the drug in the morning to prevent nocturia.

Avoid sudden posture changes and rise slowly to avoid orthostatic hypotension.

Use sunscreen.

Monitor serum creatinine and BUN levels regularly.

Monitor blood uric acid, especially with history of gout.

Check insulin requirements in diabetic patients.

Geriatric Considerations

Elderly patients are often more sensitive to the effects of diuretics than younger adults so observe for signs of excessive diuresis and electrolyte imbalance.

Dosage may need to be decreased.

Monitor BP carefully.

Implement safety precautions to prevent injury due to orthostatic hypotension.

Counseling with regard to diet may be necessary to maintain potassium balance.

Generic Name
Levothyroxine sodium

Trade Name
Synthroid, Levothroid, Levoxyl

Class
Thyroid hormone (T4)

Action
Acts at cellular level, principally through triiodothyronine to increase metabolic rate; increases cardiac output, oxygen consumption, body temperature, blood volume, growth, and development at cellular level.

Uses
Thyroid hormone replacement in the treatment of hypothyroidism, myxedema coma, cretinism, functional deficiency, and thyroid cancer.

Dosage
Hypothyroidism: Initially, 0.05 PO mg/d. Increase by 0.025 mg q 2–3 wk. Maintenance: 0.1–0.2 mg/d.

Myxedema coma: Initially, 0.4 mg IV. Follow with daily supplements of 0.1–0.2 mg. Maintenance: 0.05–0.1 mg/d.

Thyroid suppression therapy: 2.6 PO mg/kg/d for 7–10 d.

TSH suppression in thyroid cancer, nodules, euthyroid goiters: Use larger doses.

Side Effects
Most reactions are due to excessive dosage and consist of signs and symptoms of hyperthyroidism. Sweating, alopecia, anxiety, insomnia, tremor, headache, heat intolerance,

fever, coma, thyroid storm, tachycardia, palpitations, angina, dysrhythmia, hypertension, HF, nausea, diarrhea, increased or decreased appetite, cramps, and menstrual irregularities.

Interactions

Cholestyramine and colestipol decrease oral absorption. Thyroid hormone increases effect of oral anticoagulants. May cause an increase in the requirement for insulin or oral hypoglycemic agents in diabetics. Additive CNS and cardiac stimulation with sympathomimetic agents (amphetamines, vasopressors, decongestants). May decrease same effects of beta-adrenergic blockers. Increases effects of anticoagulants.

Nursing Implications

Check pulse and BP before each dose.

Measure I & O. Weigh qd in same clothing, using same scale, at same time of day.

Monitor levels of T3 and T4, which are decreased if patient is on too low a dose of medication.

Administer at same time each day to maintain drug level, preferably before breakfast to prevent insomnia.

Geriatric Considerations

The elderly are usually more sensitive to and experience more adverse reactions to thyroid hormone than other age groups. In some patients, the dose should be 25% lower than the usual adult dose. Hypothyroidism is the second most common endocrine disorder in the elderly and is often misdiagnosed. Only one-third of the geriatric clients exhibit the typical signs and symptoms of cold intolerance and weight gain. Instead, the symptoms are usually nonspecific, such as stumbling and falling, and if neurologic involvement has occurred, the patient may be misdiagnosed as having dementia, depression, or a psychotic episode.

Generic Name
Lisinopril

Trade Name
Prinivil, Zestril

Class

Antihypertensive, angiotensin converting enzyme (ACE) inhibitor.

Action

Prevents the production of angiotensin II, a potent vaso-constrictor that stimulates the aldosterone system by blocking its conversion to the active form. The result is systemic vasodilation.

Uses

Hypertension, also used in combination with other agents in the management HF.

Dosage

Adult: PO hypertension, not using diuretics, 10 mg/d, single dose. If using diuretics, discontinue diuretics for 2–3 days if possible, 5 mg/d. Maximum 80 mg/d. PO HF, 5 mg/d, single dose. Maximum 20 mg/d.
Children: Not established.

Side Effects

Orthostatic hypotension, headache, dizziness, insomnia, fatigue, angioedema, diarrhea, nausea, hyperkalemia, cough.

Interactions

Induced hypotension with concurrent antihypertensives, nitrates, or alcohol usage. May increase serum levels of lithium. Potassium supplements, potassium-sparing diuretics may cause hyperkalemia. Decreased antihypertensive effects with indomethacin and other NSAIDs.

Nursing Implications

Monior BP prior to administration to evaluate hypertensive control.
Assess for angioedema and the presence of fluid overload.
Caution patient to change position slowly to minimize orthostatic hypotension.
Emphasize the importance of follow-up examinations.
Instruct patient to take lisinopril as directed, even if feeling well.

Advise patient that drug may alter taste perception.

Geriatric Considerations
Dosage may be lower with maximum of 40 mg/d.

Generic Name
Lorazepam

Trade Name
Alzapam, Loraz, Apo-Lorazepam, Ativan, Novolorazem

Class
Antianxiety

Action
Inhibits the ability of excitatory neurotransmitters to stimulate a nerve impulse.

Uses
Anxiety neuroses, organic disorders, anxiety, agitation, tension, irritability, insomnia, and as premedication to anesthesia.

Dosage
1–3 mg PO daily or divided doses (maximum dose is 10 mg) or 2–4 mg PO hs or 0.05 mg/kg IM or IV (maximum dose is 4 mg) over 1 min. or longer. Elderly: 1–2 mg/d PO single doses.

Side Effects
Lethargy, hangover, drowsiness, transient hypotension, fainting, abdominal discomfort, dry mouth, respiratory depression.

Interactions
Alcohol and other CNS depressants increase the CNS depression. CNS stimulants decrease the CNS effect.

Nursing Implications
Monitor for abuse as there is addiction potential with long-term usage.

Administer IM deep into muscle mass.

Administer IV with equal amount of diluent.

Use sterile water for injection, sodium chloride injection or dextrose 5% injection.

Store parenteral form in refrigerator.

Teach patients to avoid activities that require alertness until CNS effects are known; avoid combining drug with alcohol and avoid giving medication to others.

Use with caution in patients with myasthenia gravis, renal or hepatic dysfunction, and organic brain syndrome.

Do not administer to patients with psychoses, mental depression, and acute narrow-angle glaucoma.

Geriatric Considerations

Reduce dosage. If used as a premedication for patients over 50, IV dose should not exceed 2 mg.

Generic Name

Lovastatin

Trade Name

Mevacor

Class

Antilipemic

Action

Controls the production of cholesterol by decreasing liver synthesis of it.

Uses

Primary hypercholesterolemia, Types IIa and IIb, when diet and nonpharmacologic therapies have been shown to be ineffective.

Dosage

20 mg PO as initial dose daily with evening meal. If cholesterol is above 300 mg/dL, the initial dose is 80 mg. Recommended dosage range is 20–80 mg as a daily or individual dose.

Headache, blurred vision, dizziness, diarrhea, constipation, abdominal cramps, nausea, vomiting, rash, myalgia, and elevated liver function tests.

Interactions

Clofibrate and cholestyramine act to enhance lipid-reducing activity. Gemfibrozil and immunosuppressive agents increase the chances for polymyositis.

Nursing Implications

Administer daily dose with the evening meal when absorption is increased and cholesterol is being synthesized.

Store tablets in a light-resistant container and at room temperature.

Instruct patient to report muscle aches to theprescribing health care provider, to follow a diet that restricts cholesterol and fat intake; to exercise as recommended by prescribing health care provider, to control weight; to avoid alcohol and to have periodic age examinations.

Monitor liver function tests at beginning of therapy and periodically. Expect therapeutic effects of therapy within 2 weeks. Lovastatin should only be given if diet and nonpharmacologic therapies are ineffective.

Geriatric Considerations

Use with caution and monitor closely. Emphasize exercise, diet, and weight control since lovastatin causes a high likelihood of having side effects.

Generic Name
Meclizine hydrochloride

Trade Name

Antivert, Antivert/25, Ancolan, Antivert/50, Bonine, Bonamine, Dizmiss, Meni-D, Ru-Vert-M

Class

Antiemetic agent, antihistamine

Action
Inhibits the action of acetylcholine in the chemoreceptor trigger zone of the brain to prevent nausea and vomiting. Also decreases vestibular stimulation and depresses labyrinthine activity.

Uses
Treatment of dizziness and motion sickness.

Dosage
25–100 mg PO daily; for motion sickness, take 1 h before travel

Side Effects
Excessive drowsiness, dry mouth, fatigue, blurred vision, urinary retention, orthostatic hypotension. Can mask symptoms of intestinal obstruction, ototoxicity, or brain tumor.

Interactions
CNS depressants increase the risk of drowsiness. Anticholinergics enhance the anticholinergic effect. Antihypertensive agents enhance the hypotensive effect.

Nursing Implications
Instruct the patient to:
    Avoid activities that require alertness until CNS effects of the drug are known.
    Report excessive drowsiness to the prescribing health care provider.
Administer with caution in patients with glaucoma, GI and GU obstruction (benign prostatic hypertrophy).
Do not give when digitalis toxicity is present or suspected.

Geriatric Considerations
Increased risk for drowsiness.

Generic Name
Meperidine hydrochloride

Trade Name
Demerol HCl, Pethadol, Pethidine.

Class

Narcotic and opioid analgesic, Schedule II

Action

Binds with opiate receptors at many sites in the central nervous system, altering both perception of and emotional response to pain through an unknown mechanism.

Uses

Relief of moderate to severe pain; preoperative.

Dosage

Pain: 50–150 mg PO, IM, or SC q 3–4 h prn or around the clock; or 15–35 mg/h by continuous IV infusion.

Preoperatively: 50–100 mg IM or SC 30–90 min. before surgery.

Side Effects

Frequent: Sedation, somnolence, clouded sensorium, euphoria, hypotension, nausea, vomiting, constipation, urine retention.

Less frequent: Paradoxical excitement, tremor, dizziness, seizures with large doses, bradycardia, tachycardia, ileus, respiratory depression, physical dependence, muscle twitching, pain at injection site, tissue irritation and induration after subcutaneous injection, phlebitis after IV use.

Interactions

Used with meperidine, alcohol and CNS depressants have an additive effect.

Increased CNS excitation or depression can be severe or fatal when this drug is used with monoamine oxidase inhibitors, barbiturates, and isoniazid.

Decreased blood levels of meperidine when used with phenytoin.

Nursing Implications

Monitor respiratory and cardiovascular status carefully.

Hold medication if respirations are less than 12/min. or if a change in pupils is noted.

Monitor bladder function in postoperative patients.

Monitor bowel function; may need a laxative or stool softener ordered.

Administer before patient's pain is severe to provide a
better analgesic effect.

Instruct ambulatory patients to avoid activities that require alertness.

Do not administer to patients with head injuries.

Geriatric Considerations

Decreased dosage is usually required for the older adult.

Hypotension is more common in the elderly so monitor
the blood pressure frequently.

Instruct patient to avoid activities requiring alertness.

Implement safety measures to prevent injury due to falls.

Urinary retention may be more pronounced in the elderly.
Question the patient regarding any difficulty in
voiding, pain in the bladder area, or sensations of
inadequate bladder emptying. Palpate for bladder
distention.

Generic Name
Metoprolol

Trade Name
Lopressor, Toprolxl

Class
Antihypertensive, antianginal, beta-adrenergic blocker

Action
Blocks cardiac beta receptors and depresses renin secretion.

Uses
Treatment of hypertension, angina pectoris, and as early
intervention in acute myocardial infarction.

Dosage
Angina/hypertension: 100–450 mg PO qid or bid.

Acute MI: Administer 3 injections of 5-mg IV boluses q 2
min.; 15 min. after last dose, administer 50 mg PO q
6 h for 48 h. Maintenance dose is 100 mg PO bid.

Side Effects

Frequent: Bradycardia, hypotension.

Occasional: Fatigue, lethargy, nausea, vomiting, dyspnea, heart failure, bronchospasm.

Interactions

May increase cardiac effects of calcium channel blockers, digitalis.

Antagonized by nonsteroidal anti-inflammatory drugs, barbiturates, rifampin.

May cause bradycardia with catecholamine-depleting drugs.

Potentiated by felodipine.

May block epinephrine.

Nursing Implications

Check the apical pulse prior to administration and hold the drug if less than 60/min.

Monitor BP before administration and frequently thereafter until the patient's response to the drug is determined.

Administer drug IV at a rate not exceeding 1 mg/min.

Instruct patient:

   About the disease and the importance of taking drug as prescribed.

   To check with physician, other prescribing health care provider, or pharmacist before taking any over-the-counter drugs.

   To take drug consistently with meals as food may increase absorption.

   To store drug at room temperature and protect from light.

   To weigh daily and report any rapid gain or presence of edema.

Geriatric Considerations

Reduction of dosage may be necessary since older patients are more sensitive to beta blockers and the orthostatic hypotensive effects.

Observe closely for orthostatic hypotension, which could increase risk of falling.

Generic Name
Nabumetone

Trade Name
Relafen

Class
Nonsteroidal anti-inflammatory

Action
Inhibits prostaglandin synthesis.

Uses
Treatment of the signs and symptoms of rheumatoid arthritis and osteoarthritis.

Dosage
Adult: PO 1000–2000 mg/d, single dose or bid.
Children: not established.

Side Effects
Diarrhea, abdominal pain, GI bleeding, headache, drowsiness.

Interactions
Do not use with ulcer disease, GI bleeding, or other nonsteroidal anti-inflammatory agents. May increase the effects of anticoagulants and thrombolytics. May decrease the effects of antihypertensives and diuretics. May increase concentration of lithium.

Nursing Implications
Instruct patient to administer with food or antacids to decrease GI irritation.
Do not crush (chew) capsule.
Monitor stool color and report any dark, tarry stools.
Advise patient that alcohol and aspirin will increase the risk of GI irritation.

Geriatric Considerations
It is recommended that persons 65 years and over start with a lower dose.

Generic Name
Naproxen

Trade Name
Naprosyn

Class
Analgesic, nonsteroidal anti-inflammatory

Action
Inhibits prostaglandin synthesis by decreasing an enzyme needed for biosynthesis; possesses analgesic, anti-inflammatory, antipyretic properties.

Uses
Treatment of acute or long-term mild to moderate pain, osteoarthritis, rheumatoid arthritis, ankylosing spondylitis, acute gouty arthritis, bursitis, tendinitis, primary dysmenorrhea.

Dosage
PO 250–500 mg bid, not to exceed 1 g/d; naproxen sodium PO 525 mg, then 275 mg q 6–8 h prn, not to exceed 1475 mg.

Side Effects
Frequent: Nausea, dyspepsia, constipation, anorexia, vomiting, diarrhea, tinnitus, dizziness, drowsiness, fatigue, tremors, confusion, insomnia, anxiety, depression.
Less frequent: Jaundice, cholestatic hepatitis, flatulence, cramps, dry mouth, peptic ulcer, GI bleeding, tachycardia, peripheral edema, palpitations, dysrhythmias, purpura, rash, pruritus, sweating.
Rare: Dysuria, hematuria, oliguria, azotemia, blood dyscrasias, hearing loss, blurred vision.

Interactions
May increase action of heparin and toxicity of lithium. May decrease hypotensive effect of beta blockers, antihypertensive effect of ACE inhibitors, and diuretic effect of furosemide.

Nursing Implications
Assess renal, liver, and blood studies: BUN, creatinine, AST, ALT, Hgb before treatment.

Schedule audiometric and ophthalmic exams before, during, and after treatment.

Administer with food to decrease GI symptoms.

Geriatric Considerations

The elderly are more susceptible to this drug and the side effects of dizziness, fainting episodes, and falls. Caution should be used in elderly patients who have hepatic and renal impairment.

Generic Name
Nifedipine

Trade Name
Procardia, Adalat, Novo-NiFedin, Procardia XL

Class
Calcium channel blocker, antianginal, coronary vasodilator

Action
Inhibits calcium ion influx across cell membrane during cardiac depolarization; produces relaxation of coronary vascular smooth muscle, dilates coronary arteries; increases myocardial oxygen delivery in patients with vasospastic angina; dilates peripheral arteries, causing the greatest fall in BP of all the calcium channel blockers. Exerts minimal cardiac depressant action and has no tendency to slow SA nodal activity or prolong AV nodal conduction, unlike the other members of its class.

Uses
Used in the management of classic angina (chronic stable angina or effort angina), treatment of vasospastic angina (Prinzmetal's, variant, or at rest angina), and control of hypertension (investigational). Also used to treat Raynaud's phenomenon.

Dosage
Initially, 10 mg PO tid or qid for angina. Dosage is gradually increased over 7–14 d as needed and tolerated. Capsule may be administered buccally or sublingually by

piercing the capsule and squirting under the tongue. This method produces a more rapid effect than oral administration. Extended release: 30–60 mg qd, maximum 120 mg qd.

Side Effects

Lightheadedness, dizziness, giddiness, nausea, headache, flushing or feeling of warmth, occasional edema of extremities, palpitations, transient hypotension, symptoms of HF, muscle cramps, nasal congestion, sore throat, wheezing, mood changes, and nervousness. May alter Coombs' test.

Interactions

Nicotine may reduce effectiveness. Alcohol, antihypertensives, and beta-adrenergic blocking agents, including ophthalmic preparations, may enhance hypotensive effects. Serum levels of carbamazepine, cyclosporine, digitalis glycosides, and theophyllines may be increased leading to toxicity when given with Procardia. May decrease effects of quinidine.

Nursing Implications

Check BP and TPR immediately before giving medication.
Do not administer to patients who have sick sinus syndrome/second- or third-degree AV block (except in presence of pacemaker).
Monitor renal and hepatic blood work closely.
Tell patient and family to limit caffeine consumption.
Observe for giddiness and assist with ambulation if lightheadedness and dizziness occur.
Assess for peripheral edema and for flushing of the skin.
Observe for drug interactions and recognize that treatment is defibrillation for overdose, atropine for AV block and vasopressor for hypotension.

Geriatric Considerations

The elderly are more susceptible to this drug and the side effects of increased weakness, dizziness, fainting episodes, and falls. Maximum daily dosage is 180 mg.

Generic Name
Nortriptyline hydrochloride

Trade Name
Pamelor, Aventyl

Class
Tricyclic antidepressant

Action
Blocks the reuptake of norepinephrine or serotonin, or both, in the presynaptic neurons in the CNS.

Uses
Depression.

Dosage
25–40 mg PO individual doses then gradually increase to 100–150 mg/d.

Side Effects
Dizziness, drowsiness, ECG changes, tachycardia, blurred vision, constipation, dry mouth, sweating, urinary retention, and hypotension.

Interactions
Methylphenidate and cimetidine increase nortriptyline levels; barbiturates and nicotine promote a decrease in serum TCA levels; MAO inhibitors can cause the development of seizures, hyperpyrexia, and severe excitation. Use cautiously. Norepinephrine and epinephrine enhance the hypertensive effect. Antihistamines enhance the anticholinergic effect.

Nursing Implications
Do not expect a noticeable change in behavior for 2 weeks or more.
Monitor for an increase in psychotic signs, which would require a dosage reduction.
Assess for urine retention and constipation.
Instruct patient to:
   Eat sugarless hard candy or gum for dry mouth.

Avoid activities that require alertness until CNS effects are known.

Avoid taking alcohol or any OTC drugs unless approved by physician.

Take full dose at bedtime.

Take with food if GI distress occurs.

Increase fluid intake to prevent urinary retention.

Take stool softener as directed.

Never stop taking the drug without the physician's approval.

Administer with caution in patients with urine retention, thyroid and cardiovascular disease, glaucoma, impaired liver function, blood dyscrasias, or patients at risk for suicide, or receiving electroshock therapy or elective surgery.

Do not give to patients recovering from a myocardial infarction or to those with prostatic hypertrophy, or seizure disorders.

Geriatric Considerations

Reduction of dose is necessary, then gradually increase dose over several weeks. Increased risk of experiencing confusion, sedation, hypertension, and anticholinergic effects.

Generic Name
Ofloxacin

Trade Name
Floxin, Ocuflox

Class
Antiinfective (quinoline, antibiotic)

Action
Inhibits bacterial DNA synthesis; bactericidal.

Uses
Urinary tract and skin/skin structure infections, sexually transmitted diseases, lower respiratory tract infections, urinary tract infections, prostatitis, prostatitis, bacterial conjunctivitis.

Dosage

Adult: PO and IV 200–400 mg q 12 h for 3–10 d. For uncomplicated gonorrhea, 400 mg single dose.

Children: Not recommended.

Ophthalmic (adult and children): 1–2 drops q 2–4 h for the first 2 d, then qid for up to 5 d.

Side Effects

PO and IV — seizures, headaches, restlessness, nausea, diarrhea, vomiting, abdominal pain.

Ophthalmic — local burning, itching, tearing, bad taste in mouth.

Interactions

Antacids, sucralfate, iron, and zinc may decrease absorption. Increases serum theophylline levels. May increase the effects of oral anticoagulants.

Nursing Implications

Instruct patient to take on an empty stomach.

Instruct patient regarding the importance of completing the full course of therapy as prescribed, even if the signs and symptoms of the infection subside.

Assess patient for infection at the beginning and throughout the course of therapy.

Obtain specimens for culture and sensitivity tests prior to beginning therapy.

Encourage liberal fluid intake (1200–1500 mL/d).

Do not give antacids, iron, or zinc preparations within 2 hours before or 2 hours after administration of ofloxacin.

Geriatric Considerations

May consider a lower dose.

Generic Name
Oxaprozin

Trade Name
Daypro

Class
Nonsteroidal anti-inflammatory

Action
Inhibits prostaglandin synthesis.

Uses
Reduce pain and inflammation, management of osteoar-thritis and rheumatoid arthritis.

Dosage
Usual dose 1200 mg PO qd. Not to exceed 1800 mg/d. Patients with osteoarthritis and low body weight or mild disease may be started at 600 mg/d.

Side Effects
Nausea, dyspepsia, abdominal pain, GI bleeding, dizzi-ness, headache, tinnitus.

Interactions
Increased risk of adverse GI effects when used with other NSAIDs, aspirin, potassium, alcohol, or glucocorticoids. May decrease the effectiveness of diuretics or antihy-pertensives. May increase the hypoglycemic effects of insulin or oral hypoglycemic agents. Patients with asthma, aspirin-induced allergy, and nasal polyps are at an in-creased risk for developing hypersensitivity reactions.

Nursing Implications
Monitor bleeding times as oxaprozin may prolong bleed-ing.
Evaluate liver function tests for those patients receiving prolonged courses of therapy.
Instruct patient to take with food or antacids to decrease GI irritation.
Monitor stool color and report any dark, tarry stools.
Take with a full glass of water and have the patient remain upright for 15–30 minutes.

Geriatric Considerations
It is recommended that persons 65 years and over start with a lower dose.

Generic Name
Paroxetine hydrochloride

Trade Name
Paxil

Class
Antidepressant

Action
Selective inhibition of serotonin reuptake in the CNS.

Uses
Treatment of depression.

Dosage
PO 20 mg/d in the morning. Dosage should be increased gradually over weeks. Maximum 50 mg/d.

Side Effects
Somnolence, dizziness, headache, insomnia, tremor, nausea, dry mouth, constipation, diarrhea, ejaculatory disorders, sweating.

Interactions
MAO inhibitors and cimetidine may increase Paxil levels. Paxil increases serum levels of procyclidine, tryptophanase, and warfarin. Phenobarbital and phenytoin may decrease the effectiveness of Paxil. Concurrent use with alcohol is not recommended.

Nursing Implications
Inform patients that the therapeutic effects may take 1–4 weeks to be evident.
Monitor suicidal patients closely at the beginning of therapy.
Emphasize the importance of follow-up examination.
Stress to the patient Paxil should be taken only as prescribed.

Geriatric Considerations
Initial dosage should be 10 mg/d with the maximum 40 mg/d.

Generic Name
Penicillin V Potassium

Trade Name
Betapen-VK, Pen-Vee K, Beepen-VK, Robicillin VK, V-Cillin K, VC-K, Veetids

Class
Penicillins (antimicrobial and antiparasitic agents)

Action
Inhibits cell wall synthesis during active multiplication (bactericidal effect).

Uses
Mild to moderate systemic infections that are penicillin sensitive. Endocarditis prophylaxis for dental surgery.

Dosage
Infections: 250–500 mg (400,000–800,000 U) PO q 6 h.
Endocarditis prophylaxis: 2 g PO q 30–60 min. before
    procedure, then 1 g 6 h after.

Side Effects
Frequent: Epigastric distress, nausea.
Less frequent: Blood dyscrasias, neuropathy, vomiting,
    diarrhea, hypersensitivity (rash, urticaria, chills,
    fever, edema, anaphylaxis).

Interactions
Avoid concomitant tetracyclines.
Absorption decreased with neomycin.
Increased blood levels with probenecid.

Nursing Implications
Obtain specimen for culture and sensitivity tests prior to
    administering first dose.
Instruct patient to:
    Take medication exactly as prescribed and to finish the
        full course of treatment, even if feeling better.
    Call the prescribing health care provider if any rash,
        fever, or chills develop.
    Take medication 1–2 hours before meals or 2–3 hours after
        meals to avoid food interfering with the absorption.

Take the medication with a full glass of water (not juice or carbonated beverage as acid will inactivate the drug).

Avoid using any leftover penicillin for a new illness or sharing the drug with family or friends.

Geriatric Considerations

Observe for superinfection in the elderly as indicated by continued fever while on medication, poor wound healing, signs of sepsis.

Monitor renal function. The plasma half-life is elevated in the elderly due to decreased renal elimination so adjustment in the dosage may be necessary.

Generic Name

Pentoxifylline

Trade Name

Trental

Class

Peripheral perfusion enhancer

Action

Increases erythrocyte flexibility and lowers blood viscosity to improve capillary blood flow.

Uses

Used in intermittent claudication caused by chronic occlusive vascular disease in patients who are not good surgical candidates.

Dosage

400 mg PO tid with meals.

Side Effects

Dyspepsia, headache, dizziness, nausea, vomiting.

Interactions

Anticoagulants and antihypertensives have enhanced effects that may necessitate dosage adjustments.

Instruct the patient to:

> Take with meals to minimize GI upset.
>
> Swallow whole; do not break, crush, or chew.
>
> Report GI or CNS adverse reactions as a reduction in dose may be needed.
>
> Avoid smoking since the vasoconstrictive effect of nicotine can worsen the condition.
>
> Not discontinue taking medication unless directed by physician since it may take up to 8 weeks to achieve therapeutic effects.

Do not administer to patients who cannot take methylxanthines such as caffeine, theophylline, and theobromine.

Geriatric Considerations

May be more sensitive to adverse effects.

Generic Name

Phenobarbital

Trade Name

Barbita, Gardenal, Luminal Sodium, Solfoton

Class

Anticonvulsant agent, sedative-hypnotic

Action

Decreases monosynaptic and polysynaptic transmission in the CNS to increase the seizure threshold in the motor cortex. The sedation effects result from Inhibition of nerve impulse transmission to the cortex of the brain.

Uses

Treatment of tonic-clonic epilepsy, status epilepticus, temporal lobe partial seizures, and febrile seizures in children. Also used as a sedative-hypnotic.

Dosage

Epilepsy: 100–300 mg PO, IM, IV, bid, tid, or given as a single dose hs.

Status epilepticus: 10 mg/kg, IV infusion rate no faster than 50 mg/min. Maximum dose is 20 mg/kg total. Sedation: 30–120 mg PO, IM, IV, daily, bid, or tid. Insomnia: 100–300 mg PO, IM, or IV. Therapeutic blood levels are 15–40 mg/mL.

Side Effects

Drowsiness, hangover, sedation, diplopia, lethargy, nausea, vomiting, anorexia, rash, urticaria, anemia, hepatitis symptoms.

Interactions

Alcohol, CNS depressants, and narcotic analgesics cause excessive drowsiness. Diazepam and phenobarbital are mutually potentiating. Griseofulvin absorption is decreased. MAO inhibitors potentiate CNS and respiratory depression. TCAs, oral anticoagulants, estrogens, oral contraceptives, doxycycline, and corticosteroids decrease blood levels, as may rifampin. Primidone and valproic acid increase phenobarbital blood levels, increasing risk of toxicity.

Nursing Implications

Instruct patient to:

Avoid activities that require alertness and psychomotor coordination until CNS effects are known.

Contact prescribing health care provider if adverse reactions are experienced. Don't stop the drug. Recognize that therapeutic effects do not occur for 2–3 weeks except with a loading dose.

Administer IM phenobarbital deeply as superficial injection can cause pain, abscess development, and tissue sloughing at the site.

Administer IV, in emergencies, 60 mg/min. and only with resuscitation equipment available to combat respiratory depression.

Do not use a cloudy injectable solution.

Use a diluent that is nonacidic to prevent precipitation.

Monitor for signs of barbiturate toxicity such as coma, asthmatic breathing, cyanosis, clammy skin, and hypotension.

Administer with caution to patients with hyperthyroidism, diabetes mellitus, and anemia.

Do not administer to patients with barbiturate hypersensitivity, porphyria, hepatic dysfunction, respiratory disease with dyspnea or obstruction, nephritis, or to breastfeeding women.

Increased risk of adverse effects and toxicity due to age-related or other decline of kidney and liver function.

Generic Name
Piroxicam

Trade Name
Feldene, Apo-Piroxicam, Novopirocam

Class
Nonsteroidal anti-inflammatory agent

Action
Inhibits prostaglandin synthesis with resultant anti-inflammatory, analgesic, and antipyretic effects.

Uses
Osteoarthritis and rheumatoid arthritis.

Dosage
20 mg PO daily (dose may be divided).

Side Effects
Prolonged bleeding time, nausea, diarrhea, bruises, petechiae, hematuria, anemia, epigastric distress, headache, drowsiness, dizziness, peripheral edema, peptic ulceration.

Interactions
Aspirin decreases plasma levels of piroxicam. Piroxicam enhances the hypoglycemic effect of oral hypoglycemics and increases plasma lithium levels. Oral anticoagulants enhance the risk of bleeding.

Nursing Implications
Instruct the patient to:
    Take with meals or milk as GI distress is a problem.
    Report signs of GI bleeding to the prescribing health
       care provider immediately.

Remember that the therapeutic effect may not be achieved for 2–4 weeks.

Return for periodic checks of renal, hepatic, and auditory function, as scheduled, during long-term therapy.

Administer with caution in patients with angioedema, GI disorders, history of renal dysfunction, peptic ulcers, cardiac disease, or with hypersensitivity to NSAIDs.

Do not administer to asthmatics with nasal polyps.

Geriatric Considerations

Increased risk of nephrotoxicity.

Generic Name

Potassium chloride

Trade Name

K-Lor, K-Lyte/CL, Klotrix, K-Dur, Micro-K, Slow-K

Class

Electrolyte/electrolyte modifer, potassium replenisher

Action

Primary intercellular action. Increases serum potassium concentration. Improves nerve impulse transmission, contraction of skeletal, cardiac, and smooth muscle. Maintains intracellular isotonicity, acid-base balance.

Uses

Treatment of potassium deficiency found in severe vomiting, diarrhea, loss of GI secretions, malnutrition, prolonged diuresis, debilitation, poor GI absorption, metabolic alkalosis, prolonged parenteral alimentation.

Dosage

Dosage is individualized.
PO: Prevention: 20 mEq/d.
Treatment: 40–100 mEq/d.
IV: Individualized based on ECG, serum potassium concentrations.

Side Effects

Occasional: Nausea, vomiting, diarrhea, flatulence, abdominal discomfort, abdominal distention, phlebitis with IV administration.

Rare: Rash.

Interactions

ACE inhibitors and potassium-sparing diuretics may cause hyperkalemia.

Nursing Implications

Give oral dose with food or after meals with full glass of water or fruit juice.

Dilute preparation further or give with meals if GI disturbances occur.

Always dilute IV doses; never give directly into the venous system.

Monitor frequency and consistency of bowel movements.

Observe for signs of hyperkalemia (pale cold skin, paresthesias of extremities, feeling of heaviness of legs).

Monitor serum potassium level, particularly with impaired renal function.

Geriatric Considerations

Instruct the elderly not to chew or crush tablets, they must be swallowed whole. If patient cannot swallow whole tablet, inform prescribing health care provider and suggest a liquid preparation.

Generic Name
Prednisone

Trade Name
Deltasone, Orasone, Prednicen-M

Class
Corticosteroids

Action
Stabilizes leukocyte lysosomal membranes, which decreases inflammation. Suppresses the immune response,

stimulates bone marrow, and influences protein, fat, and carbohydrate metabolism.

Uses

Severe inflammation or immunosuppression; acute exacerbations of multiple sclerosis.

Dosage

Inflammation/immunosuppression: 2.5–15 mg PO bid, tid, or qid. Maintenance dosage: give once daily or qod. Dosage must be individualized.

Multiple sclerosis: 200 mg PO daily for 1 w, then 80 mg qod for 1 m.

Side Effects

Frequent: Euphoria, insomnia, peptic ulcer.

Less frequent: GI irritation, congestive heart failure, delayed wound healing, edema, possible hypokalemia, hyperglycemia and carbohydrate intolerance, cataracts, glaucoma, acne, various skin eruptions, muscle weakness, pancreatitis, hirsutism, and susceptibility to infection. Acute adrenal insufficiency may occur with increased stress (surgery, infection, trauma) or abrupt withdrawal after prolonged therapy.

Interactions

Decreased corticosteroid effect with barbiturates, phenytoin, and rifampin.

Increased risk of gastrointestinal distress and bleeding with indomethacin and aspirin.

Decreased antibody response and increased risk of neurologic complications with live attenuated virus vaccines.

Enhanced potassium-wasting effects of prednisone with potassium-depleting drugs such as thiazide diuretics.

Altered dosage requirements with oral anticoagulants.

Nursing Implications

Monitor patient's blood pressure, sleep patterns, and potassium.

Weigh patient daily and report any sudden weight gain to the prescribing health care provider.

Monitor for depression or psychotic episodes, especially with high-dose therapy.

Instruct patient:

Do not discontinue taking the drug abruptly or without physician or prescribing health care provider consent.

To report any slow healing to the doctor.

To take daily dosage in the morning for better results and less toxicity.

Report early signs of adrenal insufficiency: fatigue, muscular weakness, joint pain, fever, anorexia, nausea, dyspnea, dizziness, fainting.

Carry a card identifying the need for supplemental systemic glucocorticoids during stress.

Istruct patients on long-term therapy about Cushingoid symptoms.

Instruct diabetic patients that they may require more insulin; monitor blood glucose.

Geriatric Considerations

Use cautiously in patients with osteoporosis.

Titrate to lowest possible dose to decrease untoward side effects.

Avoid contact with individuals with active infections due to its increasing the susceptibility to infection.

Generic Name

Propoxyphene hydrochloride

Trade Name

Darvon, Duraphen, Dilene, Dixaphene, Propox, Norvo-propoxyn, Propoxycon

Class

Narcotic analgesic, Schedule IV

Action

Blocks perception and emotional response to painful stimuli by binding with opiate receptors in the CNS.

Uses

Mild to moderate pain; not given for narcotic addiction, used in conjunction with aspirin or acetaminophen to enhance analgesic effect.

Dosage
65 mg PO q 4 h prn.

Side Effects
Dizziness, drowsiness, sedation, paradoxical excitement, constipation, nausea, vomiting, hypotension, physical and psychological dependence.

Interactions
CNS depressants and alcohol enhance the CNS effects; diuretics may increase the chance of orthostatic hypotension.

Nursing Implications
Instruct patient to:
    Avoid activities that need alertness until the effects are known.
    Never exceed the prescribed dose.
    Limit alcohol intake while taking propoxyphene hydrochloride.
    Eat a diet high in fiber to prevent constipation.
Reverse respiratory depression with Narcan 0.9 IV push.

Geriatric Considerations
Administer small doses at longer intervals. Risk of side effects like respiratory depression and sedation are increased.

Generic Name
Propoxyphene napsylate

Trade Name
Darvocet-N 50, Darvocet-N 100

Class
Narcotic analgesic (Opioid), Schedule IV

Action
Binds with the opiate receptors at many sites in the CNS (brain, brain stem, spinal cord), altering both the perception of and emotional response to pain.

Uses
Mild to moderate pain.

Dosage
100 mg PO q 4 h prn.

Side Effects
Side effects are not common at analgesic doses but may include: dizziness, sedation, nausea, vomiting, rash, constipation, respiratory depression, hepatotoxicity with overdosage.

Interactions
Potentiation with alcohol and CNS depressants.

Nursing Implications
Instruct patient to avoid activities requiring alertness until CNS effects are determined.
Warn patient not to exceed recommended dosage.
Advise patient to limit alcohol intake with this drug.
Use with aspirin or acetaminophen to increase analgesia.

Geriatric Considerations
Monitor level of consciousness and mental status as changes may be due to pain, hypoxia, or a reaction to the medication.
Supervise ambulation and implement safety precautions to prevent injury.

Generic Name
Ranitidine

Trade Name
Zantac

Class
Histamine (H_2) antagonist, gastrointestinal-antiulcer

Action
Inhibits the action of histamine at the H_2 receptor site located primarily in gastric parietal cells. Inhibits gastric acid secretion, which leads to healing and prevention of ulcers.

Uses

Used in treatment (short-term) and prevention of active
duodenal ulcers. Short-term treatment of benign gastric
ulcers. Management of gastroesophageal reflux disease
(GERD). Treatment of gastric hypersecretory states
(Zollinger-Ellison syndrome).

Dosage

Short-term treatment of active ulcers:
    PO: 150 mg bid or 300 mg at bedtime.
    IM: 50 mg q 6–8 h (up to 400 mg/d).
    IV: 50 mg q 6–8 h or 6.25 mg/h infusion.
Prevention of duodenal ulcers:
    PO: 150 mg once daily at bedtime.
Management of gastroesophageal reflux:
    PO: 150 mg bid.
Gastric hypersecretory conditions (Zollinger-Ellison syn-
    drome):
    PO: 150 mg bid (up to 6 g/d).
    IV: 50 mg/kg/h initially by continuous infusion. Based
      on gastric acid output after 4 h, may increase by 0.5
      mg/kg/h up to 2.5 mg/kg/h.

Side Effects

Occasional: Severe headache, confusion, dizziness, headache, malaise, drowsiness.
Rare: Bradycardia, tachycardia, premature ventricular
contractions, rashes, ocular pain, blurred vision,
gynecomastia, nausea, constipation, hepatitis, abdominal pain, diarrhea, and impotence.

Interactions

Antacids may decrease the absorption of ranitidine. Smoking may decrease the effectiveness of ranitidine. Reduces
absorption of ketoconazole.

Nursing Implications

Do not confuse medication with alprazolam (Xanax).
Assess patient routinely for epigastric or abdominal pain
and frank or occult blood in the stool, emesis, or
gastric aspirate.
Monitor severely ill patients and those with impaired
renal or hepatic function for confusion.

Assess the elderly for confusion and notify the prescribing health care provider promptly should this occur. Acute mental changes in the elderly may indicate the need for lowering the drug dose and discontinuing the medication. Gastrointestinal complaints are very common in the elderly. Pain is less frequently the initial complaint while melena is the more frequent presentation and indication of ulcer disease. Every complaint should be properly evaluated before instituting drug therapy.

Generic Name
Sertraline hydrochloride

Trade Name
Zoloft

Class
Antidepressant

Action
Selectively blocks reuptake of the neurotransmitter serotonin within the CNS.

Uses
Treatment of depression.
Unlabeled use: Treatment of obsessive-compulsive disorders.

Dosage
50 mg PO qd (AM or PM) to start. May be gradually increased every week. Maximum 200 mg per day.

Side Effects
Headache, dizziness, agitation, sweating, male sexual dysfunction, insomnia, nausea, diarrhea.

Interactions
MAO inhibitors may cause fatal reactions if taken concurrently. Use caution with other CNS agents. Tolbutamide and diazepam clearance may be reduced. Concurrent use with alcohol is not recommended.

Nursing Implications

Inform patient that the therapeutic effects may take 1–4 weeks to be evident.

Monitor suicidal patients closely at the beginning of therapy.

Instruct patient to take Zoloft as prescribed every day.

Emphasize the importance of follow-up examinations.

Withdraw gradually.

Geriatric Considerations

Use a smaller dose initially and adjust dosage to response.

Generic Name
Tetracycline hydrochloride

Trade Name
Achromycin, Panmycin, Sumycin, Tetracap, Tetralan

Class
Anti-infective

Action
Inhibits protein synthesis. Bactericidal or bacteriostatic, depending upon the concentration.

Uses
Treatment of tetracycline-sensitive infections, including those caused by rickettsiae, *Mycoplasma pneumoniae*, and *Chlamydia trachomatis*; uncomplicated urethral, endocervical, or rectal infection caused by *Chlamydia trachomatis*; brucellosis; gonorrhea and syphilis in patients sensitive to penicillin; acne; shigellosis.

Dosage
Trachoma, rickettsiae, mycoplasma, chlamydia: 250–500 mg PO q 6 h; 250 mg d/IM or 150 mg IM q 12 h; or 250–500 mg IV q 8–12 h.

Uncomplicated urethral, endocervical, or rectal infection: 500 mg PO qid for at least 7 days.

Brucellosis: 500 mg PO q 6 h for 3 weeks with streptomycin, 1 g IM q 12 h week 1 and daily week 2.

Gonorrhea: Initially, 1.5 g PO, then 500 mg q 6 h for a total
dose of 9 g.
Syphilis: 30–40 g PO total in equally divided doses over
10–15 d.
Shigellosis: 2.5 g PO in a single dose.

Side Effects

Frequent: Epigastric distress, nausea, diarrhea, increased
BUN, maculopapular and erythematous rashes,
urticaria, photosensitivity, increased pigmentation,
irritation after IM injection, thrombophlebitis.

Less frequent: Vaginal candidiasis, colitis, hepatic
cholestasis, anemia, leukopenia, neutropenia, thrombocytopenia, eosinophilia, anaphylaxis, intracranial
hypertension, hepatoxicity with large doses given
IV.

Interactions

Increase in serum digoxin levels may occur.

Reduced absorption with antacids, iron, zinc, calcium,
magnesium, dairy products, urinary alkalinizers,
and food.

Use with anticoagulants may cause increase in prothrombin time.

Decreased effects of penicillins when used concomitantly.

Nursing Implications

Obtain specimen for culture and sensitivity tests prior to
administering first dose.

Instruct patient to:

Take each dose with a full glass of water on an empty
stomach, at least 1 hour before bedtime to prevent
esophagitis.

Avoid taking medication with milk or dairy products,
food, antacids, or iron products as these decrease
the effectiveness.

Take medication exactly as prescribed and finish the
course of the medication.

Avoid direct sunlight and ultraviolet light.

Check patient's tongue for signs of monilial infection.

Inject IM dose deeply and rotate injection sites.

Observe for signs and symptoms of superinfection (tongue
discoloration, candidal infections, or diarrhea)

Avoid mixing tetracycline solution with any other additive.

Although tetracyclines are considered safe for elderly patients, it is important to reinforce the importance of taking the medication at the prescribed time as well as scheduling it appropriately around meals and other drugs with which it might cause an interaction.

Generic Name
Timolol maleate

Trade Name
Blocadren, Timoptic (usually ophthalmic agent)

Class
Beta-adrenergic blocker and nonselective antihypertensive

Action
Blocks stimulation of $beta_1$ (myocardial) and $beta_2$ receptor sites (pulmonary, vascular, or uterine). Effect of beta-$blockade_1$ includes slowed heart rate and decreased CO and contractility; effect of beta $blockade_2$ includes bronchoconstriction and increased airway resistance in those with asthma or COPD.

Uses
Treatment of mild to moderate hypertension, sinus tachycardia, persistent atrial extrasystole, tachydysrhythmias, hypertrophic cardiomyopathy, mitral valve prolapse, anxiety. Also used for prophylaxis of angina pectoris and migraine and reduction of mortality after MI.

Dosage
Hypertension: PO 10 mg bid to start. Increase at 7-d intervals as necessary, Not to exceed 60 mg/d.
Myocardial infarction: PO 10 mg bid.
Migraine prophylaxis: PO 10 mg bid initially, may be given as 20 mg qd during maintenance (range 10 mg qd to 10–15 mg bid).

Side Effects

More frequent: Fatigue, dizziness, weakness, depression, insomnia, diarrhea, nausea, vomiting.

Less frequent: Hypotension, bradycardia, HF, edema, chest pain, bradycardia, claudication, insomnia, dizziness, hallucinations, anxiety, ischemic colitis, diarrhea, abdominal pain, mesenteric arterial thrombosis, rash, alopecia, pruritus, fever, agranulocytosis, thrombocytopenia, purpura, visual changes, sore throat, double vision, dry burning eyes, impotence, frequency, bronchospasm, dyspnea, cough, crakles, hypoglycemia, joint pain, and muscle pain.

Interactions

Increased hypotension and bradycardia when given with: reserpine, hydralazine, methyldopa, prazosin, and anticholinergics. Decreased antihypertensive effects when given with indomethacin. Increased hypoglycemic effects when given with insulin. Decreased bronchodilation when given with theophyllines.

Nursing Implications

Assess: I & O, daily weight, BP during initial treatment and periodically thereafter.

Take pulse q 4 h; note rate, rhythm, quality and apical/radial pulse before administration. Notify prescribing health care provider of any significant changes.

Schedule renal and liver function tests for baseline before therapy begins.

Administer: PO ac and/or hs, crush tablet prn.

Geriatric Considerations

The elderly are more susceptible to this drug and the side effects of increased weakness, dizziness, fainting episodes and falls. May be given without regard to meals. May be crushed and mixed with food if elderly client has difficulty swallowing.

Generic Name
Triamcinolone

Trade Name
Aristocort, Atolone, Kenacort, Tricilone, Azmacort, Kenalog

Class
Corticosteroid agent

Action
Stabilizes leukocyte lysosomal membrane to decrease inflammation. Also suppresses the immune response; stimulates bone marrow and influences protein, fat, and carbohydrate metabolism.

Uses
Treatment of severe inflammation and asthma. Also used for immunosuppression.

Dosage
4–48 mg PO bid, tid, or qid, 40 mg IM weekly or 2–40 mg into joints and soft tissues, 5–48 mg into lesions, up to 0.5 mg per square inch of affected skin intralesional, or 20–40 mg intra-arterial or intrasynovial into soft tissue or into joint or lesion. Two inhalations tid to qid. Maximum of 16 inhalations daily. Not used for alternative day therapy. PO dose is titrated to lowest effective dose. Topical: Use sparingly bid–qid.

Side Effects
Euphoria, insomnia, psychotic behavior, hypertension, edema, cataracts, glaucoma, peptic ulcer, GI irritation, increased appetite, hypokalemia, hyperglycemia, delayed wound healing, acne, various skin eruptions, muscle weakness, hirsutism, susceptibility to infections. Topical preparations may cause contact dermatitis.

Interactions
Barbiturates, antihistamines, phenytoin, chloral hydrate, rifampin, glutethimide decrease corticosteroid effect. Indomethacin, phenylbutazone, and aspirin increase the risk of GI distress and bleeding. Effectiveness of oral anticoagulants is altered. A decline in antibody response

and an increased risk of neurological complications occurs following administration of live attenuated virus vaccine. Potassium-depleting drugs like the thiazide diuretics enhance the potassium-wasting effects. Adrenergics, TCAs (tricyclic antidepressants), antihistamines, anticholinergics, and meperidine can increase the risk of increased intraocular pressure.

Nursing Implications

Instruct the patient to:

> Never stop taking the drug abruptly without prescribing health care provider's approval. Sudden withdrawal can be fatal.
>
> Report slow wound healing to the prescribing health care provider.
>
> Carry an identification card for supplemental steroids during stressful periods.
>
> Recognize symptoms of adrenal insufficiency and adrenal toxicity.
>
> Practice safety measures to avoid falls and soft tissue injuries.

Administer drug in morning for better results and less toxicity.

Administer PO drug with foods to prevent GI irritation.

Administer IM deeply and rotate sites to prevent muscle atrophy.

Dilute medication using a preservative-free solution.

Monitor blood pressure, weight, serum potassium and other electrolytes.

Monitor serum glucose levels for steroid-induced hyperglycemia.

Monitor for depression or psychotic episodes when taking high-dose therapy.

Give a diet low in sodium and high in potassium and protein if ordered.

Instruct the patient taking **triamcinolone inhalation** to:

> Use bronchodilator first, wait a minute, then give the triamcinolone.
>
> Report a decrease in response to medication as dosage readjustment may be necessary.
>
> Do not use for emergency asthmatic attacks or status asthmaticus.
>
> Check oral mucosa for signs of fungal infection.
>
> Follow inhalations with a glass of water.
>
> Keep inhaler clean and unobstructed.

Administer with caution to patients with GI ulceration, renal disease, hypertension, osteoporosis, varicella, vaccinia, exanthema, diabetes mellitus, Cushing's syndrome, thromboembolic disorders, seizures, myasthenia gravis, metastatic cancer, HF, tuberculosis, ocular herpes simplex, hypoalbuminemia, emotional instability, and psychotic tendencies.

Do not administer to patients with systemic fungal or viral infections, or tubercular hypersensitivity to components of the injectable form, which contain sulfites that cause allergic responses.

Geriatric Considerations
Administer with caution to elderly persons with HF, diabetes, hypertension, and arthritis. Usually lower doses are given.

Generic Name
Triamterene

Trade Name
Dytac, Dyrenium

Class
Potassium-sparing diuretic agent

Action
Blocks the reabsorption of sodium and excretion of potassium by directly acting upon the distal tubule.

Uses
Treatment of edema. May be used in conjunction with potassium-wasting diuretics.

Dosage
100–300 mg PO daily or bid initially after meals. Maximum dose should not exceed 300 mg.

Side Effects
Hypotension, dizziness, dehydration, dry mouth, rash, photosensitivity, ECG changes, dysrhythmias, and hyperkalemia.

Interactions

NSAIDs and indomethacin increase the risk for nephro-toxicity. Avoid using together. Quinidine may have falsely high or low serum levels. Potassium supplements and ACE inhibitors enhance the chances for hyperkalemia. Don't administer together.

Nursing Implications

Instruct the patient to:

    Take after meals to prevent nausea.

    Avoid foods rich in potassium and potassium-containing salt substitutes, which can lead to hyperkalemia.

Monitor BP, daily weight, amount of edema, I & O, color and appearance of urine, BUN and serum electrolytes levels.

Withdraw the medications slowly to prevent potassium excretion.

Administer with caution in patients who have diabetes mellitus, liver dysfunction, pregnancy, and lactation.

Do not give to patients with renal disease or dysfunction, liver disease, anuria, and hyperkalemia.

Geriatric Considerations

Increased risk of hyperkalemia due to renal impairment in the older adult.

Generic Name

Verapamil hydrochloride

Trade Name

Calan, Isoptin, Verelan

Class

Calcium channel blocker, antianginal, antiarrhythmic, antihypertensive

Action

Inhibits calcium movement across cardiac and vascular smooth muscle (depresses mechanical contraction). Decreases myocardial contractility. Prolong AV conduction; increases/decreases HR, CO; dilates systemic blood vessels and decreases the oxygen demands of the heart; and decreases peripheral vascular resistance.

Uses

Effective parenterally to slow heart rate in tachydys-rhythmias and for temporary control of rapid ventricular rate in atrial flutter and atrial fibrillation. Effective orally in management of spastic (Prinzmetal's, variant) angina, unstable (crescendo, preinfarction) angina, chronic stable angina (effort-associated angina), hypertension, prevention or recurrent PSVT, and (with digoxin) control of ventricular resting rate in those with atrial flutter and/or fibrillation. Also used for treatment of hypertension.

Dosage

Supraventricular tachydysrhythmias: IV: Initially, 5–10 mg, repeat in 30 min. with (calan) 10 mg dose.

Dysrhythmias: PO: 240–480 mg/d in 3–4 divided doses.

Angina: PO: Initially, 80–120 mg tid (40 mg for elderly and those patients with liver dysfunction). Titrate to optimal dose. Maintenance: 240–480 mg/d in 3–4 divided doses.

Hypertension: PO: Initially, 40–80 mg tid. Maintenance: Up to 480 mg/d. Extended release tablets: 120–240 mg/d up to 480 mg q d in 2 divided doses.

Side Effects

Frequent: Dizziness, hypotension, peripheral edema, bradycardia, headache, fatigue, and constipation.

Occasional: Nausea when given IV, hypotension, brady-cardia, dizziness.

Rare: Severe tachycardia.

Interactions

Nicotine may reduce effectiveness. Alcohol, antihyper-tensives, and beta-adrenergic blocking agents, including ophthalmic preparations may enhance hypotensive effects. Serum levels of carbamazepine, cyclosporine, digitalis glycosides, and theophylline may be increased leading to toxicity when given with calcium channel blockers. May decrease effects of quinidine. May increase levels of prazosin. Rifampin may decrease effect.

Check BP for hypotension. Assess pulse for strength/ weakness, irregular rate.

Monitor ECG for cardiac changes, particularly for prolongation of PR interval.

Notify prescribing health care provider of any significant interval changes.

Monitor for other side effects.

Geriatric Considerations

The elderly are more susceptible to this drug and the side effects of increased weakness, dizziness, fainting episodes, and falls. Maximum daily dosage is 180 mg.

Generic Name

Warfarin sodium

Trade Name

Coumadin, Carfin,

Class

Anticoagulant

Action

Interferes with blood clotting by depressing hepatic synthesis of vitamin K-dependent coagulation factors (II, VII, IX, X).

Uses

Pulmonary embolism, deep vein thrombosis, MI, atrial dysrhythmias.

Dosage

PO 10–15 mg for 3 d, then titrated to PT qd.

Side Effects

Occasional: GI distress (nausea, anorexia, abdominal cramps, diarrhea).

Rare: Hypersensitivity reaction (dermatitis, urticaria, especially in those sensitive to aspirin).

Interactions

Increased response to warfarin: Amiodarone, anabolic steroids, cimetidine, clofibrate, co-trimoxazole, dextrothyroxine, disulfiram, salicylates, sulfonamides, thyroid drugs.

Decreased response to warfarin: Barbiturates, rifampin.

Altered lab values: May increase AST, ALT; reduces thrombocyte level in differential count.

Nursing Implications

Cross-check dose with co-worker.

Determine PT before administration and daily after therapy initiated. When stabilized, follow with PT determination q 4–6 w.

Assess HCT, platelet count, urine/stool culture for occult blood, AST and ALT, regardless of route of administration.

Observe for signs of hemorrhage: Abdominal or back pain, severe headache, decreased BP, increased pulse rate.

Question about increase in menstrual flow and excessive bleeding from minor cuts and scratches.

Assess lower extremities for color, temperature and skin for bruises or petechiae.

Assess peripheral pulse, gums for erythema and gingival bleeding, and urine output for hematuria.

Geriatric Considerations

Note any changes in behavior, particularly restlessness, irritability, and confusion (earliest signs of drug toxicity). Dry mucous membranes impede swallowing, so offer water. Diminished sensation; check to see if tablet has been swallowed. Position patient so that gravity assists the drug through the esophagus and minimizes the chance of aspiration. Observe for bleeding episodes, or hemorrhage.

References

Arky,R.,et al. (1997). *Physicians' Desk Reference.* 51st ed. Montvale NJ: Medical Economics Company.

Deglin, J.H. & Vallerand, A.H. (1997). *Davis's Drug Guide for Nurses.* Fourth Edition. Philadelphia: F.A. David Company.

Edmonds, J. (1997). *Pharmacology for the Primary Care Practitioner.* St Louis: Mosby Yearbook.

Fried, J., & Petska, S. (1995). *The American Druggist's Complete Family Guide To Prescriptions, Pills, and Drugs.* New York: Hearst Books.

Griffith, H. (1996). *Complete Guide to Prescription and Nonprescription Drugs.* New York: Berkley Publishing Group.

Kee, J. & Hayes E. (1997). *Pharmacology: A Nursing Process Approach.* 2nd ed. Philadelphia: WB Saunders Company.

Lehne, RA. (1997) *Pharmacology for Nursing Care.* 3rd ed. Philadelphia: WB Saunders Company.

Nursing 96 Books. (1996). *Nursing 96 Drug Handbook.* Pennsylvania: Springhouse Corporation.

Skidmore-Roth, L. & McKenry, L. (1997). *Mosby's Drug Guide for Nurses.* St louis: CV Mosby.

Spratto, G. & Woods, A. (1996). *Delmar's NDR-96 Nurse's Drug Reference.* Albany: Delmar Publishers.

The PDR Family Guide To Prescription Drugs. (1996). New York: Medical Economics Company, Inc.

United States Pharmacopeia. (1997). *Complete Drug Reference.* Yonkers, NY : Consumer Report Books.

Appendices

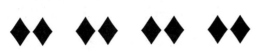

APPENDIX ONE: Standard Precautions

Use Standard Precautions, or the equivalent, for the care of all patients. *Category IB*

A. Hand-washing
  (1) Wash hands after touching blood, body fluids, secretions, excretions, and contaminated items, whether or not gloves are worn. Wash hands immediately after gloves are removed, between patient contacts, and when otherwise indicated to avoid transfer of microorganisms to other patients or environments. It may be necessary to wash hands between tasks and procedures on the same patient to prevent cross-contamination of different body sites. *Category IB*

  (2) Use a plain (nonantimicrobial) soap for routine handwashing. *Category IB*

  (3) Use an antimicrobial agent or a waterless antiseptic agent for specific circumstances (e.g., control of outbreaks or hyperendemic infections), as defined by the infection control program. *Category IB* (See Contact Precautions for additional recommendations on using antimicrobial and antiseptic agents.)

B. Gloves
  Wear gloves (clean, nonsterile gloves are adequate) when touching blood, body fluids, secretions, excretions, and contaminated items. Put on clean gloves just before touching mucous membranes and nonintact skin. Change gloves between tasks and procedures on the same patient after contact with material that may contain a high concentration of microorganisms. Remove gloves promptly after use, before touching noncontaminated items and environmental surfaces, and before going to another patient, and wash hands immediately to avoid transfer to microorganisms to other patients or environments. *Category IB*

C. Mask, Eye Protection, Face Shield
Wear a mask and eye protection or a face shield to protect mucous membranes of the eyes, nose, and mouth during procedures and patient-care activities that are likely to generate splashes or sprays of blood, body fluids, secretions, and excretions. *Category IB*

D. Gown
Wear a gown (a clean, nonsterile gown is adequate) to protect skin and to prevent soiling of clothing during procedures and patient-care activities that are likely to generate splashes or sprays of blood, body fluids, secretions, or excretions. Select a gown that is appropriate for the activity and amount of fluid likely to be encountered. Remove a soiled gown as promptly as possible, and wash hands to avoid transfer of microorganisms to other patients or environments. *Category IB*

E. Patient-Care Equipment
Handle used patient-care equipment soiled with blood, body fluids, secretions, and excretions in a manner that prevents skin and mucous membrane exposures, contamination of clothing, and transfer of microorganisms to other patients and environments. Ensure that reusable equipment is not used for the care of another patient until it has been cleaned and reprocessed appropriately. Ensure that single-use items are discarded properly. *Category IB*

F. Environmental Control
Ensure that the hospital has adequate procedures for the routine care, cleaning, and disinfection of environmental surfaces, beds, bedrails, bedside equipment, and other frequently touched surfaces, and ensure that these procedures are being followed. *Category IB*

G. Linen
Handle, transport, and process used linen soiled with blood, body fluids, secretions, and excretions in a manner that prevents skin and

mucous membrane exposures and contamination of clothing, and that avoids transfer of microorganisms to other patients and environments. *Category IB*

H. Occupational Health and Bloodborne Pathogens

   (1) Take care to prevent injuries when using needles, scalpels, and other sharp instruments or devices; when handling sharp instruments after procedures; when cleaning used instruments; and when disposing of used needles. Never recap used needles, or otherwise manipulate them using both hands, or use any other technique that involves directing the point of a needle toward any part of the body; rather, use either a one-handed "scoop" technique or a mechanical device designed for holding the needle sheath. Do not remove used needles from disposable syringes by hand, and do not bend, break, or otherwise manipulate used needles by hand. Place used disposable syringes and needles, scalpel blades, and other sharp items in appropriate puncture-resistant containers, which are located as close as practical to the area in which the items were used, and place reusable syringes and needles in a puncture-resistant container for transport to the reprocessing area. *Category IB*

   (2) Use mouthpieces, resuscitation bags, or other ventilation devices as an alternative to mouth-to-mouth resuscitation methods in areas where the need for resuscitation is predictable. *Category IB*

I. Patient Placement
Place a patient who contaminates the environment or who does not (or cannot be expected to) assist in maintaining appropriate hygiene or environmental control in a private room. If a private room is not available, consult with infection control professionals regarding pa-

tient placement or other alternatives. *Category
IB*

From Garner JS, Hospital Infection Control Practices Advisory
Committee. Guideline for *Isolation Precautions in Hospitals.* Public
Health Service, US Dept. of Health and Human Services, Centers for
Disease Control and Prevention, Atlanta, GA, 1996.

APPENDIX TWO: Temperature Conversion Table (Centigrade to Fahrenheit)

Celsius (C°)	Fahrenheit (F°)	Celsius (C°)	Fahrenheit (F°)
34.0	93.2	38.6	101.4
34.2	93.6	38.8	101.8
34.4	93.9	39.0	102.2
34.6	94.3	39.2	102.5
34.8	94.6	39.4	102.9
35.0	95.0	39.6	103.2
35.2	95.4	39.8	103.6
35.4	95.7	40.0	104.0
35.6	96.1	40.2	104.3
35.8	96.4	40.4	104.7
36.0	96.8	40.6	105.1
36.2	97.1	40.8	105.4
36.4	97.5	41.0	105.8
36.6	97.8	41.2	106.1
36.8	98.2	41.4	106.5

Celsius	Fahrenheit		Celsius	Fahrenheit
37.0	98.6		41.6	106.8
37.2	98.9		41.8	107.2
37.4	99.3		42.0	107.6
37.6	99.6		42.2	108.0
37.8	100.0		42.4	108.3
38.0	100.4		42.6	108.7
38.2	100.7		42.8	109.0
38.4	101.0		43.0	109.4

Conversion of Celsius (Centigrade) to Fahrenheit: (9/5 × temperature + 32

Conversion of Fahrenheit to Celsius (Centigrade): (Temperature − 32) × 5/9

APPENDIX THREE: Reference Values for Laboratory Tests

REFERENCE VALUES FOR HEMATOLOGY

	Conventional Units	SI Units
Acid hemolysis (Ham test)	No hemolysis	No hemolysis
Aklaline phosphatase leukocyte	Total score 14–100	Total score 14–100
Cell counts		
Erythrocytes		
Males	4.6–6.2 million/mm^3	4.6–6.2 × 10^{12}/L
Females	4.2–5.4 million/mm^3	4.2–5.4 × 10^{12}/L
Children (varies with age)	4.5–5.1 million/mm^3	4.5–5.1 × 10^{12}/L
Leukocytes, total	4500–11,000/mm^3	4.5–11.0 × 10^9/L
Leukocytes, differential counts*		
Myelocytes	0%	0/L
Band neutrophils	3–5%	150–400 × 10^6/L
Segmented neutrophils	54–62%	3000–5800 × 10^6/L
Lymphocytes	25–33%	1500–3000 × 10^6/L
Monocytes	3–7%	300–500 × 10^6/L
Eosinophils	1–3%	50–250 × 10^6/L

Basophils	0–1%	15–50×10^6/L
Platelets	150,000–400,000/mm^3	150–400×10^9/L
Reticulocytes	25,000–75,000/mm^3	25–75×10^9/L
	(0.5–1.5% of erythrocytes)	
Coagulation tests		
Bleeding time (template)	2.75–8.0 min	2.75–8.0 min
Coagulation time (glass tube)	5–15 min	5–15 min
D-Dimer	<0.5 μg/mL	<0.5 μg/mL
Factor VIII and other coagulation factors	50–150% of normal	0.5–1.5 of normal
Fibrin split products (Thrombo-Welco test)	<10 μg/mL	<10 mg/L
Fibrinogen	200–400 mg/dL	2.0–4.0 g/L
Partial thromboplastin timet (PTT)	20–35 sec	20–35 sec
Prothrombin time (PT)	12.0–14.0 sec	12.0–14.0 sec
Coombs' test		
Direct	Negative	Negative
Indirect	Negative	Negative

(continued)

---

*Conventional units are percentages; SI units are absolute counts.

REFERENCE VALUES FOR HEMATOLOGY *(continued)*

	Conventional Units	SI Units
Corpuscular values of erythrocytes		
Mean corpuscular hemoglobin (MCH)	26–34 pg/cell	26–34 pg/cell
Mean corpuscular volume (MCV)	80–96 μm^3	80–96 fL
Mean corpuscular hemoglobin concentration (MCHC)	32–36 g/dL	320–360 g/L
Erythrocyte sedimentation rate (ESR)		
Wintrobe		
Males	0–5 mm/h	0–5 mm/h
Females	0–15 mm/h	0–15 mm/h
Westergren		
Males	0–15 mm/h	0–15 mm/h
Females	0–20 mm/h	0–20 mm/h
Haptoglobin	20–165 mg/dL	0.20–1.65 g/L
Hematocrit		
Males	40–54 mL/dL	0.40–0.54
Females	37–47 mL/dL	0.37–0.47

Newborns	49–54 mL/dL	0.49–0.54
Children (varies with age)	35–49 mL/dL	0.35–0.49
Hemoglobin		
Males	13.0–18.0 g/dL	8.1–11.2 mmol/L
Females	12.0–16.0 g/dL	7.4–9.9 mmol/L
Newborns	16.5–19.5 g/dL	10.2–12.1 mmol/L
Children (varies with age)	11.2–16.5 g/dL	7.0–10.2 mmol/L
Hemoglobin, fetal	<1.0% of total	<0.01 of total
Hemoglobin A_{1c}	3–5% of total	0.03–0.05 if total
Hemoglobin A_2	1.5–3.0% of total	0.015–0.03 if total
Hemoglobin, plasma	0.0–5.0 mg/dL	0.0–3.2 µmol/L
Methemoglobin	30–130 mg/dL	19–80 µmol/L

REFERENCE VALUES* FOR BLOOD, SERUM, AND PLASMA

	Conventional Units	SI Units
Acetoacetate plus acetone		
Qualitative	Negative	Negative
Quantitative	0.3–2.0 mg/dL	30–200 µmol/L
Acid phosphatase, serum (Thymolphthalein monophosphate substrate)	0.1–0.6 U/L	0.1–0.6 U/L
ACTH (see Corticotropin)		
Alanine aminotransferase (ALT, SGPT), serum	1–45 U/L	1–45 U/L
Albumin, serum	3.3–5.2 g/dL	33–52 g/L
Aldolase, serum	0.0–7.0 U/L	0.0–7.0 U/L
Aldosterone, plasma		
Standing	5–30 ng/dL	140–830 pmol/L
Recumbent	3–10 ng/dL	80–275 pmol/L
Alkaline phosphatase (ALP), serum		
Adult	35–150 U/L	35–150 U/L
Adolescent	100–500 U/L	100–500 U/L
Child	100–350 U/L	100–350 U/L

	Conventional Units	SI Units
Ammonia nitrogen, plasma	10–50 μmol/L	10–50 μmol/L
Amylase, serum	25–125 U/L	25–125 U/L
Anion gap, serum, calculated	8–16 mEq/L	8–16 mmol/L
Ascorbic acid, blood	0.4–1.5 mg/dL	23–85 μmol/L
Aspartate aminotransferase (AST, SGOT), serum	1–36 U/L	1–36 U/L
Base excess, arterial blood, calculated	0 ± 2 mEq/L	0 ± 2 mmol/L
β-carotene, serum	60–260 μg/dL	1.1–8.6 μmol/L
Bicarbonate		
Venous plasma	23–29 mEq/L	23–29 mmol/L
Arterial blood	21–27 mEq/L	21–27 mmol/L
Bile acids, serum	0.3–3.0 mg/dL	0.8–7.6 μmol/L
Bilirubin, serum		
Conjugated	0.1–0.4 mg/dL	1.7–6.8 μmol/L
Total	0.3–1.1 mg/dL	5.1–19.0 μmol/L
Calcium, serum	8.4–10.6 mg/dL	2.10–2.65 mmol/L
Calcium, ionized, serum	4.25–5.25 mg/dL	1.05–1.30 mmol/L
Carbon dioxide total, serum or plasma	24–31 mEq/L	24–31 mmol/L
Carbon dioxide tension (PCO_2), blood	35–45 mmHg	35–45 mmHg
Ceruloplasmin, serum	23–44 mg/dL	230–440 mg/L

(continued)

465

REFERENCE VALUES* FOR BLOOD, SERUM, AND PLASMA (continued)

	Conventional Units	SI Units
Chloride, serum or plasma	96–106 mEq/L	96–106 mmol/L
Cholesterol, serum or EDTA plasma		
Desirable range	<200 mg/dL	<5.20 mmol/L
LDL cholesterol	60–180 mg/dL	1.55–4.65 mmol/L
HDL cholesterol	30–80 mg/dL	0.80–2.05 mmol/L
Copper	70–140 µg/dL	11–22 µmol/L
Corticotropin (ACTH), plasma, 8 AM	10–80 pg/mL	2–18 pmol/L
Cortisol, plasma		
8:00 AM	6–23 µg/dL	170–630 nmol/L
4:00 PM	3–15 µg/dL	80–410 nmol/L
10:00 PM	<50% of 8:00 AM value	<50% of 8:00 AM value
Creatine, serum		
Males	0.2–0.5 mg/dL	15–40 µmol/L
Females	0.3–0.9 mg/dL	25–70 µmol/L
Creatine kinase (CK), serum		
Males	55–170 U/L	55–170 U/L
Females	30–135 U/L	30–135 U/L

Creatine kinase MB isoenzyme, serum	<5% of total CK activity	<5% of total CK activity
	<5% ng/mL by immunoassay	<5% ng/mL by immunoassay
Creatinine, serum	0.6–1.2 mg/dL	50–110 µmol/L
Estradiol-17β, adult		
Males	10–65 pg/mL	35–240 pmol/L
Females		
Follicular phase	30–110 pg/mL	110–370 pmol/L
Ovulatory phase	200–400 pg/mL	730–1470 pmol/L
Luteal phase	50–140 pg/mL	180–510 pmol/L
Ferritin, serum	20–200 ng/mL	20–200 µg/L
Fibrinogen, plasma	200–400 mg/dL	2.0–4.0 g/L
Folate, serum	2.0–9.0 ng/mL	4.5–20.4 nmol/L
erythrocytes	170–700 ng/mL	385–1590 nmol/L
Follicle-stimulating hormone (FSH), plasma		
Males	4–25 mU/mL	4–25 U/L
Females, premenopausal	4–30 mU/mL	4–30 U/L
Females, postmenopausal	40–250 mU/mL	40–250 U/L
γ-glutamyltransferase (GGT), serum	5–40 U/L	5–40 U/L

(continued)

REFERENCE VALUES* FOR BLOOD, SERUM, AND PLASMA (*continued*)

	Conventional Units	SI Units
Gastrin, fasting, serum	0–110 pg/mL	0–110 mg/L
Glucose, fasting, plasma or serum	70–115 mg/dL	3.9–6.4 nmol/L
Growth hormone (hGH), plasma, adult, fasting	0–6 ng/mL	0–6 µg/L
Haptoglobin, serum	20–165 mg/dL	0.20–1.65 g/L
Immunoglobulines, serum (see Reference Values for Immunologic Procedures)		
Insulin, fasting, plasma	5–25 µU/mL	36–179 pmol/L
Iron, serum	75–175 µg/dL	13–31 µmol/L
Iron binding capacity, serum		
Total	250–410 µg/dL	45–73 µmol/L
Saturation	20–55%	0.20–0.55
Lactate		
Venous whole blood	5.0–20.0 mg/dL	0.6–2.2 mmol/L
Arterial whole blood	5.0–15.0 mg/dL	0.6–1.7 mmol/L
Lactate dehydrogenase (LDH), serum	110–220 U/L	110–220 U/L
Lipase, serum	10–140 U/L	10–140 U/L

Lutropin (LH) serum		
Males	1–9 U/L	1–9 U/L
Females		
Follicular phase	2–10 U/L	2–10 U/L
Midcycle peak	15–65 U/L	15–65 U/L
Luteal phase	1–12 U/L	1–12 U/L
Postmenopausal	12–65 U/L	12–65 U/L
Magnesium, serum	1.3–2.1 mg/dL	0.65–1.05 mmol/L
Osmolality	275–295 mOsm/kg water	275–295 mOsm/kg water
Oxygen, blood, arterial, room air		
Partial pressure (PaO_2)	80–100 mm Hg	80–100 mm Hg
Saturation (SaO_2)	95–98%	95–98%
pH, arterial blood	7.35–7.45	7.35–7.45
Phosphate, inorganic serum		
Adult	3.0–4.5 mg/dL	1.0–1.5 mmol/L
Child	4.0–7.0 mg/dL	1.3–2.3 mmol/L
Potassium		
Serum	3.5–5.0 mEq/L	3.5–5.0 mmol/L
Plasma	3.5–4.5 mEq/L	3.5–4.5 mmol/L

(continued)

REFERENCE VALUES* FOR BLOOD, SERUM, AND PLASMA (continued)

	Conventional Units	SI Units
Progesterone, serum, adult		
Males	0.0–0.4 ng/mL	0.0–1.3 mmol/L
Females		
Follicular phase	0.1–1.5 ng/mL	0.3–4.8 mmol/L
Luteal phase	2.5–28.0 ng/mL	8.0–89.0 mmol/L
Prolactin, serum		
Males	1.0–15.0 ng/mL	1.0–15.0 µg/L
Females	1.0–20.0 ng/mL	1.0–20.0 µg/L
Protein, serum, electrophoresis		
Total	6.0–8.0 g/dL	60–80 g/L
Albumin	3.5–5.5 g/dL	35–55 g/L
Globulins		
Alpha$_1$	0.2–0.4 g/dL	2.0–4.0 g/L
Alpha$_2$	0.5–0.9 g/dL	5.0–9.0 g/L
Beta	0.6–1.1 g/dL	6.0–11.0 g/L
Gamma	0.7–1.7 g/dL	7.0–17.0 g/L
Pyruvate, blood	0.3–0.9 mg/dL	0.03–0.10 mmol/L

Rheumatoid factor	0.0–30.0 IU/mL	0.0–30.0 kIU/L
Sodium, serum or plasma	135–145 mEq/L	135–145 mmol/L
Testosterone, plasma		
Males, adult	300–1200 ng/dL	10.4–41.6 nmol/L
Females, adult	20–75 ng/dL	0.7–2.6 nmol/L
Pregnant females	40–200 ng/dL	1.4–6.9 nmol/L
Thyroglobulin	3–42 ng/mL	3–42 µg/L
Thyrotropin (hTSH), serum	0.4–4.8 µIU/mL	0.4–4.8 mIU/L
Thyrotropin-releasing hormone (TRH)	5–60 pg/mL	5–60 ng/L
Thyroxine (FT$_4$), free, serum	0.9–2.1 ng/dL	12–27 pmol/L
Thyroxine (T$_4$), serum	4.5–12.0 µg/dL	58–154 nmol/L
Thyroxine-binding globulin (TBG)	15.0–34.0 µg/mL	15.0–34.0 mg/L
Transferrin	250–430 mg/dL	2.5–4.3 g/L
Triglycerides, serum, after 12-hour fast	40–150 mg/dL	0.4–1.5 g/L
Triiodothyronine (T$_3$), serum	70–190 ng/dL	1.1–2.9 nmol/L
Triiodothyronine uptake, resin (T$_3$RU)	25–38%	0.25–0.38
Urate		
Males	2.5–8.0 mg/dL	150–480 µmol/L
Females	2.2–7.0 mg/dL	130–420 µmol/L

(continued)

REFERENCE VALUES* FOR BLOOD, SERUM, AND PLASMA (continued)

	Conventional Units	SI Units
Urea, serum or plasma	24–49 mg/dL	4.0–8.2 nmol/L
Urea nitrogen, serum or plasma	11–23 mg/dL	8.0–16.4 nmol/L
Viscosity, serum	1.4–1.8 × water	1.4–1.8 × water
Vitamin A, serum	20–80 µg/dL	0.70–2.80 µmol/L
Vitamin B_{12}, serum	180–900 pg/mL	133–664 pmol/L

*Reference values may vary depending on the method and sample source used.

REFERENCE VALUES FOR THERAPEUTIC DRUG MONITORING (SERUM)

	Therapeutic Range	Toxic Concentrations	Proprietary Names
ANALGESICS			
Acetaminiphen	10–20 μg/mL	>250 μg/mL	Tylenol Datril
Salicylate	100–250 μg/mL	>300 μg/mL	Aspirin Bufferin
ANTIBIOTICS			
Amikacin	25–30 μg/mL	Peak >35 μg/mL Trough >10 μg/mL	Amikin
Chloramphenicol	10–20 μg/mL	>25 μg/mL	Chloromycetin
Gentamicin	5–10 μg/mL	Peak >10 μg/mL Trough >2 μg/mL	Garamycin
Tobramycin	5–10 μg/mL	Peak >10 μg/mL Trough >2 μg/mL	Nebcin
Vancomycin	5–10 μg/mL	Peak >40 μg/mL Trough >10 μg/mL	Vancocin

(continued)

473

REFERENCE VALUES FOR THERAPEUTIC DRUG MONITORING (SERUM) *(continued)*

	Therapeutic Range	Toxic Concentrations	Proprietary Names
ANTICONVULSANTS			
Carbamazepine	5–12 µg/mL	>15 µg/mL	Tegretol
Ethosuximide	40–100 µg/mL	>150 µg/mL	Zarontin
Phenobarbital	15–40 µg/mL	40–100 ng/mL (varies widely)	Luminal
Phenytoin	10–20 µg/mL	>20 µg/mL	Dilantin
Primidone	5–12 µg/mL	>15 µg/mL	Mysoline
Valproic acid	50–100 µg/mL	>100 µg/mL	Depakene
ANTINEOPLASTICS AND IMMUNOSUPPRESSIVES			
Cyclosporine	50–400 ng/mL	>400 ng/mL	Sandimmune
Methotrexate, high dose, 48-hour	Variable	>1 µmol/L 48 hr after dose	Mexate
			Folex
Tacrolimus (FK-506), whole blood	3–10 µg/L	>15 µg/L	Prograf
BRONCHODILATORS AND RESPIRATORY STIMULANTS			
Caffeine	3–15 ng/mL	>30 ng/mL	

Drug	Therapeutic Range	Toxic Level	Trade Name
Theophylline (Aminophylline)	10–20 µg/mL	>20 µg/mL	Elixophyllin, Quibron

CARDIOVASCULAR DRUGS

Drug	Therapeutic Range	Toxic Level	Trade Name
Amiodarone	1.0–2.0 µg/mL	>2.0 µg/mL	Cordarone
(Obtain specimen more than 8 h after last dose)			
Digitoxin	15–25 ng/mL	>35 ng/mL	Crystodigin
(Obtain specimen 12–24 h after last dose)			
Digoxin	0.8–2.0 ng/mL	>2.4 ng/mL	Lanoxin
(Obtain specimen more than 6 h after last dose)			
Disopyramide	2–5 µg/mL	>7 µg/mL	Norpace
Flecainide	0.2–1.0 ng/mL	>1 ng/mL	Tambocor
Lidocaine	1.5–5.0 µg/mL	>6 µg/mL	Xylocaine
Mexiletine	0.7–2.0 ng/mL	>2 ng/mL	Mexitil
Procainamide	4–10 µg/mL	>12 µg/mL	Pronestyl
Procainamide plus NAPA	8–30 µg/mL	>30 µg/mL	
Propranolol	50–100 ng/mL	Variable	Inderal
Quinidine	2–5 µg/mL	>6 µg/mL	Cardioquin, Quinaglute

(continued)

REFERENCE VALUES FOR THERAPEUTIC DRUG MONITORING (SERUM) *(continued)*

	Therapeutic Range	Toxic Concentrations	Proprietary Names
Tocainide	4–10 ng/mL	>10 ng/mL	Tonocard
PSYCHOPHARMACOLOGIC DRUGS			
Amitriptyline	120–150 ng/mL	>500 ng/mL	Elavil Triavil
Bupropion	25–100 ng/mL	Not applicable	Wellbutrin
Desipramine	150–300 ng/mL	>500 ng/mL	Norpramin Pertofrane Tofranil
Imipramine	125–250 ng/mL	>400 ng/mL	Janimine
Lithium (Obtain specimen 12 h after last dose)	0.6–1.5 mEq/L	>1.5 mEq/L	Lithobid
Nortriptyline	50–150 ng/mL	>500 ng/mL	Aventyl Pamelor

REFERENCE VALUES FOR URINE

	Conventional Units	SI Units
Acetone and acetoacetate, qualitative	Negative	Negative
Albumin		
Qualitative	Negative	Negative
Quantitative	10–100 mg/24 h	0.15–1.5 μmol/d
Aldosterone	3–20 μg/24 h	8.3–55 nmol/d
δ-Aminolevulinic acid (δ-ALA)	1.3–7.0 mg/24 h	10–53 μmol/d
Amylase	<17 U/h	<17 U/h
Amylase/creatinine clearance ratio	0.01–0.04	0.01–0.04
Bilirubin, qualitative	Negative	Negative
Calcium (regular diet)	<250 mg/24 h	<6.3 nmol/d
Catecholamines		
Epinephrine	<10 μg/24 h	<55 nmol/d
Norepinephrine	<100 μg/24 h	<590 nmol/d
Total free catecholamines	4–126 μg/24 h	24–745 nmol/d
Total metanephrines	0.1–1.6 mg/24 h	0.5–8.1 μmol/d

(continued)

477

REFERENCE VALUES FOR URINE *(continued)*

	Conventional Units	SI Units
Chloride (varies with intake)	110–250 mEq/24 h	110–250 mmol/d
Copper	0–50 µg/24 h	0.0–0.80 µmol/d
Cortisol, free	10–100 µg/24 h	27.6–276 nmol/d
Creatine		
Males	0–40 mg/24 h	0.0–0.30 mmol/d
Females	0–80 mg/24 h	0.0–0.60 mmol/d
Creatinine	15–25 mg/kg/24 h	0.13–0.22 mmol/kg/d
Creatinine clearance (endogenous)		
Males	110–150 mL/min/1.73m^2	110–150 mL/min/1.73m^2
Females	105–132 mL/min/1.73m^2	105–132 mL/min/1.73m^2
Cystine or cysteine	Negative	Negative
Dehydroepiandrosterone		
Males	0.2–2.0 mg/24 h	0.7–6.9 µmol/d
Females	0.2–1.8 mg/24 h	0.7–6.2 µmol/d
Estrogens, total		
Males	4–25 µg/24 h	14–90 nmol/d
Females	5–100 µg/24 h	18–360 nmol/d

Glucose (as reducing substance)	<250 mg/24 h	<250 mg/d
Hemoglobin and myoglobin, qualitative	Negative	Negative
Homogentisic acid, qualitative	Negative	Negative
17-Hydroxycorticosteroids		
Males	3–9 mg/24 h	8.3–25 µmol/d
Females	2–8 mg/24 h	5.5–22 µmol/d
5-Hydroxyindoleacetic acid		
Qualitative	Negative	Negative
Quantitative	2–6 mg/24 h	10–31 µmol/d
17-Ketogenic steroids		
Males	5–23 mg/24 h	17–80 µmol/d
Females	3–15 mg/24 h	10–52 µmol/d
17-Ketosteroids		
Males	8–22 mg/24 h	28–76 µmol/d
Females	6–15 mg/24 h	21–52 µmol/d
Magnesium	6–10 mEq/24 h	3–5 mmol/d
Metanephrines	0.05–1.2 ng/mg creatinine	0.03–0.70 mmol/mmol creatinine
Osmolality	38–1400 mOsm/kg water	38–1400 mOsm/kg water

(continued)

479

REFERENCE VALUES FOR URINE *(continued)*

	Conventional Units	SI Units
pH	4.6–8.0	4.6–8.0
Phenylpyruvic acid, qualitative	Negative	Negative
Phosphate	0.4–1.3 g/24 h	13–42 mmol/d
Porphobilinogen		
Qualitative	Negative	Negative
Quantitative	<2 mg/24 h	<9 µmol/d
Porphyrins		
Coproporphyrin	50–250 µg/24 h	77–380 nmol/d
Uroporphyrin	10–30 µg/24 h	12–36 nmol/d
Potassium	25–125 mEq/24 h	25–125 mmol/d
Pregnanediol		
Males	0.0–1.9 mg/24 h	0.0–6.0 µmol/d
Females		
Proliferative phase	0.0–2.6 mg/24 h	0.0–8.0 µmol/d
Luteal phase	2.6–10.6 mg/24 h	8–33 µmol/d
Postmenopausal	0.2–1.0 mg/24 h	0.6–3.1 µmol/d

Pregnanetriol	0.0–2.5 mg/24 h	0.0–7.4 µmol/d
Protein, total		
Qualitative	Negative	Negative
Quantitative	10–150 mg/24 h	10–150 mg/d
Protein/creatinine ratio	<0.2	<0.2
Sodium (regular diet)	60–260 mEq/24 h	60–260 mmol/d
Specific gravity		
Random specimen	1.003–1.030	1.003–1.030
24-hour collection	1.015–1.025	1.015–1.025
Urate (regular diet)	250–750 mg/24 h	1.5–4.4 mmol/d
Urobilinogen	0.5–4.0 mg/24 h	0.6–6.8 µmol/d
Vanillylmandelic acid (VMA)	1.0–8.0 mg/24 h	5–40 µmol/d

REFERENCE VALUES FOR TOXIC SUBSTANCES

	Conventional Units	SI Units
Arsenic, urine	<130 µg/24 h	<1.7 µmol/d
Bromides, serum, inorganic	<100 mg/dL	<10 mmol/L
Toxic symptoms	140–1000 mg/dL	14–100 mmol/L
Carboxyhemoglobin, blood	% Saturation	Saturation
Urban environment	<5%	<0.05
Smokers	<12%	<0.12
Symptoms		
Headache	>15%	>0.15
Nausea and vomiting	>25%	>0.25
Potentially lethal	>50%	>0.50
Ethanol, blood	<0.05 mg/dL	<1.0 mmol/L
	<0.005%	
Intoxication	>100 mg/dL	>22 mmol/L
	>0.1%	
Marked intoxication	300–400 mg/dL	65–87 mmol/L
	0.3–0.4%	

Alcoholic stupor	400–500 mg/dL 0.4–0.5%	87–109 mmol/L
Coma	>500 mg/dL >0.5%	>109 mmol/L
Lead, blood		
Adults	<25 µg/dL	<1.2 µmol/L
Children	<15 µg/dL	<0.7 µmol/L
Lead, urine	<80 µg/24 hr	<0.4 µmol/d
Mercury, urine	<30 µg/24 hr	<150 nmol/d

REFERENCE VALUES FOR CEREBROSPINAL FLUID

	Conventional Units	SI Units
Cells	<5/mm³ all mononuclear	<5 × 10⁶/L all mononuclear
Glucose	50–75 mg/dL (20 mg/dL less than in serum)	2.8–4.2 mmol/L (1.1 mmol less than in serum)
IgG		
Children under 14	<8% of total protein	<0.08% of total protein
Adults	<14% of total protein	<0.14% of total protein
IgG $\left(\dfrac{\text{CSF/serum IgG ration}}{\text{CSF/serum albumin ratio}}\right)$	0.3–0.6	0.3–0.6
Oligoclonal banding on electrophoresis	Absent	Absent
Pressure, opening	70–180 mmH2O	70–180 mmH2O
Protein, total	15–45 mg/dL	150–450 mg/L
Protein electrophoresis	Albumin predominant	Albumin predominant

REFERENCE VALUES FOR TESTS OF GASTROINTESTINAL FUNCTION

	Conventional Units		Conventional Units
Bentiromide	6-hour urinary arylamine excretion greater than 57% excludes pancreatic insufficiency	Maximum (after histamine or pentagastrin)	
		Males	9.0–48.0 mmol/h
β-Carotene, serum	60–250 ng/dL	Females	6.0–31.0 mmol/h
Fecal fat estimation		Ratio: basal/maximum	
Qualitative	No fat globules seen by high-power microscope	Males	0.0–0.31
		Females	0.0–0.29
Quantitative	<6g/24h (>95% coefficient of fat absorption)	Secretin test, pancreatic fluid	
Gastric acid output		Volume	>1.8 mL/kg/h
Basal		Bicarbonate	>80 mEq/L
Males	0.0–10.5 mmol/h		
Females	0.0–5.6 mmol/h	D-Xylose absorption test, urine	>20% of ingested dose excreted in 5 h

REFERENCE VALUES FOR IMMUNOLOGIC PROCEDURES

	Conventional Units	SI Units
Complement, serum		
C3	85–175 mg/dL	0.85–1.75 g/L
C4	15–45 mg/dL	150–450 mg/L
Total hemolytic (CH$_{50}$)	150–250 U/mL	150–250 U/mL
Immunoglobulins, serum, adult		
IgG	640–1350 mg/dL	6.4–13.5 g/L
IgA	70–310 mg/dL	0.70–3.1 g/L
IgM	90–350 mg/dL	0.90–3.5 g/L
IgD	0.0–6.0 mg/dL	0.0–60 mg/L
IgE	0.0–430 ng/dL	0.0–430 μg/L

LYMPHOCYTE SUBSETS, WHOLE BLOOD, HEPARINIZED

Antigen	Cell Type	Percentage	Absolute
CD3	Total T cells	56–77	860–1880
CD19	Total B cells	7–17	140–370
CD3 and CD4	Helper-inducer cells	32–54	550–1190

CD3 and CD8	Suppressor-cytotoxic cells	24–37	430–1060
CD3 and DR	Activated T cells	5–14	70–310
CD2	E rosette T cells	73–87	1040–2160
CD16 and CD56	Natural killer (NK) cells	8–22	130–500

Helper/suppressor ratio: 0.8–1.8

REFERENCE VALUES FOR SEMEN

	Conventional Units	SI Units
Volume	2–5 mL	2–5 mL
Liquefaction	Complete in 15 min	Complete in 15 min
pH	7.2–8.0	7.2–8.0
Leukocytes	Occasional or absent	Occasional or absent
Spermatozoa		
Count	$60–150 \times 10^6$/mL	$60–150 \times 10^6$/mL
Motility	>80% motile	>0.80 motile
Morphology	80–90% normal forms	>0.80–0.90 normal forms
Fructose	>150 mg/dL	>8.33 mmol/L

Tables from Rakel RE (ed). *Conn's current therapy 1997.* Philadelphia: WB Saunders, 1997.

487

APPENDIX FOUR: Acid-Base

Respiratory Acid-Base Disorders

Disorder	pCO$_2$	HCO$_3$	pH
Respiratory Acidosis Uncompensated	⇑	Normal	⇑
Respiratory Acidosis	⇑	⇑	Normal
Respiratory Acidosis Compensated in Part	⇑	⇑	(Slightly) ⇓
Respiratory Alkalosis Uncompensated	⇓	Normal	⇑
Respiratory Alkalosis Compensated	⇓	⇓	Normal
Respiratory Alkalosis Compensated in Part	⇓	⇓	(Slightly) ⇑

Metabolic Acid-Base Disorders

Disorder	pCO$_2$	HCO$_3$	pH
Metabolic Acidosis Uncompensated	Normal	⇓	⇓
Metabolic Acidosis Compensated	⇓	⇓	Normal
Metabolic Acidosis Compensated in Part	Normal	⇓	(Slightly) ⇓
Metabolic Alkalosis Uncompensated	⇑	⇑	⇑
Metabolic Alkalosis Compensated	⇑	⇑	Normal
Metabolic Alkalosis Compensated in Part	⇑	⇑	(Slightly) ⇑

Normal Values:

pH   7.35–7.45
pCO_2 35–45 mm Hg
HCO_3 22–28 mEq./L.

APPENDIX FIVE: Electrolytes: Normal Values and Imbalances

Electrolyte	Normal Value	Imbalance
Sodium	137–147 mEq./L.	Hyponatremia <137 mEq./L. S/S: irritability, weakness, dizziness, confusion, cramps Management: replace losses and remove underlying cause Hypernatremia >147 mEq./L. S/S: restlessness, increased thirst, lethargy, loss of consciousness Management: water replacement, diuretics, and removal of underlying cause
Potassium	3.5–5.0 mEq./L.	Hypokalemia <3.5 mEq.L. S/S: muscle weakness, fatigue, nausea, vomiting, ECG changes Management: replace losses by PO or IV supplements, treat underlying cause, observe for digitalis toxicity Hyperkalemia >5.0 mEq./L. S/S: anxiety, irritability, diarrhea, cramps, weakness, pulse irregularities, ECG changes Management: reduce intake of potassium, oral Kayexalate or IV calcium gluconate and sodium bicarbonate to shift potassium into the cells

Calcium	4.5–5.5 mEq./L.	Hypocalcemia <4.5 mEq./L. S/S: numbness, tingling, tetany, convulsions, increased reflexes, positive Chvostek's and Trousseau's signs Management: oral or IV calcium and vitamin D supplements, removal of underlying cause Hypercalcemia >5.5 mEq./L. S/S: fatigue, weakness, lethargy, nausea, pathologic fracture, pain Management: IV phosphates, low-calcium diet, increases physical activity, treatmnet of underlying cause
Magnesium	1.5–2.5 mEq./L.	Hypomagnesemia <1.5 mEq./L. S/S: agitation, cramps, confusion, tremors, tetany, nausea, vomiting, convulsions, positive Chvostek's and Trousseau's signs Management: increased dietary intake and oral magnesium supplements Hypermagnesemia >2.5 mEq./L. S/S: nausea, vomiting, dizziness, diaphoresis, decreased level of consciousness, hypotension Management: removal of underlying cause, IV calcium, dialysis, if severe

Index

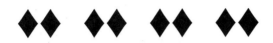

A

Abdominal hysterectomy, 277–280
ABGs (arterial blood gases), 214–216
Acetaminophen/codeine, 343
Achromycin, 441–443
Acid-base balance
arterial blood gases and, 214–216
disorders of, 488–489
Acidosis, 214
Acquired immunodeficiency syndrome (AIDS), 203, 220
Acute idiopathic pericarditis, 83
Acute renal failure (ARF), 3–5
Adalat, 421–423
Adapin, 377–378
Adenocarcinomas, of lung, 125
Adult respiratory distress syndrome (ARDS), 5–7
Advil, 404–405
Aerolate, 346–348
AIDS. *See* Acquired immunodeficiency syndrome.
Albuterol, 344–345
Alkalosis, 214
Alpha-antitrypsin deficiency, 80
Alprazolam, 345–346
Alzapam, 412–413
Alzheimer's disease, 7–10
Aminophylline, 22, 346–348
Amoxicillin trihydrate, 348–349
Amoxil, 348–349
Ampicillin, 349–351
Ampicin, 349–351
Amputation, 209–214

Anaphylaxis, 10–11
Ancolan, 414–415
Anemias, 11–13
Aneurysm, 13–17
Angina, 17–19
  verapamil dosages for, 449
Angiography, 217–218
Antiestrogen therapy, for breast cancer, 36
Antiplatelet therapy, for carotid arterial occlusion, 25
Antivert, 414–415
Antivert/25, 414–415
Antivert/50, 414–415
Apo-Diazepam, 370–372
Apo-Erythrobase, 382–383
Apo-Hydro, 399–400
Apo-Lorazepam, 412–413
Apo-Piroxicam, 432–433
Apo-Sulfatrim, 369–370
Appendicitis, 19–22
ARDS (adult respiratory distress syndrome), 5–7
ARF (acute renal failure), 3–5
Aristocort, 445–447
Arrhythmias. *See* Cardiac dysrhythmias
Arterial blood gases (ABGs), 214–216
Arterial lines, 216–217
Arterial occlusive disease, chronic, 51–52
Arteriography, 217–218
Arteriosclerosis obliterans, 51–52
Arthritis
  osteoarthritis, 140
  rheumatoid, 171–175
Arthroscopy, 218
Aspiration, signs of, 265
Aspiration biopsy, 218. *See also* Biopsy
Aspiration pneumonia, 164
Asthma, 22–25
Atenolol, 351–352
Atherosclerosis, 25–30, 51–52
Ativan, 412–413
Atolone, 445–446
Atropine sulfate, 353–354

Autoimmune disorders
  Graves' disease, 109–112
  pericarditis, 76–79
Aventyl, 423–424
Azithromycin, 354–355

B

Bactrim, 369–370
Bactrim DS, 369–370
Barbita, 430–432
Beepen-VK, 428–429
Benadryl, 10
Bence-Jones protein, 134
Benign prostatic hyperplasia (BPH), 30–31
Beta-hemolytic streptococcus infection, 86
Betapen-VK, 428–429
Biaxin, 367–368
Biaxin Filmtabs, 367–368
Bicarbonate, 214. *See also* Arterial blood gases
Biopsy, 219–220
Bleeding disorders, disseminated intravascular
  coagulation, 71
Blocadren, 443–444
Blood tests, reference values for, 464–472
Blood transfusions, 220–223
Body fluids, Standard Precautions for, 454
Bonamine, 414–415
Bone tumors, 31–35
Bonine, 414–415
BPH (benign prostatic hyperplasia), 30
Bradycardia, 42. *See also* Dysrhythmias
Brain tumor, 35
Breast cancer, 36
Bronchial toilet, 23
Bronchitis, chronic, 52–56
Bronchoscopy, 223–224
Bronchospasm
  acute, aminophylline dosage for, 347
  chronic, aminophylline dosage for, 347
Buerger's disease, 183–185
Burns, 36–40

Bu Spar, 355–356
Buspirone, 355–356
Bypass grafting, for aneurysm management, 13–14

C

CAD (coronary artery disease), 62–63
Calan, 448–450
Calcilean, 395–397
Calciparine, 395–397
Calcium
  imbalances, 491
  normal values, 491
Cancer, 40–42. *See also* Carcinomas
  breast, 36
  cervical, 47–50
  colorectal, 62
  endometrial, 80
  gastric, 85
  laryngeal, 120
  liver, 125–126
  lung, 126
  pancreatic, 147
  prostate, 168–169
  testicular, 179–180
  thyroid, 189–190
Capoten, 357–358
Captopril, 357–358
Carbon dioxide
  narcosis, signs of, 74
  partial pressure of, 214. *See also* Arterial blood
gases
Carcinomas, 40. *See also* Cancer
  squamous cell, 47, 125
  thryroid, 189–190
Cardiac catheterization, 224–226
Cardiac disease, ischemic, 119
Cardiac dysrhythmias, 42–43
  verapamil dosages for, 449
Cardiogenic shock, 175–176
Cardizem/Cardizem SR, 375–376
Cardizem CD, 375–376

Carfin, 450–451
Carotid arterial occlusion, 25
Casts, 227–232
Catecholamines, pheochromocytomas and, 161
Catheterization, cardiac, 224–226
Ceclor, 359–360
Cefaclor, 359–360
Cefanex, 363–364
Cefadroxil monohydrate, 360–361
Ceflin, 361–363
Cefuroxime sodium, 361–363
Centigrade temperature conversion table, 458–459
Cephalexin, 363–364
Cerebrospinal fluid tests, reference values for, 484
Cerebrovascular accident (CVA), 44–47
Cervical cancer, 47–50
Cervical disk, herniated, symptoms of, 94. *See also* Herniated disk disease
Chemotherapy, 232–243
Chest drainage, 243–245
Chest pain. *See* Angina
CHF. *See* Heart failure (HF)
Cholecystectomy, 51, 245–249
Cholecystitis, 50–51
Choledocholithotomy, 245–246
Cholelithiasis, 50–51
Chondrosarcoma, 31
Chronic arterial occlusive disease, 51
Chronic bronchitis, 52–56
Chronic obstructive pulmonary disease (COPD). *See* Chronic bronchitis; Pulmonary emphysema
Chronic renal failure (CRF), 56–59
Ciloxan, 365–367
Cimetidine, 364–365
Cipro, 365–367
Ciprofloxacin, 365–367
Cirrhosis, 59–61
Clarithromycin, 367–368
Claudication, intermittent, 51
Closed fracture, 81
Coagulation test, 461
Co-Trimoxazele, 369–370

Collateral vessels, 134
Colonoscopy, 245
Colorectal cancer, 62
Colostomy, 250–256
Compound fracture, 80
Computed tomography (CT), 257–258
COPD (chronic obstructive pulmonary disease). *See*
  Chronic bronchitis; Pulmonary emphysema
Coronary artery disease (CAD), 62–63
Cortef, 402–404
Cortenema, 402–404
Costovertebral angle, 196
Cotrim, 369–370
Cotrim DS, 369–370
Co-trimoxazole, 369–370
Coumadin, 450–451
Craniotomy, 259–261
Crohn's disease, 63–66
Cromolyn sodium, 22
CT (computed tomography), 257–258
CVA (cerebrovascular accident), 44–47
Cystitis, 195. *See also* Urinary tract infections
Cystoscopy, 262–263

D

Darvocet-N 50, 437–438
Darvocet-N 100, 437–438
Darvon, 436–437
Daypro, 425–426
D&C (dilation and curettage), 263–264
Degenerative joint disease, 139
Deltasone, 434–436
Demerol, 415–417
Diabeta, 393–395
Diabetes mellitus, 66–71
Diazepam, 370–372
Diazepam Intensol, 370–372
DIC (disseminated intravascular coagulation), 77
Dichlotride, 399–400
Diclofenac sodium, 372–373
Digoxin, 373–375

Dilacor XR, 375–376
Dilation and curettage (D&C), 263–264
Dilene, 436–437
Diltiazem hydrochloride, 375–376
Disseminated intravascular coagulation (DIC), 71
Diuchlor, 399–400
Diverticular disease, 72–74
Diverticulitis, 72
Diverticulosis, 72
Dixaphene, 436–437
Dizmiss, 414–415
Doryx, 378–380
Doxepin hydrochloride, 377–378
Doxy-100, 378–380
Doxy-200, 378–380
Doxy-Caps, 378–380
Doxychel, 378–380
Doxycycline hyclate, 378–380
Doxy-Tabs, 378–380
Drainage, chest, 243–245
Drugs. *See also* specific drugs
    therapeutic monitoring of, 473–476
Duodenal ulcers, 156–158
Duractin, 364–365
Duraphen, 436–437
Duricef, 360–361
Dyrenium, 447–448
Dysplasia, 47
Dysrhythmias, cardiac, 42–43
    verapamil dosages for, 449
Dytac, 447–448

E

Edema, pulmonary, 306
Electrocardiography (ECG; EKG), 264
Electrolytes
    imbalances of, 490–491
    normal values, 490–491
Embolism, pulmonary, 170–171
Emphysema, 74
E-Mycin, 382–383

Enalopril maleate, 380–382
Encephalitis, 75–76
Endocarditis, 76–79
Endocrine therapy, for prostate cancer, 170
Endometrial cancer, 80
Endoscopy, 265
Enteral nutrition, 265–268
Environment, Standard Precautions for, 455
E-Pam, 370–372
Epilepsy, phenobarbital dosage for, 430
Epinephrine, for bronchospasm, 10
Equipment, Standard Precautions for, 455
Eryc, 382–383
ErycSprinkle, 382–383
Ery-Tab, 382–383
Erythrocyte sedimentation rate, 462–463
Erythromid, 382–383
Erythromycin base, 382–383
Esidrix, 399–400
Esophagogastroduodenoscopy, 268–269
Etodolac, 383–385
Ewing's sarcoma, 31
Excisional biopsy, 218. *See also* Biopsy
Exercise stress testing, 336–338
External fixation devices, 269–274

F

Fahrenheit temperature conversion table, 458–459
False aneurysms, 13
Famotidine, 385–386
Feldene, 432–433
Feosol, 386–387
Fer-Iron, 386–387
Ferralyn, 386–387
Ferrous sulfate, 386–387
Fibrosarcoma, 31
Fixation devices, 269–274
Floxin, 424–425
Fluid volume. *See* under specific disorders
    excess, signs/symptoms of, 57
Fluoxetine hydrochloride, 387–388

Follicular thryroid carcinoma, 189–190
Foods, high-fiber, 73
Fractures, 80–85
Full thickness burns, 36
Furosemide, 388–390

G

Gallstones, 50–51
Gangrene, 182, 201
Gardenal, 430–432
Gastrectomy, 274–277
Gastric cancer, 85
Gastric ulcers, 155–158
Gastrointestinal functions, reference values for, 485
Gemfibrozil, 390–392
Glipizide, 392–393
Glomerulonephritis, 85–88
Glucose blood levels, in diabetes, 66
Glucotrol, 392–393
Glyburide, 393–395
Glynase, 393–395
Grading, of tumor cells, 40
Grafts
    for aneurysm management, 13
    skin, for wound closure, 339–340
Granulation, 339
Graves' disease, 109–112

H

HAV (hepatitis A), 203. *See also* Viral hepatitis
HBV (hepatitis B), 203. *See also* Viral hepatitis
HCTZ, 399–400
HCV (hepatitis C), 203. *See also* Viral hepatitis
HDV (hepatitis D), 203. *See also* Viral hepatitis
Handwashing, 454
Haplock, 395–397
Heart. *See* cardiac entries
Heart failure (HF), 88–93
Hematology tests, reference values for, 460–463
Hemolytic anemia, 11–13

Hemopneumothorax, 166–168
Hemorrhagic anemia, 11–13
Hemothorax, 166–168
Heparin, 395–397
Hepatic tumors, malignant, 125–126
Hepatitis, viral, 202–205
Hep Lock, 395–397
Herniated disk disease, 94–97
Herpes simplex encephalitis, 75–76
HEV (hepatitis E), 203. *See also* Viral hepatitis
HHNS (hyperglycemic hyperosmolar non-ketotic syndrome), 102–103
High-fiber foods, 73
Histiocytoma, 31
HIV. *See* Acquired immunodeficiency syndrome (AIDS)
Hodgkin's disease, 97–101
Homan's sign, 187, 278
Human insulin, 397–399
Hycodan, 401–402
Hycomine, 401–402
Hycort, 402–404
Hydration, of burn patient, 37
Hydrocet, 401–402
Hydrochlorothiazide, 399–400
Hydrocodone bitartrate, 401–402
Hydrocortisone, 402–404
Hydrocortone, 402–404
Hydrodiuril, 399–400
Hydronephrosis, 101
Hyperalimentation, 327–330
Hypercalcemia, 491
Hypercapnia, 213
Hyperglycemia, signs of, 328
Hyperglycemic hyperosmolar non-ketotic syndrome (HHNS), 101-103
Hyperkalemia, 490
Hypermagnesemia, 491
Hypernatremia, 490
Hypertension, 103–109
Hypertensive vascular disease, 103–109
Hyperthyroidism, 109–112

Hypocalcemia, 491
Hypoglycemia, signs of, 328
Hypokalemia, 490
Hypomagnesemia, 491
Hyponatremia, 490
Hypoproliferative anemia, 11–13
Hypothyroidism, 112–115
Hypovolemia, signs of, 118–119
Hypovolemic shock, 175–176
Hypoxemia, 213
Hypoxia, 23, 213
Hysterectomy, 277–280
Hytone, 402–404

I

IBD (inflammatory bowel disease). *See* Crohn's disease; Ulcerative colitis
Ibuprofen, 404–405
ICP (intracranial pressure), increased, 115–117
IDDM (insulin-dependent diabetes mellitus), 72. *See also* Diabetes mellitus
Idiopathic thrombocytopenic purpura (ITP), 184
IgE antibody, anaphylaxis and, 10
Ileostomy, 280–281
Ileus, mechanical, 117–118
Ilotycin, 382–383
Imipramine, 406–407
Immunologic procedures, reference values for, 486
Incisional biopsy, 218. *See also* Biopsy
Indopamide, 407–409
Infarction, myocardial, 134–138
Infective waste, Standard Precautions for, 455
Inflammatory bowel disease (IBD). *See* Crohn's disease; Ulcerative colitis
Inguinal orchiectomy, 180
Insulin-dependent diabetes mellitus (IDDM), 72. *See also* Diabetes mellitus
Intensol, 370–372
Intermittent claudication, 51
Internal fxation devices, 269–274
Internal radiation, for cervical cancer, 47

Intestinal obstruction, 117–118
Intestinal resection, 281–284
Intracavitary radiation, for cervical cancer, 47
Intracranial pressure (ICP), increased, 115–117
Intubation, nasogastric, 302–305
Invasive procedures, Standard Precautions for, 455
Ischemic cardiac disease, 119
Isoptin, 448–450
ITP (idiopathic thrombocytopenic purpura), 184

J

Janimine. 406–407
Joint disease, degenerative, 139
Joint replacement, 284–288

K

K-Dur, 433–434
Keflet, 363–364
Keflex, 363–364
Keftab, 363–364
Kefurox, 361–363
Kenacort, 445–447
Kenalog, 445–447
Kernig's sign, 128
Kidney disorders. *See* specific disorders
Kidney failure
    acute, 3-5
    chronic, 56–59
K-Lor, 433–434
Klotrix, 433–434
K-Lyte-CL, 433–434

L

Laboratory tests, reference values for, 460–487
Laennec's cirrhosis, 59
Lanoxicaps, 373–375
Lanoxin, 373–375
Laparoscopy, 289
Laryngeal cancer, 119

Lasix, 388–390
Left-sided heart failure, 62
Leukemias, 40, 119-124
Levothyroid, 409–410
Levothyroxine, 425-427
Levoxyl, 409–410
Linen, soiled, Standard Precautions for, 455–456
Liquaemin sodium, 395–397
Lisinopril, 410–412
Liver cancer, 124–125
Lobectomy, 290–292
Lodine, 383–385
Lopid, 390–392
Lopressor, 417–418
Loraz, 412–413
Lorazepam, 412–413
Lorcet, 401–402
Lortab, 401–402
Lovastatin, 413–414
Lozd, 407–409
Lumbar disk, herniated, symptoms of, 94. *See also*
    Herniated disk disease
Lumbar puncture, 292
Luminal, 430–432
Lung cancer, 125
Lymphomas, 40

M

Magnesium
    imbalances, 491
    normal values, 491
Magnetic resonance imaging (MRI), 293
Malignant hepatic tumors, 124–125
Manual traction, 333. *See also* Traction
Mastectomy, modified radical, 298–302
Mechanical ileus, 118–119
Mechanical ventilation, 293–298
Meclizine hydrochloride, 414–415
Mediastinal shift, signs and symptoms of, 306
Meni-D, 414–415
Medipren, 404–405

Medullary thryroid carcinoma, 190–191
Meningeal irritation, signs of, 128
Meningitis, 127–129
Mental deterioration, signs of, 7
Meperidine hydrochloride, 415–417
Metabolic acid-base disorders, 488–489
Metoprolol, 417–418
Mevacor, 413–414
Meval, 370–372
MI (myocardial infarction), 134–138
Micro-K, 433–434
Micronase, 393–395
Mictrin, 399–400
Minidiab, 392–393
Mitral valve
  prolapse, 130
  stenosis, 130–132
Modified radical mastectomy, 298–302
Motrin, 404–405
MRI (magnetic resonance imaging), 293
Multiple myeloma, 132–134
Myelomas, 40
Myocardial infarction (MI), 134–138
Myocarditis, 76–79
Myrosemide, 388–390

N

Nabumetone, 419
NANB (non-A,non-B hepatitis), 203
Naprosyn, 420–421
Naproxen, 420–421
Nasogastric intubation, 302–305
Natrimax, 399–400
Navodipam, 370–372
Nephrotic syndrome, 138–139
NIDDM (non-insulin-dependent diabetes mellitus),
  72. See also Diabetes mellitus
Nifedipine, 421–422
Non-A, non-B hepatitis (NANB), 203
Non-insulin-dependent diabetes mellitus (NIDDM),
  72. See also Diabetes mellitus

Nortriptyline hydrochloride, 423–424
Norvopropoxyn, 436–437
Novohydrazide, 399–400
Novolin, 397–399
Novolorazem, 412–413
Novo-NiFedin, 421–422
Novopirocam, 432–433
Novorythro, 382–383
Nuprin, 404–405

O

Ocuflox, 424–425
Ofloxacin, 424–425
Omnipen, 350–351
Open fracture, 86
Orasone, 434–436
Oretic, 399–400
Osteoarthritis, 139
Osteomalacia, 139–140
Osteomyelitis, 141–144
Osteoporosis, 144–147
Oxaprozin, 425–426
Oxygen, partial pressure of, 214. *See also* Arterial
   blood gases
Oxygen saturation levels, 214. *See also* Arterial blood
   gases
   pulse oximetry of, 321–322

P

Pain management. *See* under specific disorder
Pamelor, 423–424
Pancreatic cancer, 147
Pancreatitis, 147–150
Panmycin, 441–443
Panwarfin, 450–451
Papillary thryroid carcinoma, 189–190
Parkinson's disease, 150–155
Paroxetine, 427
Partial thickness burns, 36
Patch grafting, for aneurysm management, 13

Paxil, 427
PCE Disperstabs, 382–383
Penicillin V potassium, 428–429
Pentoxifylline, 429–430
Pen Vee K, 428–429
Pepcid, 385–386
Pepcidine, 385–386
Peptic ulcer disease, 156–158
Perforation, of ulcer, 156
Pericardiocentesis, 77
Pericarditis, 76–79
Peripheral vascular disease (PVD), 159
Peritonitis, 126, 159–160
Pethadol. 415–417
Pethidine, 415–416
pH, blood, 214. *See also* Arterial blood gases
Phenaphen with codeine, 343
Phenobarbital, 430–432
Pheochromocytoma, 161–163
Physical deterioration, signs of, 7
Piroxicam, 432–433
Plasma tests, reference values for, 464–472
Pneumonectomy, 305–309
Pneumonia, 163–166
Pneumothorax, 166–168
Polymox, 348–349
Postnecrotic cirrhosis, 59
Postoperative nursing care, 310–312
Potassium
    imbalances of, 490
    normal values, 490
Potassium chloride, 433–434
Prednicen-M, 434–436
Prednisone, 434–436
Preoperative nursing care, 310–312. *See also* under
    specific surgical procedures
PresTab, 393–395
Primary biliary cirrhosis, 59
Principen, 349–351
Priniril, 410–412
Procardia, 421–422
Procardio XL, 421–422

Propox, 436–437
Propoxycon, 436–437
Propoxyphene napsylate, 436–437
Propoxyphine hydrochloride, 436–437
Prorentil, 344–345
Prostate cancer, 168–169
Prostatectomy, 315–320
Prozac, 387–388
Pulmonary edema, signs and symptoms of, 306
Pulmonary embolism, 169–170
Pulmonary emphysema, 80
Pulmonary function studies, 321
Pulse oximetry, 321–322
PVD (peripheral vascular disease), 159
P wave, 264
Pyelonephritis, 195. *See also* Urinary tract infections

Q

Q-Pam, 370–372
QRS complex, 264

R

Radiation therapy, 322–325
Radical mastectomy, modified, 298–302
Radical pancreatoduodenectomy (Whipple procedure), 147
Ranitidine, 438–440
Raynaud's disease, 199
Reed-Sternberg cells, 97
Reference values, for laboratory tests, 460–487
Relafen, 419
Respiratory acid-base disorders, 488
Respiratory irritation/infection, prevention and treatment of, 55–56
Respolin, 344–345
Resting tremors, 151
Rheumatoid arthritis, 170–174
Right-sided heart failure, 62
Rival, 370–372
Robicillin VK, 428–429

Robimycin, 382–383
Rufen, 404–405
Ru-vert M, 414–415z

S

Salbutamol, 344–345
Sarcomas, 40
Semen tests, reference values for, 487
Seminomas, 179
Senile osteoporosis, 144
Septra, 369–370
Septra DS, 369–370
Septrin, 369–370
Sertraline, 440–441
Serum tests, reference values for, 464–472
Shock, 174–176
Sinequan, 377–378
Skin flaps, 339
Skin grafts, 339–340
Skin integrity impairment. *See* under specific
    disorders
Skin traction, 344. *See also* Traction
Slo-Bid, 346–348
Slo-Phyllin, 346–348
Slow-Fe, 386–387
Slow-K, 433–434
Sodium
    imbalances of, 490
    normal values, 490
Sofarin, 450–451
Solfoton, 430–432
Spinal cord injury, 176–179
Squamous cell carcinomas
    of cervix, 47–48
    of lung, 125
ST segment, 264
Standard Precautions, 454–457
Substernal pain, in myocardial infarction, 134
Sufamethoprim, 369–370
Sulfa, 369–370
Sulfamethoprim, 369–370

Sulfamethoprim DS, 369–370
Sulfamethoxazole-trimethoprim, 369–370
Sulmeprim, 369–370
Sumycin, 441–443
Surgical risk, evaluation of, 312–313
Synthroid Levothyroid, 409–410
Systolic hypertension, 103–104

T

Tachycardia, 42. *See also* Dysrhythmias
Tagamet, 364–365
Temperature conversion table, 458–459
Tenormin, 351–352
Tension pneumothorax, 166
Testicular cancer, 180–183
Testicular self-examination (TSE), 181–182
Tetracap, 441–443
Tetracycline, 441–443
Tetralan, 441–443
Theo-24, 346–348
Theo-Dur,346–348
Theolair,346–348
Theophylline, 27,346–348
Therapeutic drug monitoring, 473–476
Thiuretic, 399–400
Thoracentesis, 325
Thromboangiitis obliterans, 182–184
Thrombocytopenic purpura, 184–186
Thrombophlebitis, 186–189
    signs of, 278
Thrombosis, venous, 186–189
Thyroid cancer, 189–190
Thyroidectomy, 325–327
Thyroid storm, symptoms of, 110
Timolol, 443–444
Timoptic, 443–444
TNM staging system, 40–41
Tofranil, 406–407
Toprolxi, 417–418
Total parenteral nutrition (TPN), 327–330
Toxicology tests, reference values for, 482–483

TPN (total parenteral nutrition), 327–330
Tracheostomy, 330–333
Traction, 333–336
Transfusion reactions, 222–223
Transfusions, blood, 220–223
Transurethral prostatectomy (TURP), 315
Treadmill testing, 336–338
Trendar, 404–405
Trental, 429–430
Triamcinolone, 445–447
Triaminic expectorant, 401–402
Triamterene, 447–448
Tricilone, 445–447
Triggers, asthmatic, 22, 24
Trimox, 348–349
Tripramine, 406–407
True aneurysms, 13
TSE (testicular self-examination), 181–182
Tube feedings, 265–268
Tuberculosis, 190–194
Tumors. *See also* Cancer; Carcinoma
    bone, 31–35
    brain, 35
    malignant hepatic, 124–125
TURP (transurethral prostatectomy), 315
Tussionex, 401–402
T wave, 264
Tylenol with codeine, 343

U

Ulcerative colitis, 194–195
Ulcers, peptic, 155–158
Ultracef, 360–361
Ultradol, 383–385
Ultrasonography, 338–339
Undifferential thyroid carcinoma, 190
Uniphyl, 346–348
Urethritis, 197. *See also* Urinary tract infections
Urinary tract infections, 195–198
Urine tests, reference values for, 477–481

Uroplus S, 369–370
Urozide, 399–400
UTI (urinary tract infections), 195–198

V

Vaginal hysterectomy, 277–280
Valium, 370–372
Valrelease, 370–372
Varicose veins, 198–199
Vascular disease, hypertensive, 103–109
Vasepam, 370–372
Vasogenic shock, 175
Vasospastic disorder, 199–202
Vasotec, 380–382
V-Cillin K, 428–429
VC-K Veetids, 428–429
Veins, varicose, 198–199
Venous thrombosis, 186–189
Ventilation, mechanical, 293–298
Verapamil hydrochloride, 448–450
Verelan, 448–450
Vibramycin, 378–380
Vibra-Tabs, 378–380
Vicodin, 401–402
Viral hepatitis, 202–204
Vitamin D, osteomalacia and, 140
Vivol, 370–372
Voltaren, 372–373
Voltaren SR, 372–373

W

Warfarin sodium, 450–451
Whipple procedure (radical pancreatoduoden-
    ectomy), 148–149
Wound closure, 339–340

X

Xanax, 345–346

Y

Yeast infection in colostomy patient, signs of, 253

Z

Zantac, 438–440
Zestril, 410–412
Zetran, 370–372
Zinacef, 361–363
Zithromax, 354–355
Zoloft, 440–441
Zonalon, 377–378
Zydone, 401–402